Amyloid Diseases

Edited by Dmitry Kurouski

Published in London, United Kingdom

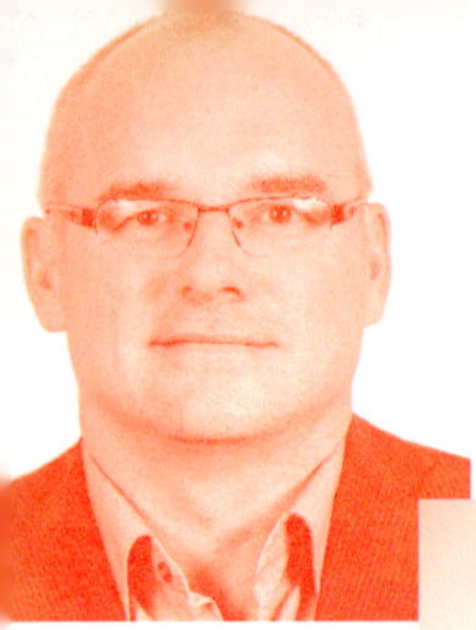
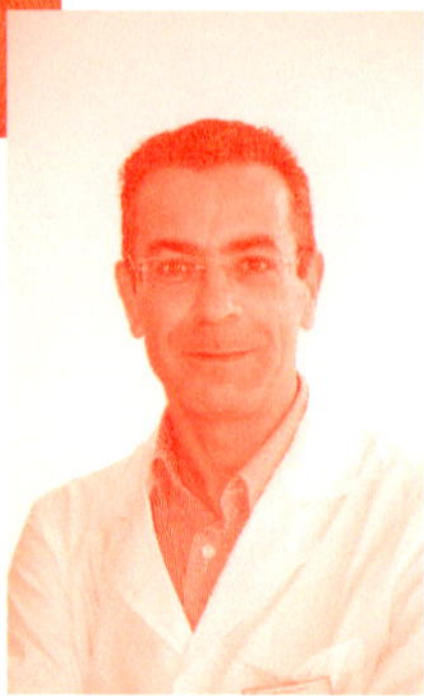
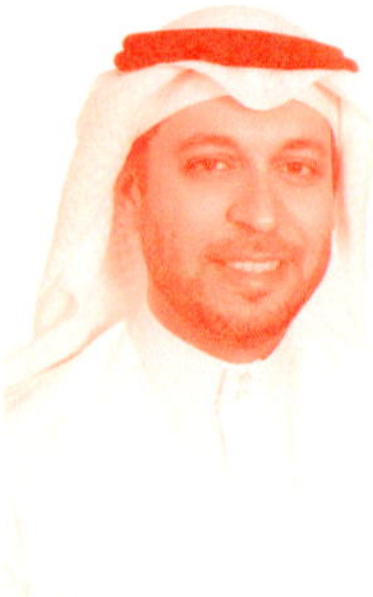
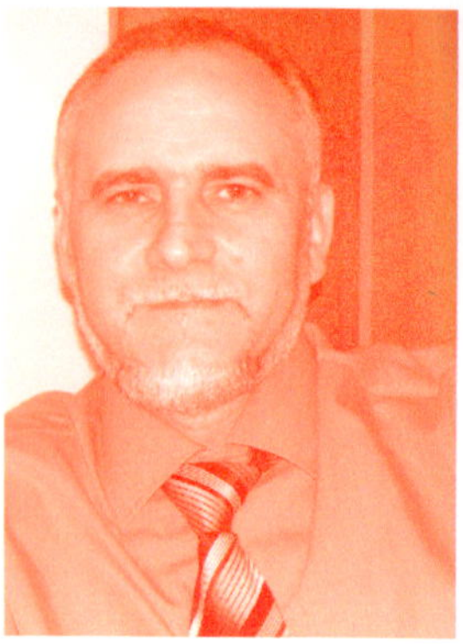
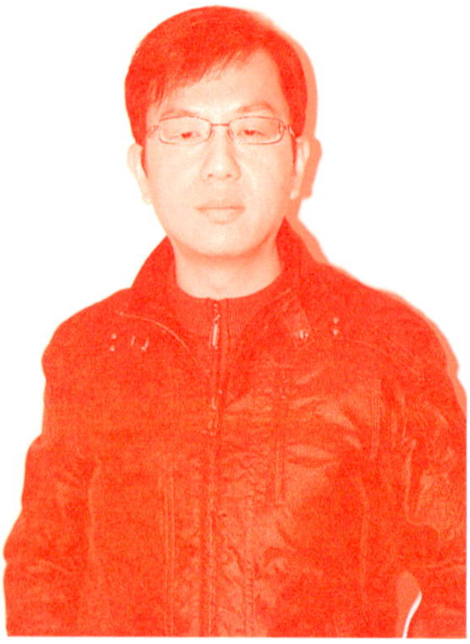
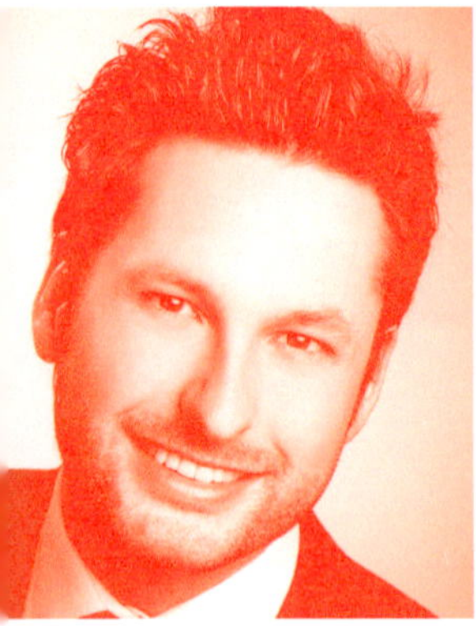
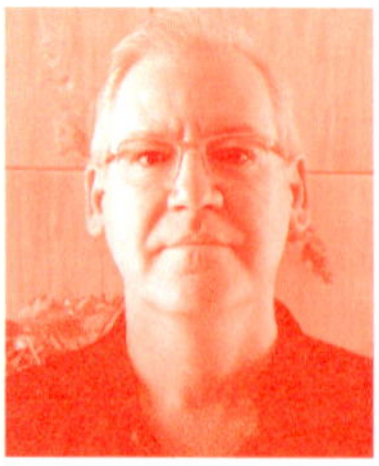

IntechOpen

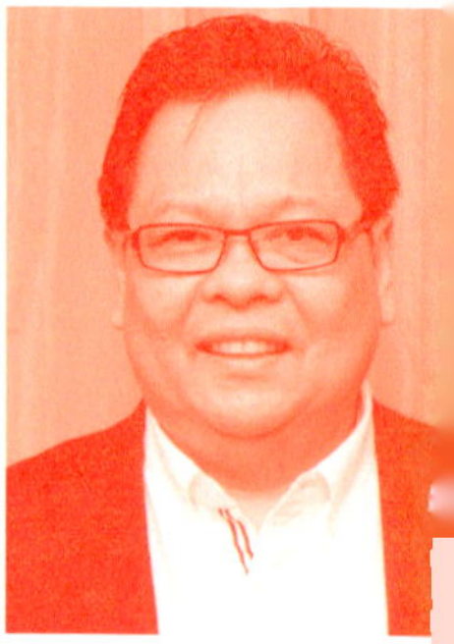
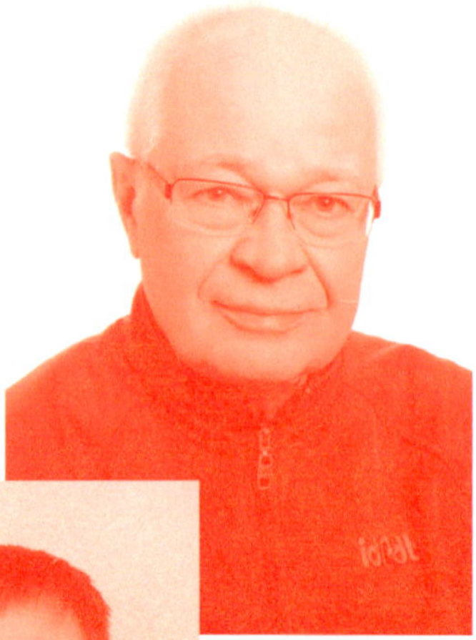
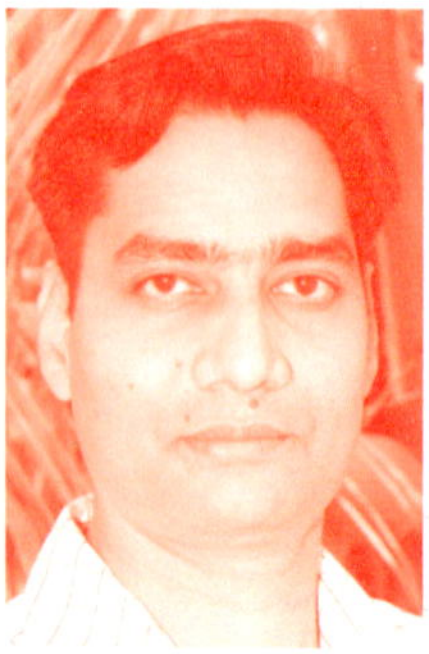
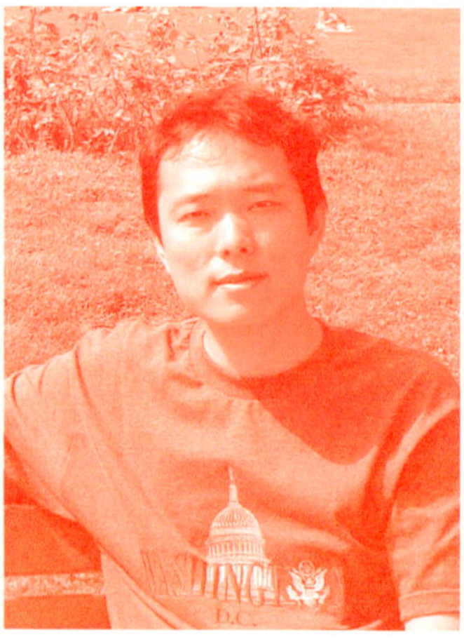
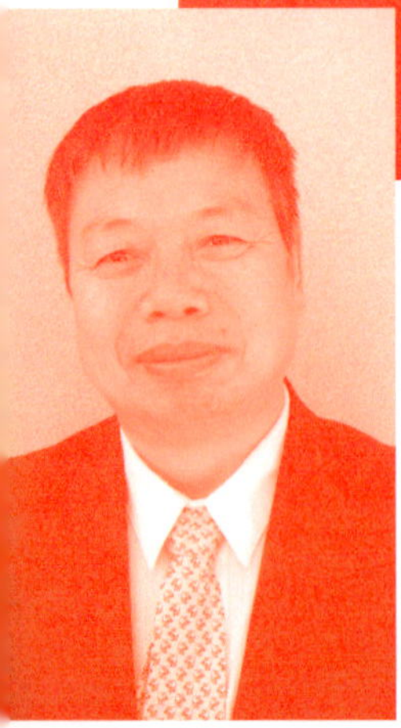
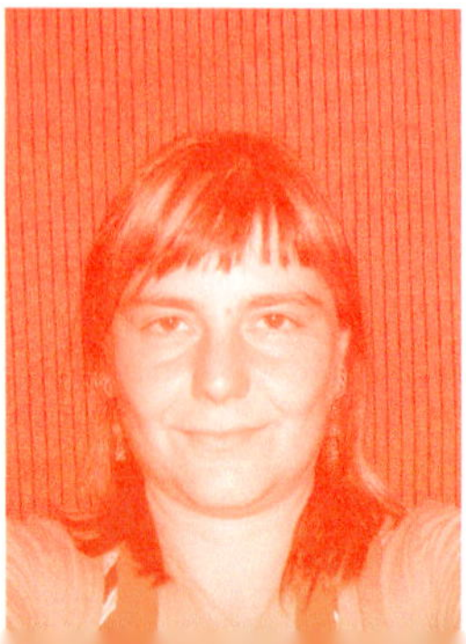

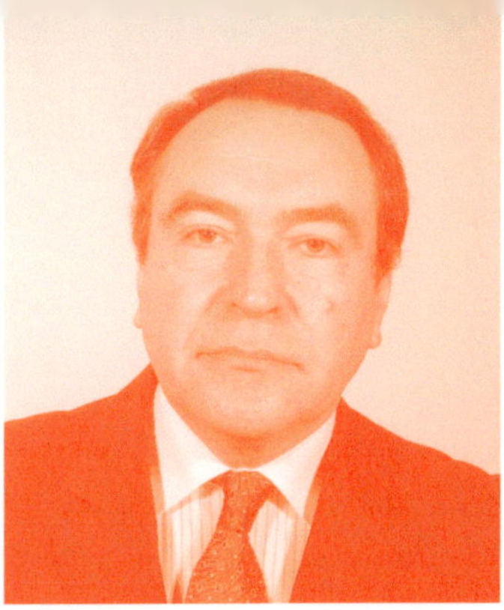
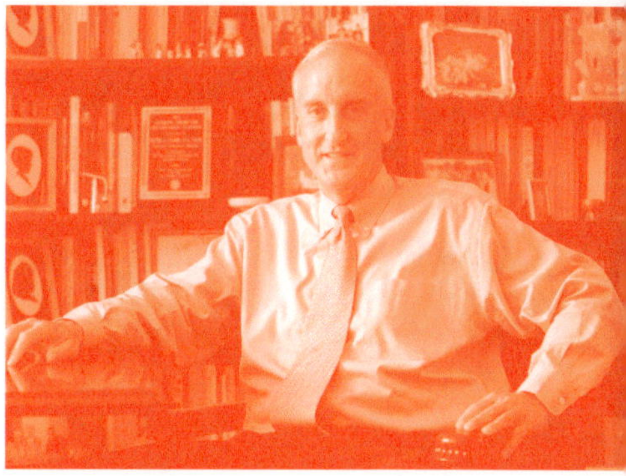
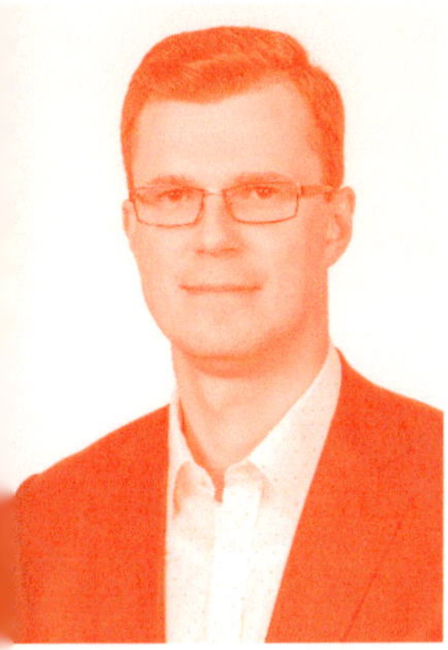
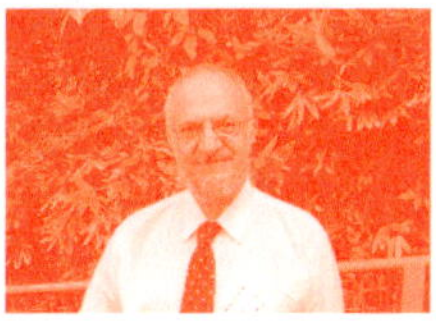
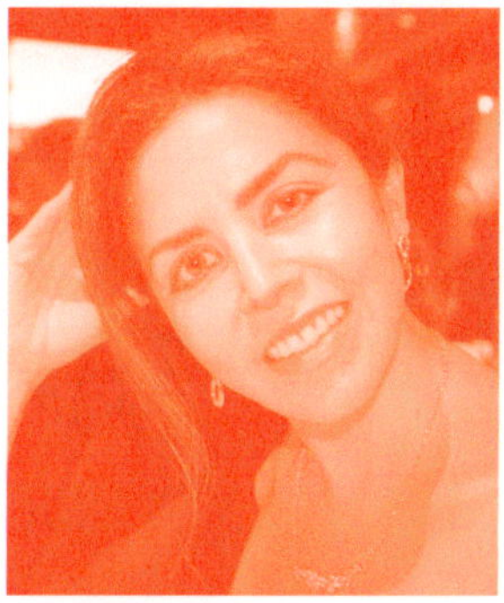

Supporting open minds since 2005

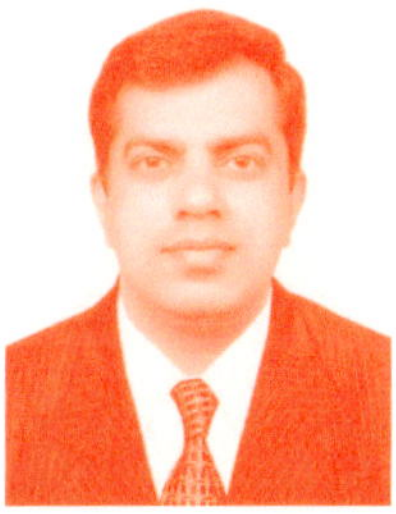
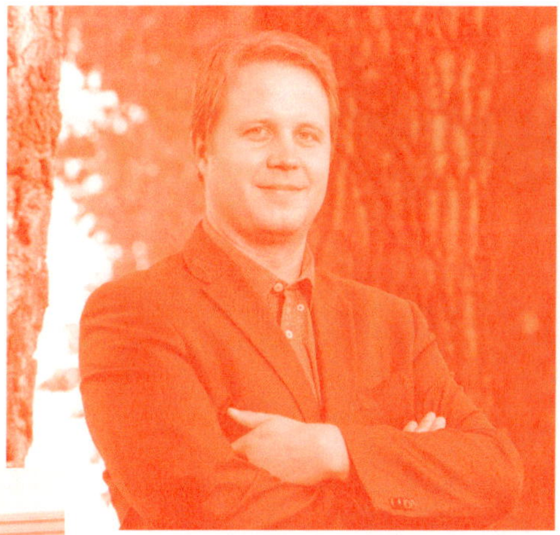
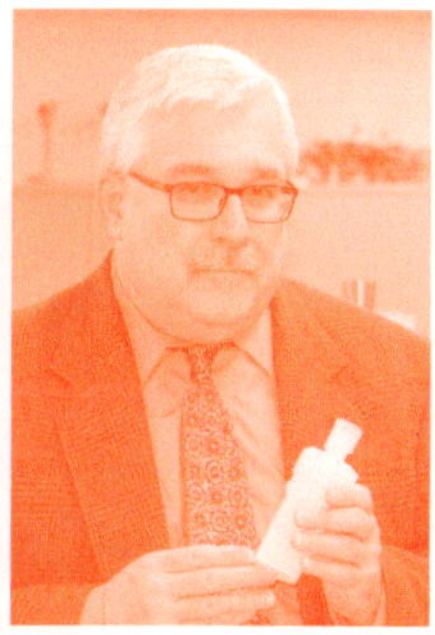
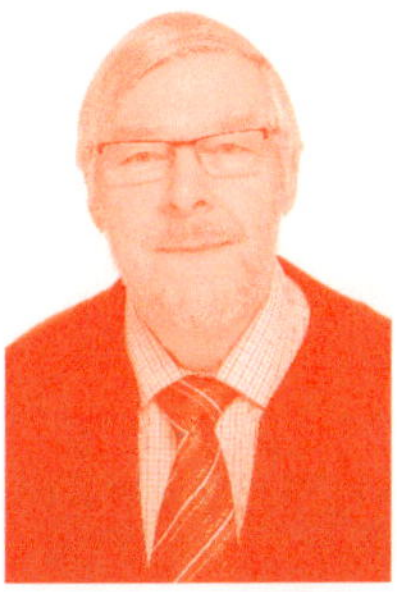
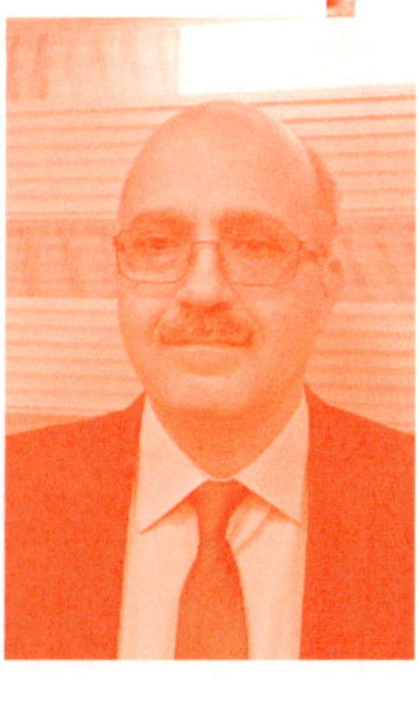
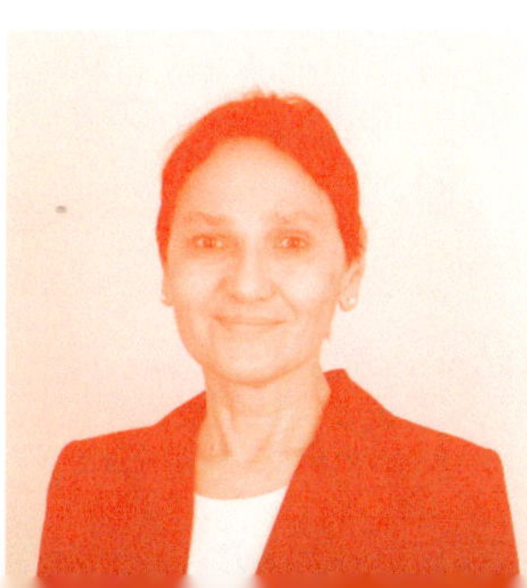
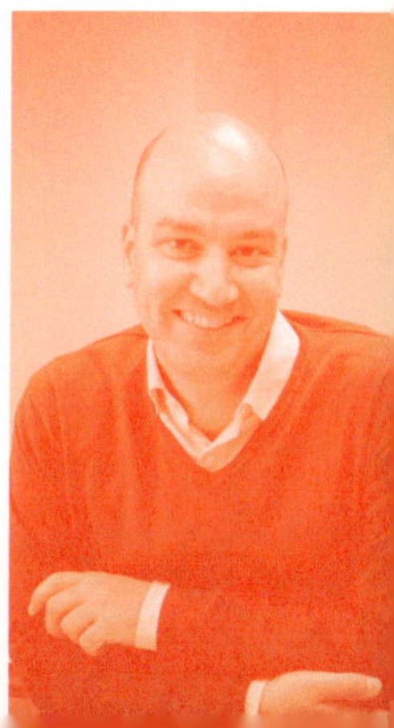

Amyloid Diseases
http://dx.doi.org/10.5772/intechopen.73821
Edited by Dmitry Kurouski

Contributors
Estefania Azevedo, Debora Foguel, Matthew Zabel, Kayla Sheehan, Yasmeen Alhomsy, Quinto Gesiotto, Eileen Ly, Anu Stephen, Asal Homayouni, Joshua Fisher, Prashanth Venkataraman, Matthew Habib, Jonathan Harrison, Aswanth Reddy, Enrique Ballesteros, Elena Zakharova, Richard Ye, Yu Fan, Chi Teng Vong, Sonia Villapol, George Sack, Alejandra Martinez-Maldonado, Patricia Bocanegra Lopez, Teresa Ponce-Lopez, Andrew Sorsby Vargas, Miguel Angel Ontiveros Torres, José Luna-Muñoz, Ignacio Villanueva Fierro, Parmenides Guadarrama Ortiz, Juan Lopez-Garriga, Igor Lednev, Manuel Rosario-Alomar, Tatiana Quiñones-Ruiz, Leishla Marie Cruz-Collazo, Kourosh Rezania, Laleh Saadat, Moon Joo Kim, Donghwa Baek, Luan Truong, Jae Y. Ro, Bhargy Sharma, Konstantin Pervushin

First published in London, United Kingdom, 2019 by IntechOpen
IntechOpen is the global imprint of INTECHOPEN LIMITED, registered in England and Wales, registration number: 11086078, The Shard, 25th floor, 32 London Bridge Street
London, SE19SG – United Kingdom
Printed in Croatia

British Library Cataloguing-in-Publication Data
A catalogue record for this book is available from the British Library

Additional hard and PDF copies can be obtained from orders@intechopen.com

Amyloid Diseases
Edited by Dmitry Kurouski
p. cm.
Print ISBN 978-1-78985-381-0
Online ISBN 978-1-78985-382-7
eBook (PDF) ISBN 978-1-83881-132-7

For EU product safety concerns:
IN TECH d.o.o., Prolaz Marije Krucifikse Kozulić 3, 51000 Rijeka, Croatia, info@intechopen.com or visit our website at intechopen.com.

Meet the editor

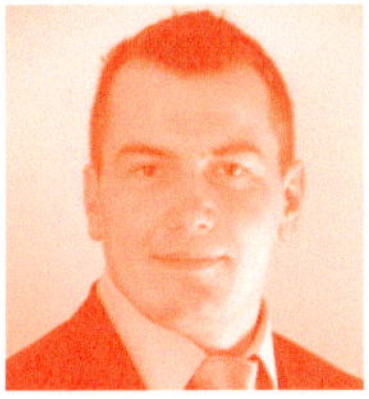

Dmitry Kurouski earned his MS in Biochemistry from Belarusian State University, Belarus, and his PhD (Distinguished Dissertation) in Analytical Chemistry from SUNY Albany, NY, USA. After a postdoc in the laboratory of Professor Richard P. van Duyne at Northwestern University, Dr. Kurouski joined Boehringer-Ingelheim Pharmaceuticals, where he worked as a senior research scientist. In 2017, Dr. Kurouski joined the Biochemistry and Biophysics Department of Texas A&M University as an assistant professor. He develops Raman spectroscopy for detection and identification of plant diseases, as well as probe structures and dynamics of biological and photocatalytic systems with nano-IR spectroscopy (infrared atomic force microscopy (AFM-IR)) and nano-Raman spectroscopy (tip-enhanced Raman spectroscopy).

Contents

Preface

There are nearly 44 million people around the world who are diagnosed with Alzheimer's disease. It is one of the most common diseases in Western Europe and the sixth leading cause of death in the United States. Every 67 seconds, someone in the United States develops Alzheimer's disease, while only 45% of these people are aware of this diagnosis. In the United Kingdom, the cost of Alzheimer's and dementia already exceeds £30 billion, while the global cost of Alzheimer's and dementia is estimated to be around $600 billion. Similar to Alzheimer's, the incidence of Parkinson's disease increases with age. There are around 5 million people living with Parkinson's disease worldwide. The combined direct and indirect cost of Parkinson's, including medical treatment, social care, and lost income from an inability to work, is estimated to be nearly $25 billion per year in the United States alone.

The most astonishing fact is that the cause of both Alzheimer's and Parkinson's diseases, as well as other neurodegenerative maladies, is still unknown. Consequently, there is no effective treatment against these diseases. Medical diagnostics are primarily based on movement disorders and signs of memory loss. Such a drastic change in behavior is associated with neuron death, change in structures, and, consequently, the physiological functions of proteins.

Postmortem microscopic examination of organs and tissues of patients diagnosed with these severe maladies reveals amyloid plaques that contain long, unbranched, rod-like protein aggregates, known as amyloid fibrils. Therefore, it is concluded that these amyloid fibrils are associated with neurodegenerative diseases. However, there is a growing body of evidence suggesting that prefibrillar oligomers rather than fibrils are responsible for the onset and progression of Alzheimer's and Parkinson's diseases.

This book provides a broad scope of research and clinical findings on amyloids. It also provides the most recent understanding of possible treatment of neurodegenerative diseases and is also an excellent summary of histological and physiological changes that are associated with amyloid diseases. I am convinced that this book will be interesting to a broad range of researchers ranging from graduate students to clinical practitioners who work in this very important and interesting area of biological research.

Dmitry Kurouski
Texas A&M University,
Department of Biochemistry and Biophysics,
TX, USA

Section 1

Clinical Diagnostics of Amyloidosis

Chapter 1

The Clinical Spectrum of Amyloidosis

Aswanth Reddy, Enrique Ballesteros and Jonathan Scott Harrison

Abstract

Amyloidosis is a group of disorders that share a common pathobiology: in each case, a protein that exhibits misfolding is deposited in one or multiple organs leading to disruption in organ function. These amyloid proteins are recognized as amorphous pink material in Hematoxylin and Eosin staining, with confirmation by staining with Congo red and yellow or green birefringence under polarized light microscope. To date at least 36 different types of amyloid proteins have been identified. Worldwide, AA amyloidosis is the most common type, and this occurs secondary to chronic inflammatory disease states—such as chronic infections and rheumatological disorders. In western countries, the incidence of AA amyloidosis is decreasing, and AL is the most common type of amyloidosis, characterized by amyloid due to light chain deposition. ATTR amyloidosis, which can be either hereditary or acquired, is a unique variant of systemic amyloidosis that results from mutations in the transthyretin (TTR) gene. Our review will focus on clinical features of the most common systemic amyloidosis, with a detailed review on evaluation and management of AA, AL and ATTR amyloidosis.

Keywords: AA amyloidosis, AL amyloidosis, ATTR amyloidosis

1. Introduction

Amyloidosis is a group of disorders that share the common feature of deposition into tissues of any one of a number of different proteins. The uniform underlying pathobiology is the finding that in each case, the protein—termed amyloid—deposited into the target organ has undergone abnormal three-dimensional folding. The abnormal folding of the peptide results in accumulation in tissues as micro-fibrillary structures. The deposition of amyloid protein, regardless of which specific protein forms the amyloid, results in disruption in the function of the organ in which the amyloid protein is deposited. The common histopathologic feature of all amyloidosis is the finding, by light microscopy, of amorphous protein in one or more organs, typically initially recognized upon histologic review of a biopsy, as an amorphous pink material on Hematoxylin and Eosin staining (**Figure 1**). Per the International Society of Amyloidosis 2016 nomenclature guidelines, amyloid fibrils must exhibit affinity for the histologic stain Congo red, showing green, yellow or orange birefringence when the Congo red-stained deposits are viewed with polarized light. At least 36 different proteins can undergo abnormal folding and result in deposition of amyloid, causing clinical disease. It is conventional to describe a particular amyloid protein as "Amyloid Protein AX," where the X is a suffix to the designation, based on the identity of the amyloid protein. The more commonly encountered subtypes are, for example Amyloid Protein AL, Amyloid Protein AA, and Amyloid Protein ATTR, as discussed below. This chapter is an overview of the different categories of amyloidosis, with a focus on the clinical features, prognosis, and management of focal or systemic amyloidosis. Symptoms depend on the type and amount of amyloid protein, and are often variable. The manifestations depend on the identity of the underlying protein that forms the amyloid fibrils, the burden of amyloid, and the organs involved, as well as comorbidities of an individual patient (see **Table 1**).

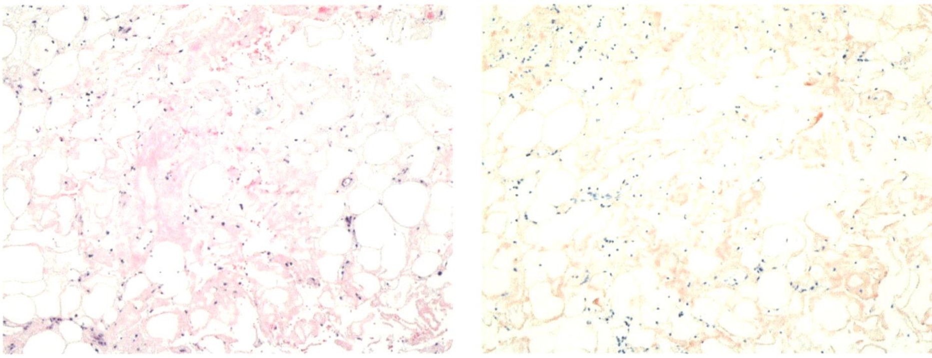

Figure 1.
Photomicrographs of a lymph node biopsy with AL amyloidosis. Panel A: 10× magnification of a left axillary lymph node biopsy stained using Hematoxylin and Eosin, demonstrating amorphous pink material typical of amyloid infiltration. White areas are fat that has been leached from the tissue in processing. Panel B: 10× magnification of the same lymph node stained using Congo red, viewed by light microscopy.

Symptoms commonly seen in systemic amyloidosis
Fatigue
Edema at one or more sites
Lightheadedness upon standing (due to orthostatic hypotension)
Diarrhea
Focal pain (due to peripheral neuropathy)
Physical signs commonly seen in systemic amyloidosis
Edema at one or more sites (due to either heart failure, nephrotic syndrome, or both)
Focal mass lesions (amyloid deposition focally)
Orthostatic hypotension (due to autonomic nerve dysfunction)
enlarged tongue (macroglossia)
Purpura (due to either coagulation disorder, skin fragility due to amyloid infiltration, or both)

Table 1.
Clinical manifestation of systemic amyloidosis.

2. Types of systemic amyloidosis

2.1 AA amyloidosis

Worldwide, AA amyloidosis is the most common type of systemic amyloidosis. Although AA amyloid currently is the most common form of amyloidosis, the incidence is decreasing over time in western countries. This has been attributed to a significant decrease in chronic infections, as well as improved therapies for inflammatory diseases. A review from the UK in 2013 estimated in excess of 8.0 per million cases of amyloidosis every year and AA being second most common (18%) [1]. The underlying causes of systemic AA amyloidosis include a wide range of inflammatory diseases, including but not limited to chronic inflammatory disorders, infections, and malignancy (**Table 2**). The amyloid fibril AA is most often a result of abnormal folding and aggregation of serum apolipoprotein A (SAA), which is an acute phase reactant—that is, the level becomes elevated in the blood in response to inflammation [2]. AA amyloid fibrils form through a process of cleavage, misfolding, and aggregation into a highly ordered abnormal β-sheet conformation. Amyloid fibrils associate anatomically with other moieties, including glycosaminoglycans and serum amyloid P component (SAP), forming deposits that disrupt the structure and function of tissues and organs [3].

In the healthy, physiological state in humans, the serum SAA concentration is relatively low, but the level increases about a thousand fold during an inflammatory reaction. In humans, SAA is expressed in three different isoforms: SAA1, SAA2 and SAA4 and are encoded by different genes. SAA1 and SAA2 are solely expressed in liver and are entirely bound to plasma High Density Lipoprotein in plasma [4]. Inflammation increases the secretion of cytokines, including IL-1, IL-6 and TNF, which in turn increases the production of SAA [5]. SAA functions to transport and recycle cholesterol from sites of tissue injury, thereby modulating the immune response. Not all individuals with high SAA levels develop amyloidosis; it appears that certain polymorphisms and mutations in the SAA genes predispose to abnormal protein folding and therefore amyloid formation [6]. The formation of amyloid fibril from precursor SAA protein is the result of complex interaction with glycosaminoglycans, including most prominently heparan sulfate [7]. Impairing this interaction or the degrading of heparan sulfate by a heparinase has been shown to prevent formation of amyloid fibrils, and this has led to an area of research for potential treatment.

More recently, a protein named A Leukocyte Chemotactic factor 2 (ALECT2) protein has been shown to be a cause of AA amyloidosis, with a propensity to cause renal amyloidosis [8]. The human ALECT2 gene, discovered only in 2008, has been localized to chromosome 5 (5q31.1-q32) [9]. ALECT2 is being increasingly recognized as a cause of AA amyloidosis.

Inherited forms of AA amyloidosis arise due to mutations in a variety of proteins that can undergo abnormal folding and consequent deposition into tissues,

Chronic disorders [64–66]	Infections	Malignancy [74]
Rheumatoid arthritis (RA) Alzheimer's disease Juvenile idiopathic arthritis Ankylosing spondylitis Psoriasis and psoriatic arthritis Still disease [67] Behçet syndrome [68] Familial Mediterranean fever Crohn's disease Castleman disease [69] Cryopyrin-associated periodic syndromes (CAPS) [70] TNF-receptor–associated periodic fever syndrome Vasculitis	Leprosy [71] Osteomyelitis Tuberculosis [72] Chronic bronchiectasis [73]	Hodgkin disease Non-Hodgkin lymphoma Renal cell carcinoma Gastrointestinal cancers Lung cancer [75] Urogenital carcinoma Mesothelioma [76]

Table 2.
Causes of AA amyloidosis.

resulting in organ dysfunction. These include mutations in the genes encoding transthyretin, the fibrinogen A α-chain, apolipoprotein A-I, apolipoprotein A-II, and lysozyme [10]. These mutations appear to account for the vast majority of relatively rare familial amyloidosis. Each of these has clinical characteristics that are somewhat peculiar to the specific etiology of the inherited disorder.

2.1.1 Clinical features of systemic AA amyloidosis

Amyloidosis may be localized, or systemic. The clinical symptoms of AA amyloidosis depend on the organ involved by the amyloid fibril. Liver and spleen are the most common sites of deposition, but they are asymptomatic until late in the course of the disease. Hepatosplenomegaly and adrenal insufficiency are common in the advanced stage of AA amyloidosis. Renal involvement damages the glomerular membrane, resulting in nephrotic syndrome and proteinuria. Proteinuria is one of the earliest signs of AA amyloidosis, and seen in approximately 95% of patients with AA amyloidosis [2, 11]. Persistent, untreated renal damage results in end stage renal disease (ESRD), requiring some form of renal substitute therapy—either dialysis or renal transplantation. Cardiac involvement is by deposition of fibrils into cardiac muscle, but clinical cardiac dysfunction is extremely rare in AA amyloidosis, occurring in only 2% of patients in most series [12]. Gastrointestinal involvement results in diarrhea, malabsorption and pseudo obstruction of the bowel. There are several reports of thyroid gland involvement, manifesting as goiter [13].

2.1.2 Treatment

Treatment of AA amyloidosis is challenging due to diverse underlying causes. Ideally, in inflammatory disorders—whether chronic infectious disease (e.g., mycobacterium tuberculosis, staphylococcal osteomyelitis, and other chronic infections), autoimmune disease (e.g., rheumatoid arthritis, scleroderma, and other immune mediated inflammatory diseases), idiopathic (e.g., sarcoidosis), and chronic low-grade malignancy (e.g., B and T cell low-grade lymphomas, Hodgkin disease) the treatment of AA amyloidosis is the treatment of the underlying disease process. The role of controlling inflammation is also essential in the management of AA amyloidosis in patients with chronic rheumatologic diseases. In the era of advanced therapies, the incidence of rheumatic arthritis leading to AA amyloidosis has declined significantly; this was at one time among the most common causes. Specific treatments such as surgical excision in Castleman disease, high dose colchicine for familial Mediterranean fever (FMF) and effective therapy for tuberculosis have shown to significantly reduce serum SAA levels thereby improvement in end organ dysfunction. Treatments of malignancy with chemotherapy and surgery have shown to reverse organ function.

Several anti-inflammatory agents have been studied as potential therapy to reduce the levels of SAA. Tocilizumab, a monoclonal antibody against IL-6 has been successful in significantly reducing circulating levels of SAA when used in autoimmune diseases. A recent series showed significant reduction in acute phase reactants as well as an improvement in proteinuria in patients treated with Tocilizumab for FMF [14].

In vitro studies have shown low molecular weight heparin to impair amyloid deposition by impeding the structural changes necessary for fibril formation. Eporsidate, a sulfonated small molecule similar to heparin sulfate binds competitively to glycosaminoglycan and reduces inflammation and amyloid deposition. This was initially studied as an agent to retard progressive renal failure, and it resulted in a favorable response in a phase II clinical trial [15]. Unfortunately, a phase III trial did not meet the targeted endpoints, and so Eporsidate has not been developed further to date [16]. Dimethyl sulfoxide (DMSO) is a derivative of intercellular low-density lipoprotein, which reduces levels of acute phase reactants including SAA, and has been shown to improve symptoms in patients with gastro-intestinal involvement by AA amyloid [17].

Anti-SAP antibody, R-1-[6-[R-2-carboxy-pyrrolidin-1-yl]-6-oxo-hexanoyl] pyrrolidine-2-carboxylic acid (CPHPC) was studied in Al and AA amyloidosis with favorable responses in an open label study [18]. A recent phase Ib trial of SAP inhibitor, Miridesap followed by humanized monoclonal antibody Dezamizumab against SAP showed clearance of amyloid fibrils in liver and spleen, confirmed by I-SAP scintigraphy [19]. Further studies are ongoing and these treatments are a real potential for future management of amyloidosis.

2.2 AL amyloidosis

AL amyloidosis results from the deposition of abnormally folded immunoglobulin light chains into tissues. The formation of amyloid fibrils from immunoglobulin light chains requires abnormal three-dimensional folding of the light chain, resulting in filaments of β-sheets of relatively insoluble protein [20]. AL amyloid may arise from either polyclonal immunoglobulin light chains or, much more commonly, from monoclonal immunoglobulin light chains. In order for polyclonal AL amyloidosis to result, however, the light chains must fold abnormally—in order to form amyloid and accumulate in target organs. Further, the local concentration of these peptides must, in general, be high. In AL amyloidosis, whether polyclonal or monoclonal, the specific light chains have a peptide sequence that results in a predisposition to abnormal folding of the peptide. In some cases, this appears to be due to genetic polymorphisms in the light chain gene structure. Among the variable regions of the light chain gene products, several (Vλ1, Vλ2, Vλ3, Vλ6, and Vκ1) are over-represented as amyloid protein, suggesting that these peptide sequences have a predilection to fold abnormally and become amyloid. In monoclonal AL amyloidosis, the tendency of monoclonal light chain to fold abnormally may be due, rather, to a mutational event attributable to genomic instability of the clone, rather than a genetic polymorphism in the light chain sequence. Several laboratories have demonstrated that peptide sequences from patients with different levels of secreted light chain have distinct differences in the location of non-conservative mutations in the light chain genes. This implies that the location of non-conservative mutations may be one determinant of the amyloidogenic propensity of light chains in some cases. Three-dimensional structure analyses and site-mutagenesis experiments indicate that both replacement of conserved polar residues in light chains, and loss of hydrogen bonding sites, are common features seen in amyloidogenic immunoglobulin light chains [21–24]. Separately, there is evidence that posttranslational modification of light chains can influence the propensity for amyloid to accumulate, including peptide glycosylation, lysine modification, and rate of proteolysis. Impaired function of metalloproteases that degrade extracellular matrix proteins have been implicated in the propensity of amyloid to accumulate. There is also strong evidence that glycosaminoglycans of the extracellular matrix—particularly heparan sulfate, but also dermatan sulfate and chondroitin sulfate, interact with amyloid protein, providing a scaffold for the polymerized amyloid fibrils [25]. The relative concentration of these glycosaminoglycans appears to impact on the propensity of amyloid to be deposited. It should be noted that in a recent series from China, Huang and Liu reported that immunoglobulin heavy chain amyloidosis accounted for 3.7% of cases of amyloidosis, as compared to AL amyloidosis accounting for 93% of cases. In that report, AA amyloidosis accounted for only 2.2% of all patients with systemic amyloidosis [26].

2.2.1 Polyclonal AL amyloidosis

The Mayo Clinic pioneered the use of Mass Spectroscopy and High Performance Chromatography to identify the specific proteins present in amyloid tissue specimens. They have applied that technology to determine, from patient samples, whether a patient's amyloid is AA or AL, and to further characterize if an AL specimen is entirely kappa or lambda light chains—consistent with a monoclonal process; or if the AL amyloid is an approximately equal mix of both kappa and lambda light chains—suggesting a polyclonal process. In a 2013 report, Grogg and colleagues identified two patients with pulmonary amyloidosis in whom Liquid Chromatography-Mass Spectroscopy documented equal amounts of kappa and of lambda light chain in the amyloid deposits. In addition, the polyclonal identity of the amyloid was demonstrated by immunohistochemical staining for kappa and lambda light chains, and polymerase chain reaction amplification of immunoglobulin gene sequence showed only a polyclonal population in these patients [27]. In 2016, the Mayo Clinic studied in detail a patient with localized amyloidosis of the oropharynx. Liquid Chromatography and Mass Spectroscopy documented polyclonal AL amyloid, with equal proportions of kappa and lambda light chains present. No monoclonal protein was identified, and no monoclonal lymphoid or plasma cell population was present. Thus, this group has well documented the process of localized amyloidosis attributable to polyclonal light chain deposition. In that report they also summarized data regarding an additional 17 patients identified from the medical literature with isolated amyloidosis of the palate [28]. In three of those seventeen cases, a plasma cell dyscrasia was present (MGUS in two and myeloma in one). Similarly, Wey and colleagues from Taiwan reported a patient with Sjogren's syndrome complicated by localized, cutaneous nodular amyloidosis of the legs. In this case, C-reactive protein 0.12 mg/dL antinuclear antibody titer, anti-centromere antibody titer, and anti-Ro/SSA antibody titer were all pathologically elevated and polyclonal gammaglobulinemia was detected by serum immune-electrophoresis [29]. Thus, multiple investigators have substantiated the observation that AL amyloid can be polyclonal. Definitive data regarding the relative incidence of monoclonal versus polyclonal AL amyloid is not available. However, it does appear from these cases that polyclonal AL amyloidosis seems to be a more indolent process and less aggressive than AL amyloidosis, and is most often a localized process. In these cases, local therapy appears likely to control the disease. Nonetheless, there are documented cases of systemic polyclonal AL amyloidosis with multi-organ involvement and relatively poor prognosis as compared to age-matched individuals without amyloidosis.

Localized amyloidosis is much rarer than systemic amyloidosis, predominantly affects the skin or mucosal tissues (86%), and is usually of the AL subtype (98%). It is generally accepted that localized AL amyloidosis results from monoclonal light chains. However, the most recent amyloid nomenclature developed by the International Society of Amyloidosis in 2014 does not distinguish between monoclonal and polyclonal sources.

2.2.2 Monoclonal AL amyloidosis

In contrast to polyclonal AL amyloidosis, monoclonal AL amyloidosis is typically an aggressive, multi-organ disease with a generally poor prognosis. The disease process is driven by production of a monoclonal immunoglobulin light chain—hence the name AL (amyloid, light chain). As noted previously, only a minority of monoclonal light chain gammopathy results in amyloidosis. The exonic coding sequence for the specific light chain will most often have either a mutation, or a polymorphism, that results in abnormal protein folding, in order for the light chain to be deposited as amyloid and cause organ dysfunction, as previously discussed. AL amyloid is found both extracellularly and intracellularly, in affected organs. Kyle and colleagues at the Mayo Clinic reported that the incidence of AL amyloid in Olmsted County, Minnesota, was in the range of 3–5 cases per million annually [30]. Others have estimated the annual incidence to be in the range of 10–14 patients per million. In contrast, it is estimated that the annual incidence of MGUS in men is 120 per 100,000 population at the age of 50 years, and increases to 530 per 100,000 population at the age of 90 years. The incidence of multiple myeloma is in the range of 85 cases per million annually in the United States. Thus, only a very small minority of patients with MGUS or overt multiple myeloma develop clinical AL amyloidosis. The average age at diagnosis of patients with AL amyloidosis is approximately 64. The disease appears to occur more commonly in males than females [31].

Presenting signs and symptoms of amyloidosis are the consequences of specific organ involvement. Cardiac involvement occurs in the majority of patients diagnosed as having AL amyloidosis, most typically presenting with symptoms and signs of heart failure syndrome but with a preserved left ventricular ejection fraction. In an excellent recent review, Gertz reported that 71% of patients with AL amyloidosis seen at the Mayo Clinic had cardiac involvement, with 58% having kidney disease [32]. Renal involvement most often includes nephrotic range proteinuria; in an early series reported by Kyle in 1975, of all patients reviewed in that series with any type of amyloidosis, approximately 90% had some degree of proteinuria. Neurologic involvement occurs in approximately 25% of patients, and may include peripheral neuropathies, including, most commonly carpet tunnel syndrome; or autonomic neuropathy—most prominently orthostatic hypotension but also including anhydrosis [33]. Organ enlargement is common, with as many as half of patients having hepatomegaly, and an enlarged tongue (macroglossia) occurs in approximately a quarter of patients. Kyle also described purpura, particularly periorbital purpura, as a notable finding.

AL amyloid is most commonly a systemic disorder. However, there are cases of AL amyloidosis localized to a single site. The sites of localized AL amyloid reported include the skin, the larynx, the gastrointestinal tract, and the urinary bladder. Diagnosis must be confirmed by tissue biopsy, in order to demonstrate the presence of the amyloid by Congo red histologic staining. When a clinician encounters a patient over the age of 60 with suspected systemic AL amyloidosis, serum protein electrophoresis is essential to determine if a monoclonal serum para-protein is present. If a monoclonal protein is either suspected or identified, then serum protein immune-electro fixation or immunoelectrophoresis is indicated. Once a monoclonal serum paraprotein is identified, bone marrow biopsy and aspirate should be obtained in order to assess the percentage of clonal plasma cells infiltrating of the marrow, and determine if the patient meets the criteria for diagnosis of multiple myeloma or a lymphoplasmacytic lymphoma. In patients with a clonal AL amyloid, treatment to eradicate the clone of plasma cells or lymphocytes producing the light chain, if successful, will prevent synthesis of new immunoglobulin light chains, and, if the patient can be supported to survive long enough, organ recovery may occur over time as the relatively insoluble amyloid is ultimately metabolized and broken down.

2.2.3 Clinical features of AL amyloidosis

The clinical features of AL amyloidosis are extremely variable from one patient to the next; nearly every organ can potentially be involved. However, the disease has a stereotypic pattern of presentation in many cases. As noted earlier, systemic AL amyloidosis involves the heart in approximately 70–80% of cases, depending on the series. The most common clinical presentation of symptomatic organic heart disease due to AL amyloidosis is heart failure syndrome, with dyspnea and often leg swelling (edema), although angina pectoris (chest pain due to ischemia) may also occur, as well as arrhythmias. Prior to onset of clinically evident heart disease, nearly all patients with cardiac involvement by amyloidosis will have an elevated serum level of N-terminal Pro-natriuretic peptide Type B (NT-ProBNP). Progressive elevation of the Pro-BNP correlates with progressively poorer prognosis, and the level of Pro-BNP is a criterion for risk stratification and prognosis in several staging systems for cardiac amyloidosis. Similarly, cardiac troponin T (cTnT) and cardiac troponin I (cTnI) are sensitive (although not specific) markers of myocardial damage. The degree of elevation of these proteins are additional markers of myocardial cell damage in cardiac amyloidosis [34]. A characteristic finding on electrocardiogram is decreased voltage in the limb leads, as compared to normal; however, this is not a consistent finding even in patients with biopsy proven cardiac amyloidosis. Imaging of the heart by echocardiogram may demonstrate the characteristic amyloidosis findings of pathologically increased ventricular wall thickness, as well as a granular, sparkling appearance of the myocardium on three-dimensional echocardiographic imaging. Again, there is the caveat that early in the disease process these findings may not be evident. A longitudinal "strain" pattern may also be present, but again is not a specific finding for amyloidosis [35]. Technetium-99 pyrophosphate scanning of the heart, particularly with single photon emission computed tomography (SPECT), is a sensitive imaging technique that will show retention of the radionuclide in cases of cardiac amyloidosis; this is widely considered a diagnostic study of choice. Technetium-99 pyrophosphate scanning of the heart can often distinguish between ATTR amyloid and AL amyloid. Magnetic Resonance Imaging of the heart using the contrast agent gadolinium for enhancement, a more costly approach than echocardiogram or Technetium-99 scan, can provide evidence of cardiac amyloidosis. Delayed enhancement pulse sequences following infusion of the gadolinium will most often demonstrate a diffuse and irregular hyper-enhancement of the myocardium in patients with cardiac amyloidosis. Subendocardial late gadolinium enhancement (LGE) occurs more commonly in AL amyloidosis, and transmural LGE more commonly in ATTR cardiac amyloidosis. In this context, even greater specificity may be achieved using a Magnetic Resonance Imaging technique termed "myocardial nulling." This technique exploits the observation that gadolinium contrast accumulates excessively and abnormally in myocardial tissue, that has accumulated amyloid, and the findings are quite specific for amyloidosis of the heart.

Several groups have developed staging systems that stratify cardiac prognosis in patients with AL amyloidosis. The Mayo Clinic group Cardiac Staging System stratifies patients based on the combination of NT-proBNP together with either the cTnT or the cTnI. These parameters may be used to assess prognosis at the time of initial diagnosis, and often form a part of eligibility criteria for clinical trials [36].

As noted, clinically evident heart disease in AL amyloidosis manifests most often as congestive heart failure syndrome, despite preservation of the left ventricular ejection fraction. The symptoms most often include fatigue and exertional dyspnea, as well as edema due to heart failure, in some cases. Signs may include a lateral shift of the cardiac point of maximal impulse, as well as adventitial heart sounds and murmurs. Cardiomegaly may be evident on chest radiogram. Due to amyloid deposition, a fraction of patients will have electrical conduction abnormalities, and resultant cardiac arrhythmias. Such arrhythmias may result in sudden cardiac death, if the abnormal rhythm does not result in non-lethal signs or symptoms first.

Second to cardiac manifestations, the most common organ clinically involved by systemic AL amyloidosis are the kidneys. Kidney disease due to amyloid seen in approximately 50–60% of patients, depending on the series. The organ tropism of AL amyloid correlates with the variable region gene sequence, and the IGLV6-57 gene sequence appears to predispose to renal involvement. Within the affected kidney, amyloid deposits are seen prominently in the glomeruli, with additional amyloid seen in blood vessels, in tubular-basement membranes, and in the interstitial space. Uptake of amyloid by mesangial cells induces a functional change in phenotype resulting in cellular dysfunction. In experimental models, uptake of amyloid results in a transformation of a mesangial cell from a smooth muscle cells to a macrophage phenotype. Renal dysfunction clinically is typically manifest first as a protein wasting process, which typically progresses to nephrotic range proteinuria. Nephrotic range proteinuria results in edema and with time leads to chronic kidney disease with progressive edema, followed by electrolyte disorders and progressively worsening glomerular filtration rate [37]. Because of urinary loss of natural anticoagulants such as Protein C, which has a relatively short half-life, venous thrombosis may occur in patients with Amyloidosis and renal disease. Both renal involvement by AL amyloidosis, and cardiac disease due to AL amyloidosis, contribute to the generalized weakness experienced by a majority of patients who have AL amyloidosis.

The nervous system is clinically involved in AL amyloidosis in approximately 20% of patients. The most common neurologic process seen is a sensory peripheral neuropathy, which is often painful. Dysautonomia is also seen, particularly manifesting as orthostatic hypotension due to amyloid damaging the autonomic regulation of blood pressure. Orthostatic hypotension can be disabling, and may result in falls and therefore fractures. Patients with severe orthostatic hypotension may remain bedridden to avoid symptoms, and are then at risk both for developing decubitus ulcers, as well as venous thromboses. Myopathy may also occur because of AL amyloid deposition, and may present as pseudo-hypertrophy, or may clinically mimic other muscle wasting diseases [38].

The gastrointestinal tract is involved by AL amyloidosis. In a recent report from Stanford University Medical Center, Yen and colleagues reported that in a retrospective analysis of 583 patients with amyloidosis, approximately 16% had gastrointestinal symptoms. They observed that 50% of patients with amyloid had nausea, vomiting, or abdominal pain. In this cohort, approximately 82% of patients had AL amyloid. A classic finding reported in the earliest descriptions of amyloidosis is macroglossia, an enlarged tongue. However, it is estimated that this is seen in only about 15% of patients [39]. Malabsorption is often seen in amyloidosis of the gastrointestinal tract, with consequence diarrhea, abdominal discomfort, and weight loss on this basis.

Patients with kappa light chain AL amyloidosis have been reported to have a greater propensity for hepatic involvement than lambda light chain amyloidosis [40]. In contrast, dominant soft-tissue and bone involvement is associated with the IGLV3-1 gene, and in some reports, the Kappa 1 light chain. Hepatic involvement is typically manifest as hepatomegaly, and biopsy typically documents the presence of amyloid [41]. Splenomegaly is also common, particularly when hepatomegaly is present, and splenomegaly may result in blood cell sequestration in the spleen, with cytopenias.

Amyloid infiltration has been reported in virtually every gland, although these reports suggest that direct endocrine dysfunction due to amyloidosis is relatively less common than involvement by the heart, kidneys, and neurologic systems [42]. Amyloidosis of the breast have been reported, as well as amyloidosis of the seminal vesicles also occurs. Amyloidosis can infiltrate the pancreas, and amyloid infiltration of the adrenal gland may result in adrenal insufficiency. Similarly, amyloid infiltration of the pituitary gland can result in polyendocrine dysfunction.

Cutaneous AL amyloidosis is well described, and most often presents as either hemorrhagic bullous lesions, or, classically, as purpura or ecchymosis. Among the early classic descriptions of cutaneous manifestations of amyloidosis is the phenomenon of periorbital purpura [43].

Patients with AL amyloidosis may have one or more acquired coagulopathies, resulting in a bleeding diathesis. This may be due to impaired synthesis of clotting proteins by a liver involved by amyloid infiltration; however, adsorption of coagulation proteins, most commonly Factor X, but other factors as well, results in increased clearance of coagulation proteins and a bleeding disorder. Other than Factor X, adsorption of Factor V and of von Willebrand factor have been reported in a number of series. In such cases, frequent infusion of the deficient factor can temporarily control bleeding [44]. An algorithm for diagnostic evaluation is seen in **Figure 2**.

2.2.4 Treatment of AL amyloidosis

Management of AL amyloidosis is, in the first instance, management of end-organ dysfunction, with the goal to support the patient. However, definitive therapy requires eradication of the clone of B cells producing the immunoglobulin light chains that are misfolded and deposited as amyloid. Clinical trials have documented that the combination of the alkylating anti-neoplastic agent L-phenylalanine mustard (Melphalan) together with a potent corticosteroid such as Prednisone or Dexamethasone, can suppress production of new light chains, and, with adequate time, alter the balance of production and very slow degradation of AL amyloid. High dose Melphalan with autologous hematopoietic rescue was compared to conventional dose Melphalan plus dexamethasone in a prospective, randomized clinical trial published in 2007 [45]. That study reported inferior survival for patients randomized to high dose chemotherapy with autologous hematopoietic rescue (autologous transplant). However, in the past decade, the morbidity and mortality from autologous transplant has declined, and the risk-benefit ratio appears to have improved. An analysis by the Center for International Blood and Marrow Transplant Research (CIBMTR) published in 2015 reported that five-year overall survival following autologous transplant for AL amyloidosis had improved from 55% during the period of 1995–2000, to 77% in the time period from 2007 to 2012. Thus, outcome for transplant now appears superior to outcome from conventional dose anti-neoplastic therapy [46]. However, there have been no new prospective randomized clinical trials of autologous transplant versus non-transplant therapy. Newer therapies that are effective in reducing the burden of neoplastic plasma cells producing AL amyloid include proteasome inhibitors, and monoclonal antibodies that target plasma cells, such as daratumumab, an anti-CD38 monoclonal antibody. There are being studied, with promising results; however, no mature randomized data is available as of this writing from use of the agents. Anti-SAP antibody is a promising modality that appears to remove AL amyloid with relative efficiency; however, this agent remains investigational as of this writing [47].

2.3 ATTR amyloidosis

Hereditary transthyretin amyloidosis is an autosomal dominant, progressive, life-threatening disease caused by mutations in the gene encoding transthyretin. Transthyretin (TTR) is a homotetramer plasma transport protein secreted primarily by liver but also in retinal pigment epithelium and choroid plexus. It functions to transport thyroxine and retinol-binding protein and hence the name transthyretin [48]. ATTR amyloidosis results from deposition of abnormal TTR protein, which is a result of destabilized TTR-tetramer misfolding and fibril formation. ATTR

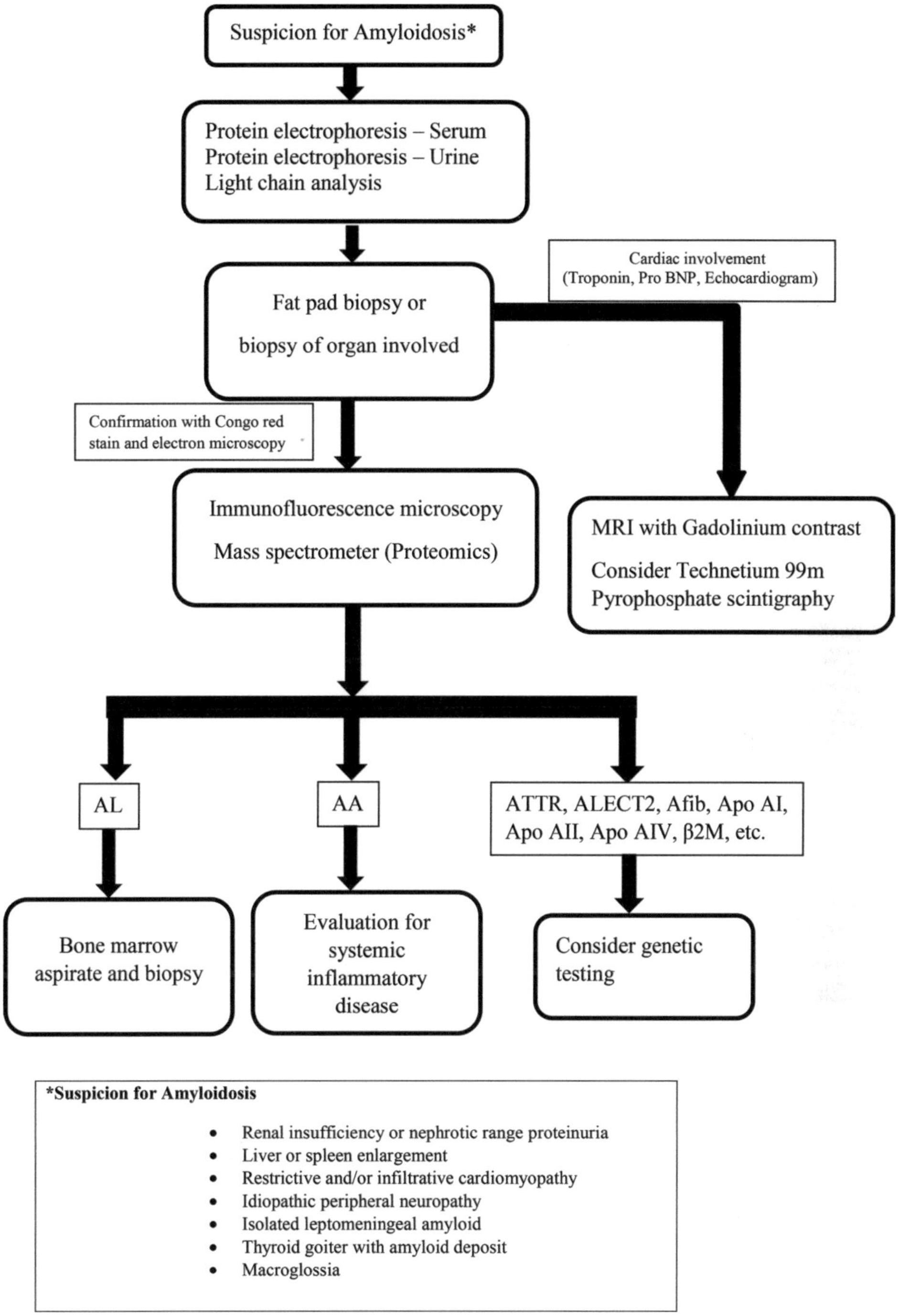

Figure 2.
Diagnostic algorithm of systemic amyloidosis.

amyloidosis can be hereditary or wild type. There are more the 130 mutations identified worldwide in the hereditary form with the most common being Val30Met mutation [49]. ATTR amyloidosis is a rare disease but recently it has been identified more commonly from advances in diagnostics. Wild type ATTR, occasionally called senile systemic amyloidosis because of the late age of onset is reported at an incidence of 10% in people more than 80 years of age [50].

2.3.1 Clinical features of ATTR amyloidosis

Phenotypically the ATTR results in clinical syndrome with respect to the organ involved. The three main clinical entities are polyneuropathy, cardiomyopathy and leptomeningeal disease. Fiber length-dependent neuropathy is pathognomonic of the disease. In the initial phase, small fiber neuropathy results in pain, paresthesia, allodynia, hyperalgesia, dysesthesia and impaired sensation to temperature. In later stages, large fiber dysfunction results in loss of vibration sense and balance, ultimately leading to difficulty with ambulation from progressive motor weakness [51]. Autonomic dysfunction results in orthostatic hypotension, neurogenic bladder, sexual dysfunction and gastrointestinal symptoms such as diarrhea and/or constipation [52]. Some patients with wild type ATTR develop carpel tunnel syndrome as their initial presentation and are also related to specific TTR mutations such as Leu58His, Ile84Ser and Tyr114His [53].

Familial amyloid cardiomyopathy occurs commonly with Val122Ile TTR mutation and they present with EKG abnormalities, heart failure, intractable arrhythmias and conduction abnormalities. Echocardiogram reveals a granular sparkling with ventricular and septal wall thickening [54]. MRI can show a classical late gadolinium enhancement but cardiac scintigraphy by Technetium-99 m pyrophosphate has the highest sensitivity and specificity in diagnosis [55]. Leptomeningeal amyloidosis occurs in patients with Asp18Gly, Ala25Thr and Tyr114Cys mutations. TTR protein is secreted by choroid plexus and gets deposited in cerebral and subarachnoid blood vessels and leptomeninges [49, 56]. Symptoms include transient ischemic attack, cerebral infarction or hemorrhage, subarachnoid hemorrhage, hydrocephalus, ataxia, spastic paralysis, convulsion, and dementia. Isolated leptomeningeal involvement is infrequent and occurs in patients harboring Val30Met mutation [57]. Ocular, renal and isolated gastrointestinal involvements are also reported in ATTR amyloidosis.

2.3.2 Treatment of ATTR amyloidosis

Once untreatable, hereditary ATTR amyloidosis is now primarily treated with liver transplantation, especially in Japan where it has shown better survival benefit and life expectancy. Liver transplantation is not widely practiced outside Japan due to low availability of living donors [58]. The transplantation replaces the abnormal TTR protein to a wild type protein. Overall studies have shown better outcomes in patients with early disease and Val30Met mutation compared to late onset and non-Val30Met patients. Leptomeningeal disease and retinal involvement do not improve by liver transplantation. Cardiac involvement continues to progress even after liver transplantation in some cases due to deposition of wild type ATTR.

Although liver transplantation has better outcome, not all patients are eligible due to advanced disease and multiple other sites of involvement. The tetramer destabilization is the initial step in the process of amyloid fibril formation and this was studied as a potential for treatment. Tafamidis, a benzoxazole derivative binds to thyroxine-binding sites of transthyretin and inhibits the dissociation of tetramers thereby blocking the rate-limiting step in monomer formation. In a randomized double-blinded phase II/III study in patients with polyneuropathy, Tafamidis did not meet the co-primary endpoints in the intention to treat population but did show significant improvement of neuropathy improvement score and quality of life in efficacy-evaluable population [59]. In another Phase III study for patients with ATTR related cardiomyopathy, Tafamidis was superior to placebo in decreasing the all-cause mortality and cardiovascular-related hospitalizations [60]. It is approved in both Europe and Japan for use in familial amyloid polyneuropathy and received

FDA approval in the United States in 2018 for treatment of transthyretin cardiomyopathy. Difunisal, a nonsteroidal anti-inflammatory drug used to treat pain and osteoarthritis was studied as an agent to stabilize the amyloid tetramer. It functions by binding to the T4 binding site in TTR. In a phase II/III study it had significant improvement in neuropathy score in patients with amyloid polyneuropathy [61].

RNA interference is a phenomenon in which the gene expression is blocked by small RNA molecules. This approach has been studied in several diseases by introducing a small RNA into the cell and obscures a gene hence forth potentially inactivating the gene. Partisan is a RNA interference molecule developed to block production of abnormal TTR protein in liver. In a phase III trial, patients with hereditary transthyretin amyloidosis neuropathy received Partisan (dose 0.3 mg/kg every 3 weeks) and had statistically significant improvement in modified Neuropathy Impairment Score+7 [62].

Antisense oligonucleotides (ASO) are chemically modified oligonucleotides designed to selectively bind the RNA in the cell and prevent the target protein expression by interfering with translation. A phase III trial is ongoing for ISIS-TTRRx, an ASO specific to TTR mRNA [63].

Author details

Aswanth Reddy, Enrique Ballesteros and Jonathan Scott Harrison*
University of Connecticut, Farmington, CT, USA

*Address all correspondence to: joharrison@uchc.edu

References

[1] Lane T, Pinney JH, Gilbertson JA, Hutt DF, Rowczenio DM, Mahmood S, et al. Changing epidemiology of AA amyloidosis: Clinical observations over 25 years at a single national referral Centre. Amyloid. 2017;**24**:162-166. DOI: 10.1080/13506129.2017.1342235

[2] Lachmann H, Goodman HJB, Gilbertson J, Gallimore R, Sabin C, Gillmore J, et al. Natural history and outcome in systemic AA amyloidosis. The New England Journal of Medicine. 2007;**356**:2361-2371. DOI: 10.1056/NEJMoa070265

[3] Obici L, Raimondi S, Lavatelli F, Bellotti V, Merlini G. Susceptibility to AA amyloidosis in rheumatic diseases: A critical overview. Arthritis and Rheumatism. 2009;**61**:1435-1440. DOI: 10.1002/art.24735

[4] Husby G, Marhaug G, Dowton B, Sletten K, Sipe JD. Serum amyloid A (SAA): Biochemistry, genetics and the pathogenesis of AA amyloidosis. Amyloid. 1994;**1**:119-137. DOI: 10.3109/13506129409148635

[5] Kisilevsky R, Manley P. Acute-phase serum amyloid A: Perspectives on its physiological and pathological roles. Amyloid. 2012;**19**:5-14. DOI: 10.3109/13506129.2011.654294

[6] Booth DR, Booth SE, Gillmore JD, Hawkins PN, Pepys MB. SAA1 alleles as risk factors in reactive systemic AA amyloidosis. Amyloid. 1998;**5**:262-265. DOI: 10.3109/13506129809007299

[7] Noborn F, Ancsin JB, Ubhayasekera W, Kisilevsky R, Li JP. Heparan sulfate dissociates serum amyloid A (SAA) from acute-phase high-density lipoprotein, promoting SAA aggregation. The Journal of Biological Chemistry. 2012;**287**:25669-25677. DOI: 10.1074/jbc.M112.363895

[8] Larsen CP, Kossmann RJ, Beggs ML, Solomon A, Walker PD. Clinical, morphologic, and genetic features of renal leukocyte chemotactic factor 2 amyloidosis. Kidney International. 2014;**86**:378-382. DOI: 10.1038/ki.2014.11

[9] Benson MD, James S, Scott K, Liepnieks JJ, Kluve-Beckerman B. Leukocyte chemotactic factor 2: A novel renal protein. Kidney International. 2008;**74**:218-222. DOI: 10.1038/ki.2008.152

[10] Das M, Gursky O. Amyloid-forming properties of human apolipoproteins: Sequence analyses and structural insights. Advances in Experimental Medicine and Biology. 2015;**855**:175-211. DOI: 10.1007/978-3-319-17344-3_8

[11] Enríquez R, Sirvent AE, Padilla S, Noguera-Pons R, Andrada E, Ardoy F, et al. Nephrotic syndrome and AA amyloidosis revealing adult-onset cryopyrin-associated periodic syndrome. Renal Failure. 2013;**35**:738-741. DOI: 10.3109/0886022X.2013.790300

[12] Dubrey S, Cha K, Simms R, Skinner M, Falk R. Electrocardiography and Doppler echocardiography in secondary (AA) amyloidosis. The American Journal of Cardiology. 1996;**77**:313-315. DOI: 10.1016/S0002-9149(97)89403-9

[13] Lagha EK, M'sakni I, Bougrine F, Laabidi B, Ghachem DB, Bouziani A. Amyloid goiter: First manifestation of systemic amyloidosis. European Annals of Otorhinolaryngology, Head and Neck Diseases. 2010;**127**:134-136. DOI: 10.1016/j.anorl.2010.02.013

[14] Ugurlu S, Hacioglu A, Adibnia Y, Hamuryudan V, Ozdogan H. Tocilizumab in the treatment of twelve cases with aa amyloidosis secondary to

familial mediterranean fever. Orphanet Journal of Rare Diseases. 2017;**12**:105. DOI: 10.1186/s13023-017-0642-0

[15] Dember LM, Hawkins PN, Hazenberg B, Gorevic PD, Merlini G, Butrimiene I, et al. Eprodisate for the treatment of renal disease in AA amyloidosis. The New England Journal of Medicine. 2007;**356**:2349-2360. DOI: 10.1056/NEJMoa065644

[16] Press Release JUNE 20, 2016. BELLUS Health Announces Top-Line Phase 3 Results of KIACTA™ for the Treatment of AA Amyloidosis

[17] Amemori S, Iwakiri R, Endo H, Ootani A, Ogata S, Noda T, et al. Oral dimethyl sulfoxide for systemic amyloid A amyloidosis complication in chronic inflammatory disease: A retrospective patient chart review. Journal of Gastroenterology. 2006;**41**:444-449. DOI: 10.1007/s00535-006-1792-3

[18] Pepys MB, Herbert J, Hutchinson WL, Tennent GA, Lachmann HJ, Gallimore JR, et al. Targeted pharmacological depletion of serum amyloid P component for treatment of human amyloidosis. Nature. 2002;**417**:254-259. DOI: 10.1038/417254a

[19] Richards DB, Cookson LM, Barton SV, Liefaard L, Lane T, Hutt DF, et al. Repeat doses of antibody to serum amyloid P component clear amyloid deposits in patients with systemic amyloidosis. Science Translational Medicine. 2018;**10**:3128. DOI: 10.1126/scitranslmed.aan3128

[20] Merlini G, Bellotti V. Molecular mechanisms of amyloidosis. The New England Journal of Medicine. 2003;**349**:583-596

[21] Perfetti V, Casarini S, Palladini G, et al. Analysis of V(lambda)-J(lambda) expression in plasma cells from primary (AL) amyloidosis and normal bone marrow identifies 3r (lambdaIII) as a new amyloid-associated germline gene segment. Blood. 2002;**100**:948-953

[22] Perfetti V, Ubbiali P, Vignarelli MC, et al. Evidence that amyloidogenic light chains undergo antigen-driven selection. Blood. 1998;**91**:2948-2954

[23] Hurle MR, Helms LR, Li L, Chan W, Wetzel R. A role for destabilizing amino acid replacements in light-chain amyloidosis. Proceedings of the National Academy of Sciences of the United States of America. 1994;**91**:5446-5450

[24] Stevens FJ. Four structural risk factors identify most fibril-forming kappa light chains. Amyloid. 2000;**7**:200-211

[25] McLaurin J, Yang D, Yip CM, Fraser PE. Modulating factors in amyloid-beta fibril formation. Journal of Structural Biology. 2000;**130**:259-270

[26] Huang X-H, Liu Z-H. The clinical presentation and management of systemic light-chain amyloidosis in China. Kidney Diseases. 2016;**2**:1-9

[27] Grogg KL, Aubry MC, Vrana JA, Theis JD, Dogan A. Nodular pulmonary amyloidosis is characterized by localized immunoglobulin deposition and is frequently associated with an indolent B-cell lymphoproliferative disorder. American Journal of Surgical Pathology. 2013;**37**:406-412

[28] Ravindran A, Grogg KL, Domaas DA, Go RS. Polyclonal localized light chain amyloidosis—A distinct entity. Clinical Lymphoma, Myeloma & Leukemia. 2016;**16**:588-592

[29] Wey SJ, Chen YM, Lai PJ, Chen DY. Primary Sjogren syndrome manifesting as localized cutaneous nodular amyloidosis. Journal of Clinical Rheumatology. 2011;**17**:368-370

[30] Kyle RA, Linos A, Beard CM, et al. Incidence and natural history of primary systemic amyloidosis in Olmsted County, Minnesota, 1950 through 1989. Blood. 1992;**79**:1817-1822

[31] Nienhuis HLA, Bijzet J, Hazenberg BPC. The prevalence and management of systemic amyloidosis in western countries. Kidney Diseases. 2016;**2**:10-19

[32] Gertz MA. Immunoglobulin light chain amyloidosis diagnosis and treatment algorithm 2018. Blood Cancer Journal. 2018;**8**:44-56

[33] Kyle RA, Bayrd ED. Amyloidosis: Review of 236 cases. Medicine (Baltimore). 1975;**54**:271-299

[34] Aimo A, Buda G, Fontana M, et al. Therapies for cardiac light chain amyloidosis: An update. International Journal of Cardiology. 2018;**271**:152-160

[35] Tuzovic M, Yang EH, Baas AS, et al. Cardiac amyloidosis: Diagnosis and treatment strategies. Current Oncology Reports. 2017;**19**:46-57

[36] Dispenzieri A, Gertz MA, Kyle RA, et al. Serum cardiac troponins and N-terminal pro-brain natriuretic peptide: A staging system for primary systemic amyloidosis. Journal of Clinical Oncology. 2004;**22**:3751-3757

[37] Zhang C, Huang X, Li J. Light chain amyloidosis: Where are the light chains from and how they play their pathogenic role? Blood Reviews. 2017;**31**:261-270

[38] Gertz MA, Kyle RA. Myopathy in primary systemic amyloidosis. Journal of Neurology, Neurosurgery, and Psychiatry. 1996;**60**:655-660

[39] Yen T, Chen FW, Witteles RM, et al. Clinical implications of gastrointestinal symptoms in systemic amyloidosis. Neurogastroenterology and Motility. 2018;**30**:e3229

[40] Rowe K, Pankow J, Nehme F, Salyers W. Gastrointestinal amyloidosis: Review of the literature. Cureus. 2017;**8**:e1228

[41] Matsuda S, Motosugi U, Kato R, et al. Hepatic amyloidosis with an extremely high stiffness value on magnetic resonance elastography. Magnetic Resonance in Medical Sciences. 2016;**15**:251-252

[42] Ozdemir D, Dagdelen S, Erbas T. Endocrine involvement in systemic amyloidosis. Endocrine Practice. 2010;**16**:1056-1063

[43] Rubinow A, Cohen AS. Skin involvement in generalized amyloidosis: A study of clinically involved and uninvolved skin in 50 patients with primary and secondary amyloidosis. Annals of Internal Medicine. 1978;**88**:781-785

[44] Harrison JS, Frazier SR, McConnell DD, et al. Evidence of both von Willebrand factor deposition and factor V deposition onto AL amyloid as the etiology of a severe bleeding diathesis. Blood Coagulation & Fibrinolysis. 2017;**28**:342-347

[45] Jaccard A, Moreau P, Leblond V, et al. High-dose melphalan versus melphalan plus dexamethasone for AL amyloidosis. The New England Journal of Medicine. 2007;**57**:1083-1093

[46] D'Souza A, Dispenzieri A, Wirk B, et al. Improved outcomes after autologous hematopoietic cell transplantation for light chain amyloidosis: A Center for International Blood and Marrow Transplant Research Study. Journal of Clinical Oncology. 2015;**33**:3741-3749

[47] Milani P, Merlini G, Palladini G. Light chain amyloidosis. Mediterranean Journal of Hematology and Infectious Diseases. 2018;**10**(1):e2018022. DOI: 10.4084/MJHID.2018.022

[48] Hamilton J, Benson M. Transthyretin: A review from a

structural perspective. Cellular and Molecular Life Sciences. 2001;**58**:1491. DOI: 10.1007-PL00000791

[49] Sekijima Y, Ueda M, Koike H, Misawa S, Ishii T, Ando Y. Diagnosis and management of transthyretin familial amyloid polyneuropathy in Japan: Red-flag symptom clusters and treatment algorithm. Orphanet Journal of Rare Diseases. 2018;**13**:6. DOI: 10.1186/s13023-017-0726-x

[50] Ueda M, Horibata Y, Shono M, Misumi Y, Oshima T, Su Y, et al. Clinicopathological features of senile systemic amyloidosis: An ante- and post-mortem study. Modern Pathology. 2011;**24**:1533-1544. DOI: 10.1038/modpathol.2011.117

[51] Koike H, Misu K, Sugiura M, Iijima M, Mori K, Yamamoto M, et al. Pathology of early- vs late-onset TTR Met30 familial amyloid polyneuropathy. Neurology. 2004;**63**:129-138

[52] Koike H, Tanaka F, Hashimoto R, et al. Natural history of transthyretin Val30Met familial amyloid polyneuropathy: Analysis of late-onset cases from non-endemic areas. Journal of Neurology, Neurosurgery, and Psychiatry. 2012;**83**:152-158. DOI: 10.1136/jnnp-2011-301299

[53] Sekijima Y, Yoshida K, Tokuda T, et al. Familial Transthyretin Amyloidosis in: GeneReviews at GeneTests: Medical Genetics Information Resource [Database Online] Copyright. Seattle: University of Washington; 1993-2014. http://www.ncbi.nlm.nih.gov/books/NBK1194

[54] Ruberg FL, Berk JL. Transthyretin (TTR) cardiac amyloidosis. Circulation. 2012;**126**:1286-1300. DOI: 10.1161/CIRCULATIONAHA.111.078915

[55] Bokhari S, Castano A, Pozniakoff T, Deslisle S, Latif F, Maurer MS. (99m)Tc pyrophosphate scintigraphy for differentiating light-chain cardiac amyloidosis from the transthyretin-related familial and senile cardiac amyloidoses. Circulation. Cardiovascular Imaging. 2013;**6**:195-201. DOI: 10.1161/CIRCIMAGING.112.000132

[56] Jin K, Sato S, Takahashi T, et al. Familial leptomeningeal amyloidosis with a transthyretin variant Asp18Gly representing repeated subarachnoid haemorrhages with superficial siderosis. Journal of Neurology, Neurosurgery & Psychiatry. 2004;**75**:1463-1466. DOI: 10.1136/jnnp.2003.029942

[57] Maia LF, Magalhaes R, Freitas J, et al. CNS involvement in V30M transthyretin amyloidosis: Clinical, neuropathological and biochemical findings. Journal of Neurology, Neurosurgery, and Psychiatry. 2014;**86**:159-167. DOI: 10.1136/jnnp-2014-308107

[58] Sekijima Y. Transthyretin (ATTR) amyloidosis: Clinical spectrum, molecular pathogenesis and disease-modifying treatments. Journal of Neurology, Neurosurgery, and Psychiatry. 2015;**86**:1036-1043. DOI: 10.1136/jnnp-2014-308724

[59] Coelho T, Maia LF, Martins da Silva A, et al. Tafamidis for transthyretin familial amyloid polyneuropathy: A randomized, controlled trial. Neurology. 2012;**79**:785-792. DOI: 10.1212/WNL.0b013e3182661eb1

[60] Maurer MS, Schwartz JH, Gundapaneni B, et al. Tafamidis treatment for patients with transthyretin amyloid cardiomyopathy. The New England Journal of Medicine. 2018;**379**:1007-1016. DOI: 10.1056/NEJMoa1805689

[61] Berk JL, Suhr OB, Obici L, Sekijima Y, Zeldenrust SR, Yamashita T, et al. Repurposing diflunisal for familial amyloid polyneuropathy: A randomized clinical trial. JAMA. 2013;**310**:2658-2667. DOI: 10.1001/jama.2013.283815

[62] Adams D, Gonzalez-Duarte A, O'Riordan WD, et al. Patisiran, an RNAi therapeutic, for hereditary transthyretin amyloidosis. New England Journal of Medicine. 2018;**379**:11-21. DOI: 10.1056/NEJMoa1716153

[63] Millns H, Bergemann R, Ackermann E, Monia B, Lukas MA. A phase 3 clinical trial with ISIS-TTRRx, a 2nd-generation antisense oligonucleotide targeting transthyretin (TTR), for the treatment of TTR amyloid cardiomyopathy. Orphanet Journal of Rare Diseases. 2015;**10**:8. DOI: 10.1186/1750-1172-10-S1-P8

[64] Girnius S, Dember L, Doros G, Skinner M. The changing face of AA amyloidosis: A single center experience. Amyloid. 2011;**18**:226-228. DOI: 10.3109/13506129.2011.574354085

[65] Simms RW, Prout MN, Cohen AS. The epidemiology of AL and AA amyloidosis. Baillière's Clinical Rheumatology. 1994;**8**:627-634. DOI: 10.1016/S0950-3579(05)80119-0

[66] Bunker D, Gorevic P. AA amyloidosis: Mount Sinai experience, 1997-2012. Mount Sinai Journal of Medicine. 2012;**79**:749-756. DOI: 10.1002/msj.21342

[67] Oh YB, Bae SC, Jung JH, Kim TH, Jun JB, Jung SS, et al. Secondary renal amyloidosis in adult onset Still's disease: Case report and review of the literature. The Korean Journal of Internal Medicine. 2000;**15**:131-134. DOI: 10.3904/kjim.2000.15.2.131

[68] Harzallah A, El Jery HK, Hajji M, Mami I, Goucha R, Turki S, et al. Amyloïdosis complicating Behcet's disease. Open Journal of Clinical Diagnostics. 2016;**6**:42-46. DOI: 10.4236/ojcd.2016.63008

[69] Gaduputi V, Tariq H, Badipatla K, Ihimoyan A. Systemic reactive amyloidosis associated with Castleman's disease. Case Reports in Gastroenterology. 2013;**12**:476-481. DOI: 10.1159/000356825

[70] Georgin-Lavialle S, Stankovic Stojanovic K, Buob D, et al. French amyloidosis CAPS study: AA amyloidosis complicating cryopyrin-associated periodic syndrome: A study on 14 cases and review of 53 cases from literature. Pediatric Rheumatology Online Journal. 2015;**13**:32. DOI: 10.1186/1546-0096-13-S1-P32

[71] Sanz-Martín N, Samillán-Sosa Kdel R, De Miguel J, Martínez-Miguel P. Renal amyloidosis in leprosy, an infrequent cause of nephrotic syndrome in Europe. BML Case Reports. 2016;**3**:bcr2016216038. DOI: 10.1136/bcr-2016-216038

[72] Balwani MR, Kute VB, Shah PR, Wakhare P, Trivedi HL. Secondary renal amyloidosis in a patient of pulmonary tuberculosis and common variable immunodeficiency. Journal of Nephropharmacology. 2015;**4**:69-71

[73] Akçay S, Akman B, Ozdemir H, Eyüboğlu FO, Karacan O, Ozdemir N. Bronchiectasis-related amyloidosis as a cause of chronic renal failure. Renal Failure. 2002;**24**:815-823

[74] Azzopardi JG, Lehner T. Systemic amyloidosis and malignant disease. Journal of Clinical Pathology. 1966;**19**:539-548

[75] Gueutin V, Langlois AL, Shehwaro N, Elharraqui R, Rouvier P, Izzedine H. Nephrotic syndrome associated with lung Cancer: A rare case of malignancy associated with AA amyloidosis. Case Reports in Nephrology. 2013;**2013**:831903 10.1155/2013/831903

[76] Husby G, Marhaug G, Sletten K. Amyloid A in systemic amyloidosis associated with cancer. Clinical investigations. AACR. 1982;**42**:1600-1603

Chapter 2

Amyloidosis: Systems-Based Therapies

Eileen Ly, Anu Stephen, Yasmeen Alhomsy, Asal Homayouni, Joshua Fisher, Kayla Sheehan, Prashanth Venkataraman, Quinto Gesiotto, Matthew Habib and Matthew Zabel

Abstract

In this chapter, the authors will discuss the epidemiology and clinical presentations of amyloidosis. The main body of this chapter will concentrate on treatment options, both FDA-approved and experimental, specific to the various forms of amyloidosis. Since this set of diseases can affect multiple organ systems, we tackle the therapeutic avenues and the current challenges in each system under clinical investigation, including neurological, psychiatric, gastrointestinal, cardiovascular, endocrine, renal and hematologic, in addition to options for palliative treatment for severe symptom management and improved quality of life. Several recent groundbreaking discoveries have opened up the potential for successful treatment of peripheral and central neurological amyloidoses making this an exciting and evolving field.

Keywords: transthyretin, antisense oligonucleotide, protein aggregation

1. Epidemiology

Amyloidosis is a rare, albeit likely underdiagnosed, disorder [1]. Claims data in the United States shows prevalence of amyloid light-chain (AL) amyloidosis increased between 2007 and 2015 from 15.5 to 45 cases per million [2]. Incidence did not significantly increase over this time period, but ranged from 9.7 to 14 cases per million-person years [2]. This equates to more than 12,000 people in the US currently living with this disorder. Older data, from 1950 to 1989, found 9 cases per million people, more evidence of an increasing prevalence over time [3]. The trend in age- and sex-adjusted incidence rate of amyloidosis per million person years from 1950 to 1989 was not found to be significant (**Figure 1**).

This phenomenon could be explained by increased detection and diagnosis. Studies in the United Kingdom and Sweden demonstrated a prevalence of 20 cases per million and incidence of 5 cases per million-person years, 3 of them being AL, and 1 amyloid A (AA) amyloidosis [1, 4]. A US study found a mean age at diagnosis of AL amyloidosis of 63 with a standard deviation of 12, 55% male [2]. International studies also show that men are slightly more likely to be diagnosed with AL, however, AA amyloidosis more commonly affects women, possibly due to higher prevalence of underlying rheumatoid arthritis [1].

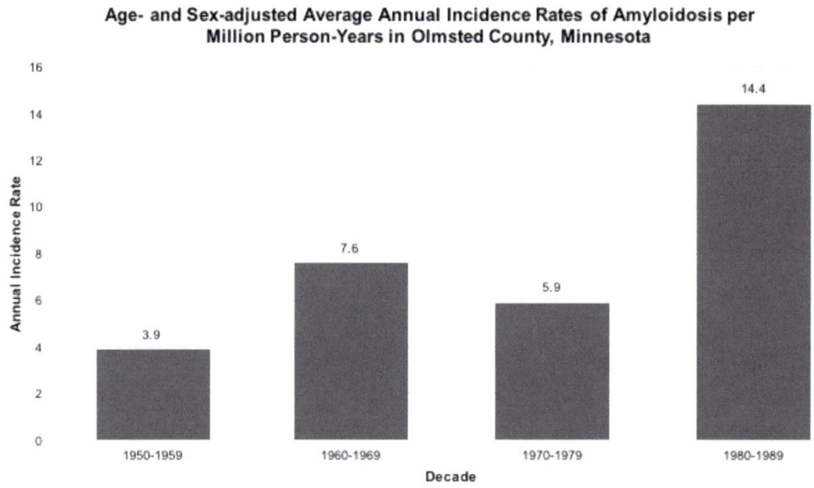

Figure 1.
Age- and sex-adjusted average annual incidence rates of amyloidosis per million person-years in Olmsted County, Minnesota from 1950 to 1989.

AL amyloidosis is more prevalent than AA amyloidosis in developed countries, however, in developing countries and some Mediterranean countries, AA is more prevalent (**Figure 2**). Other studies have shown AL to be more prevalent than AA in developed countries, but in developing nations AA has a higher prevalence than AL [1].

This follows the logic of the epidemiologic transition, since as a country develops, diseases transition from infectious to chronic disease states. In developing nations, endemic infections such as tuberculosis or leprosy lead to AA amyloidosis,

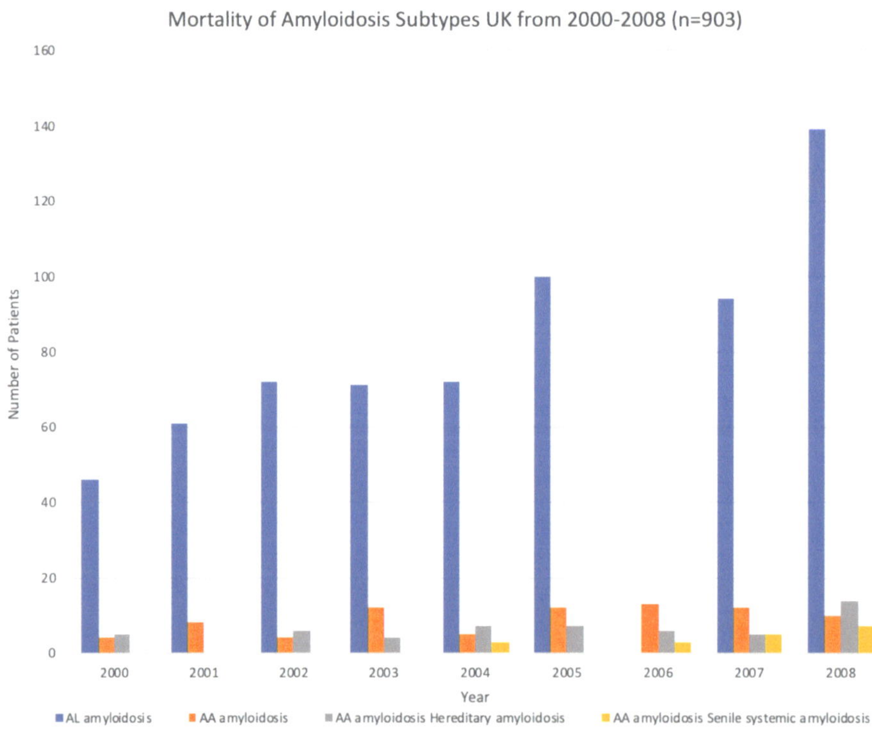

Figure 2.
Mortality of amyloidosis subtypes UK from 2000 to 2020,008 (n = 903).

while in developed nations chronic diseases lead to AL amyloidosis. The exception to this is Mediterranean nations, while developed, have a higher prevalence of AA amyloidosis. This is likely due to relatively high prevalence autoinflammatory diseases such as familial Mediterranean fever. For example, in Spain, AL amyloidosis has become the most prevalent subtype, increasing in frequency relative to other subtypes from 21% in 1977 to 44% in 2013 [5].

The prognosis for amyloidosis varies by subtype, treatment modality, extent of cardiac involvement and, to a lesser degree, hepatic and autonomic involvement [1]. A Swedish study estimated median survival to be 3, 4, and 6 years for AL, AA, and localized amyloidosis [6]. In regards to systemic amyloidosis, a median survival time of 32 months was seen in the UK [4]. Older studies found untreated median survival time ranging from 6 months to 4 years [1].

2. Palliative treatments for amyloidosis

The protein deposition and accumulation inherent in amyloidosis causes a wide range of systemic symptoms, and patients may also suffer from side effects of curative therapies. Though many mistakenly believe palliative interventions are only for end of life care, palliative treatments can be implemented at any stage of illness, and may help curb severe symptoms. In many forms of cancer, early palliative interventions have been shown to increase quality of life for both patients and caregivers [7]. While no studies have been conducted to evaluate the effectiveness of palliative therapies on amyloidosis specifically, palliative treatments for many of the common sequelae of amyloidosis have been well researched [8].

2.1 Pain

Neuropathic pain (NP) is the most common pain sensation reported in people with amyloidosis. NP is notoriously difficult to control, and is often not responsive to typical pain regimens. Antidepressants, anticonvulsants, opioids, and topical medications are the most common pharmacologic agents used. Unfortunately, many of these agents have their own side effects, and should be used with caution [8].

2.2 Depression

There has long been a link noted between depression and dementia, and depression has been viewed as both a prodrome and a risk factor for dementia. About half of patients with late-onset depression are found to have cognitive impairment, and the prevalence of dementia in depression has been reported between 9 and 68% [9]. A past history of depression is a known risk factor for developing Alzheimer's disease and vascular dementia, even when the episode of depression occurred over 10 years prior. Rather than a prodrome, depression seems to be a risk factor for Alzheimer's disease, as evidenced by a neuropathological study showing increased neurofibrillary tangles and plaques in the hippocampus in those with a history of depression [10]. Depression is linked to hypercortisolemia, which may cause prolonged damage to the hippocampus. Depression may also be a psychological reaction to the diagnosis of cognitive impairment, and may even reveal previously clinically silent cognitive impairment by depleting cognitive reserve [11]. Additionally, the use of tricyclic antidepressants in the elderly may also contribute to clinical dementia due to their anticholinergic effects.

The link between depression and Alzheimer disease may involve mechanisms in the metabolism of β-amyloid peptides in the brain. A recent study has shown significant associations between geriatric depression and β-amyloid peptide deposits in the insula, hippocampus, and amygdale [12]. Another recent study showed the link between hereditary gelsolin amyloidosis (AGel) and neuropsychiatric changes. The gelsolin mutation is associated with cerebrovascular fragility, and is an autosomal dominant form of systemic amyloidosis. The study found visuoconstructional difficulties in the AGel group in both the block design and drawing tasks. While overall processing speed was similar in both groups, the AGel group produced more errors [13]. The behavioral and psychological symptoms of people with dementia result in greater cognitive and functional impairment, and are associated with greater amyloid deposition in the neurodegenerative process leading to Alzheimer's disease [14].

2.3 Sexual dysfunction

The pathophysiology of sexual dysfunction in amyloidosis can range from medication side effects (corticosteroids, opioids), to primary hypogonadism (amyloid deposition in the testes), and depression. Determining the etiology of sexual dysfunction is key in selecting the proper treatment. For erectile dysfunction, sildenafil has been shown to be effective. Testosterone replacement may help in cases of hypogonadism, but has not been studied in patients with amyloidosis.

3. Renal amyloidosis

Renal amyloidosis is often the major cause of death for individuals with AL, AA, and hereditary amyloidosis; untreated, it usually progresses to end-stage renal disease. Understanding how amyloid fibrils form, and how the renal amyloidosis manifests are crucial in determining treatment approaches specific to each type of amyloidosis.

While amyloid can be found anywhere in the kidney, it often predominates in the glomerulus, forming nodules composed of amyloid protein that disrupt glomerular function. Consequently, patients with renal amyloidosis present with the components of nephrotic syndrome: severe proteinuria, hypoalbuminemia, edema, decreased GFR. When the amyloid protein is in the tubulointerstitium or vasculature, the patient will instead demonstrate minimal proteinuria with a decrease in GFR. (Vascular involvement may also come with HTN.) Generally, renal impairment progresses more rapidly with glomerular involvement. Patients mostly present with normal-sized kidneys but amyloidosis can cause enlargement of the kidneys.

Of the three main categories of renal amyloidoses, AL remains the most common, accounting for 81 and 68% of amyloidosis cases in two recent studies from the U.S. and Italy [15, 16]. In 50% of patients with systemic Ig-related amyloidosis, kidney disease presents as the most common manifestation [17].

3.1 Renal AL amyloidosis

Because AL amyloidosis is commonly associated with an underlying plasma cell dyscrasia, the purpose of treatment is to destroy amyloid-producing plasma cells. Therefore, treating AL amyloidosis is based on anti-myeloma therapy, which must be tailored to each patient's age, comorbidities, extent of organ involvement, and patient's wishes. The standard treatment was repeated cycles of oral melphalan and prednisone with an increase in median survival to 1.5 years [18]; however, this has changed in the past decade. In an 8 year longitudinal study by [19], 25–50% of patients who underwent high-dose intravenous melphalan followed by autologous stem cell transplantation(HDM/SCT to support bone marrow recovery demonstrated complete hematologic responses. In 2006, Seldin et al. followed 43 patients who received HDM/SCT between 1994 and 1996, and found that median survival rate of 10 years for patients with a complete hematologic response [20]. In 2011, Sanchorawala et al. followed the long-term outcome of 421 patients and reported a long-term survival of up to 20 years [19]. More research is being done on the effectiveness of repeated HDM/SCT treatments, some of them reporting favorable outcomes in patients who did not achieve a complete hematologic response the first time.

Despite the success of HDM/SCT, treatment-associated mortality is 12–14% with a higher prevalence in those with cardiac amyloidosis. Because stem cell mobilization requires high doses of growth factors, this can be complicated in patients with nephrotic syndrome or heart failure due to fluid retention. In addition to increased risks for splenic rupture (especially in patients with splenic amyloid), thrombocytopenia, and neutropenia, patients may also be subject to acute renal failure as reported by two different studies [21]. The British Journal of Hematology published guidelines in 2014 for HDM/SCT as first line treatment for selected patients up to 60–75 years of age with eGFR >50 ml/min, low cardiac biomarkers, low level plasma cell infiltration in the bone marrow, and lacking the following contraindications: cardiac amyloidosis, severe autonomic neuropathy, significant GI bleeding due to amyloid, advanced renal failure, age over 7 years, symptomatic recurrent amyloid related pleural effusions [22].

As an alternative to HDM/SCT, a combination of oral melphalan and high dose dexamethasone was shown by Pallidini et al. to have a 33% complete hematologic response in patients who are ineligible for HDM/SCT [23]. In addition to the oral melphalan and dexamethasone, patients can use proteasome inhibitor-based regimens and a bortezomib-alkylator-steroid combination for a rapid response [22].

3.2 Renal AA amyloidosis

Because AA amyloidosis is often associated with the production of serum amyloid A (SAA), an acute phase reactant protein from an underlying inflammatory disease, the goal of treatment is to treat the cause. Stopping the inflammatory processes of familial Mediterranean fever (FMF), rheumatoid arthritis (RA), and other causes of AA has been shown by several studies to prevent amyloidosis. For example, colchicine is used to inhibit Familial Mediterranean Fever-associated inflammation, which prevented amyloidosis production [24]. In a 2002 study, Elkyam et al. treated a patient with infliximab for rheumatoid arthritis, whose proteinuria resolved [25]. It is thought that these agents have additional anti-amyloid effects by suppressing cytokine production or by altering expression of specific mediators of cellular toxicity [26].

A new treatment approach involving fibrillogenic inhibition is currently underway, involving eprosidate, a sulfonated, negatively charged molecule like heparan sulfate. The molecule competitively binds to glycosaminoglycan-binding sites on SAA, and inhibits fibril polymerization and amyloid deposition. In a multicenter, randomized, double-blind, placebo controlled trial, Dember et al. demonstrated that eprodisate slowed the decline of renal function in AA amyloidosis patients [27]. The results from the second Phase III study will help determine whether eprosidate will become one of the new treatment approaches in fighting renal AA amyloidosis [28].

3.3 Dialysis and kidney transplantation

For patients with renal amyloidosis who are in ESRD, dialysis or kidney transplantation is other options. Currently, the literature for dialysis differs for AL amyloidosis patients and AA amyloidosis patients, but the consensus is a poor prognosis for AL amyloidosis patients on dialysis, especially those with cardiac involvement. For AA amyloidosis patients on dialysis, Guillaume et al. reported a 15% mortality rate, a better prognosis overall [29]. Treating patients who are on dialysis with HDM/SCT has shown no difference between the hematologic response rate and treatment -associated mortality are similar in dialysis-dependent patients compared with the overall population of patients who undergo this treatment [27].

Kidney transplantation is a good option for patients who have a complete hematologic response in AL amyloidosis and do not have significant extrarenal disease. In 2012, Gurusu et al. examined survival rates of 44 patients with amyloidosis who had undergone kidney transplantation and found the same outcomes with patients with other kidney diseases [30]. This indicates that amyloidosis patients should be accepted as transplant candidates.

3.4 Bortezomib, a game changer for multiple myeloma and AL amyloidosis

Monoclonal antibody therapy has become a mainstay of treatment in plasma cell disorders such as multiple myeloma and primary systemic (AL) amyloidosis. Bortezomib (Velcade), a proteasome inhibitor, has shown effectiveness as an initial therapy of multiple myeloma in stem cell transplant (SCT) eligible patients [31, 32]. Bortezomib has been especially effective in younger patients and contributed significantly to improvements in survival seen in the early 2000s [33]. Bortezomib and other proteasome inhibitors are associated with less cardiotoxic risk than chemotherapeutics such as melphalan, cyclophosphamide, and doxorubicin [34]. Modern induction therapy for multiple myeloma now consists a combination of bortezomib and dexamethasone (BD), plus thalidomide or melphalan for both transplant-eligible and SCT ineligible patients. A phase IIIB study found no difference in outcomes or survival between BD, BD plus thalidomide, or BD plus melphalan in transplant-ineligible patients [35]. Bortezomib is also effective as a consolidation

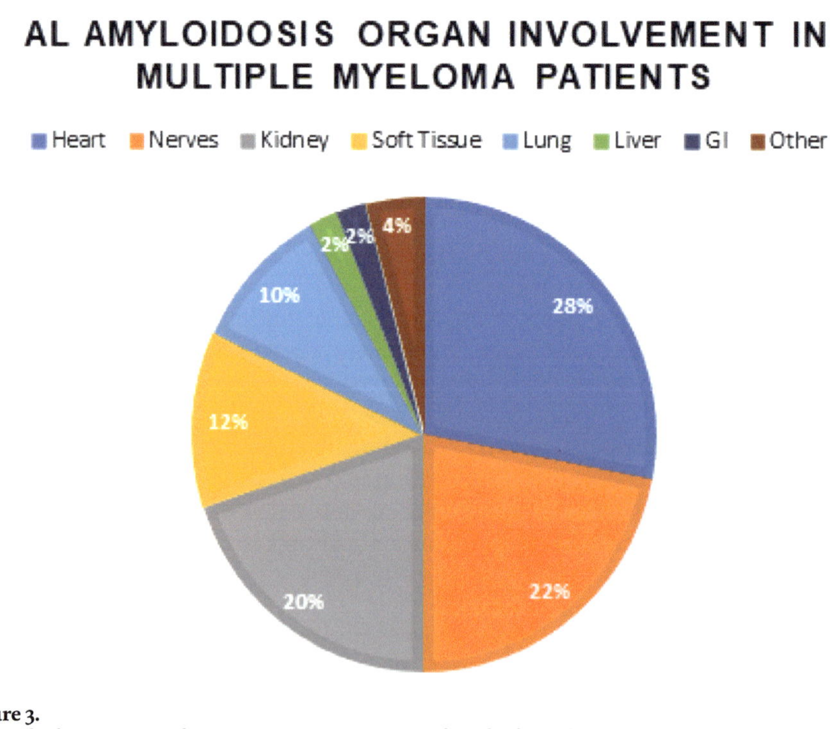

Figure 3.
AL amyloidosis organ involvement pattern in patients with multiple myeloma.

and maintenance therapy, prolonging progression-free survival and overall survival in patients with partial or very good partial response following induction/consolidation therapy [36].

AL amyloidosis can present spontaneously or in association with other blood cell disorders such as multiple myeloma and lymphoplasmocytic lymphoma. AL amyloidosis is a well-recognized complication of multiple myeloma in particular, occurring in approximately 10–15% of patients (**Figure 3**) [37]. Not surprisingly, bortezomib therapy is now a recommended treatment for primary AL amyloidosis both in SCT ineligible patients and post SCT patients [38, 39]. Reece et al. showed bortezomib to be a particularly effective and well-tolerated therapy in relapsed AL amyloidosis patients, evidenced by once and twice-weekly treatments both effectively inducing a hematological response in this population [40, 41]. A randomized phase III trial showed more profound and frequent hematological responses to bortezomib versus melphalan plus dexamethasone in patients with newly diagnosed AL amyloidosis, indicating bortezomib as a promising initial therapy [42].

4. Amyloidosis and the nervous system

Neurologic involvement of systemic amyloidosis has been observed in over 20% of cases, and the median duration of neuropathic symptoms prior to diagnosis is 2 years [43]. The pathophysiology of amyloid deposition contributing to the clinical manifestation of neurodegenerative disorders, including Alzheimer's Dementia, Parkinson's Disease, and Huntington's Disease, has been well-documented [44]. Furthermore, cerebral amyloid angiopathy is a well-known cause/risk factor for intracerebral hemorrhage in the elderly [45]. Lastly, systemic amyloidosis (classically, primary amyloidosis) affects not only the central nervous system, but is a well-known cause of peripheral and autonomic neuropathy [46]. Thus, the deposition of abnormally folded proteins has not only been linked to progressive and acute devastating CNS disorders, but also to neurologic sequelae throughout the body. In this section, we describe some of the novel treatments and their mechanisms of action for both CNS and PNS manifestations of the illness.

4.1 Amyloid beta: Alzheimer's dementia, and cerebral amyloid angiopathy

There are no current therapies that modify the deposition of A beta amyloid in the CNS. Therefore the focus of treatment has been mainly symptomatic with acetylcholinesterase inhibitors, antidepressants and antipsychotics. However, new research focusing on monoclonal antibodies reducing plaque load prove to have promising results in the mice model [47]. Modest levels of peripherally administration antibodies against the amyloid beta-peptide crossed the blood brain barrier entering the CNS and inducing clearance of preexisting amyloid via activation of microglial cells [48]. Bapineuzumab, Solanezumab, Gantenerumab, Crenezumab, Ponezumab, BAN2401, and Aducaumab are anti-amyloid beta monoclonal antibodies that have progressed to human trials and paved the pathway for the development of more effective therapies.

The mechanism of Bapineuzumab, one of the first humanized monoclonal IgG1 antibody used in humans, attaches to soluble and fibrillar amyloid beta via the five N-terminal residues inducing Fc receptor-mediated microglial phagocytosis of amyloid beta deposits. In phase 1, 30 patients were divided into low dose (0.5 mg/kg), medium (1.5 mg/kg) and high dose (5 mg/kg), and overall the drug was considered to be safe. 3/10 participants in the high dose category developed MRI findings typical of vasogenic edema that eventually resolved. Amyloid-related imaging abnormalities

(ARIA) were coined to describe imaging abnormalities as a result of treatment, for example ARIA-H for microhemorrhage and hemosiderosis and ARIA-E for effusion or vasogenic edema. IV infusion in phase 2 of the trial showed no significant treatment differences in patients with mild to moderate Alzheimer's disease. A parallel phase 2, as well as retrospective study done by neuroradiologists resulted in the conclusion that there is an increased occurrence of ARIA-E in carriers of APOE4, necessitating the incorporation of biomarkers to qualify for treatment, but increased numbers of symptomatic ARIA-E resulted in discontinuation of bapineuzumab trials.

Solanezumab, another humanized IgG1 monoclonal antibody, completed phase 3 testing without meeting efficacy requirements. It binds the mid-domain of amyloid beta residues to increase clearance of monomers, and continues in preclinical Alzheimer's disease trials to see if there is a benefit to earlier intervention. Phases 1 and 2 showed a relationship between dose and CSF Amyloid-beta protein. In phase 3 studies, termed EXPEDITION 1 and EXPEDITION 2, 18 month trials of IV solanezumab 400 mg against IV placebo, did not demonstrate any significant benefit. However, it demonstrated the drugs favorable safety profile with only 0.9% incidence of ARIA-E compared to 0.4% seen in the placebo. A third phase 3 trial, EXPEDITION 3, also showed nonsignificant results with solanezumab and eventually led to the drug's discontinuation for dementia.

As opposed to the previously mentioned therapies, Gantenerumab was the first fully human IgG1 antibody against the conformational epitope expressed on amyloid beta fibrils that contain both the N-terminal and central amino acids. Phase 1 trials with patients who had mild to moderate Alzheimer's disease showed that seven IV infusions (60–200 mg) every 4 weeks reduced brain burden. It also showed the drug's favorable safety profile. 2 out of 6 patients in the high dose group experienced ARIA-E. Initial phase 2 trials included 360 participants and doses of subcutaneous 105 mg or 225 mg every 4 weeks for 2 years, but was later expanded to a phase 2/3 with 799 participants showed no significant treatment effects for CDE-SB or changes in the amount of brain amyloid beta. Currently Gantenerumab, like solanezumab, is being explored for patients with fast progression and autosomal dominant Alzheimer's disease.

Other therapies that have proven to have non-significant results in the treatment of amyloid beta deposition within the CNS include Crenezumab, Ponezumab, BAN2401, and Aducaumab. Despite these findings, the tolerability of monoclonal antibodies lends hope for developing therapies for this pathology. Moreover, future studies should focus on the importance of brain entry of anti-amyloid beta monoclonal antibodies, as it is not currently clear whether therein lies any benefit as only 0.1% cross the blood brain barrier. Dosage and stage of disease are two other important points for consideration in improving the efficacy of these therapies, and whether the lack of efficacy was due to insufficient amounts of drug or late stage disease [49].

4.2 Transthyretin amyloidosis

Transthyretin is a liver-derived protein, that when misfolded can accumulate in the liver, kidney, GI tract, and the peripheral nerves. Multiple genetic abnormalities have been shown to contribute to increased predisposition and familial forms of transthyretin amyloidosis. These have led to syndromes such as familial amyloidotic cardiomyopathy and familial amyloidotic polyneuropathy [49, 50].

Familial amyloidotic polyneuropathy (FAP) is a fatal condition that is caused by the substitution of a methionine residue for a valine residue at the 30th position of the TTR gene [51]. In this section, we briefly discuss the role of liver transplantation and more thoroughly introduce the use of RNA interference molecules to decrease transthyretin production.

5. Liver transplantation

Around 95% of transthyretin is produced by the liver, and thus, it was postulated that liver transplantation would provide great benefit for patients with transthyretin amyloidosis. The first liver transplantation for transthyretin amyloidosis was done in 1990 in Sweden and showed promising results. Since then, liver transplantation has been a standard treatment for this devastating disorder [51].

Liver transplantation has been shown to be of benefit if intervention is taken earlier in the disease course. The risks and prognostic factors for liver transplantation have been well-documented, including the long wait times for an available transplantable organ. However, additional prognostic factors for survival post liver transplantation in patients with amyloidotic polyneuropathy include hereditary and geographic factors, duration of the disease, initial degree of polyneuropathy, presence of autonomic dysfunction, co-morbid cardiac, kidney/bladder, and GI impairment, and prior nutritional status. Liver transplantation is usually not a procedure that will improve the patient's condition, but rather, prevent further decline.

5.1 IDOX, doxycycline, and RNAi therapy

Since the difficulties associated with liver transplantation prevented adequate treatment of FAP patients, new non-surgical treatment methods were researched. It was initially shown that 4′iodo′4′-doxy-doxorubicin (IDOX) inhibits amyloid formation and promotes the resorption of amyloid deposits. Initially shown that IDOX can induce amyloid resorption in patients with immunoglobulin light chain amyloidosis, it was further studied for all types of amyloid deposition disorders. It is hypothesized that IDOX exerts its effects by inhibiting fibril growth and increasing the solubility of amyloid deposits. This, in turn, facilitates amyloid clearance. These results have been consistent in both in vivo and in vitro studies through two distinct binding sites between IDOX and amyloid fibrils [52].

At around the same time as IDOX was being investigated, Doxycycline became the next promising medication that showed similar success in both FAP transgenic mice and phase II human trials with transthyretin amyloidosis. It's theorized mechanism of action involves amyloid fibril destructuration and promotion of amyloid deposition. In one phase II trial, doxycyclin plus tauroursodeoxycholic acid resulted in stable cardiac and neuropathy symptoms after 1 year of treatment. When used in conjunction with TTR stabilizers, therapy could both block formation and promote clearance of existing amyloid simultaneously [53, 54].

The most recent research for transthyretin amyloidosis treatment has surrounded RNA interference (RNAi) therapy. RNAi therapy decreases transthyretin production from the liver by directly suppressing mRNA transcription of the gene that codes for the transthyretin protein. Due to the specific nature of this pharmacology, long-term side-effects of RNAi therapy have not been reported. Two medications, Patisiran and Inotersen, have become FDA approved in the past 5 years after studies have shown a dose-dependent reduction of both mutant and nonmuntant tranthyretin production and deposition. This RNAi therapy has been shown to cause between 50 and 80% reduction in transthyretin levels as early as 2–3 weeks after therapy initiation. Furthermore, these medications have provided significant neurologic symptomatic benefit in a majority of patients when compared to placebo therapy. Since these medications affect both mutant and non-mutant transthyretin production, they have been shown to not only have decreased side-effects to liver transplantation, but better long-term efficacy. The most common side effect to the medication reported has been transfusion-related reactions in 8–20% of patients [49, 55, 56].

6. Cardiac amyloidosis

Along with the kidneys, the heart is one of the most commonly affected organs in cases of amyloidosis, as amyloid fibrils deposit in its parenchyma and impair it from functioning optimally. The deposition of either light chain amyloid (AL) or transthyretin (TTR) in the cardiac myocardium is responsible for the vast majority (>95%) of cases of amyloid cardiomyopathy [57]. This infiltration of the myocardial tissue essentially results in a clinical presentation of heart failure with preserved ejection fraction; therefore, the treatment is twofold and is targeted at both the primary, underlying disease process and at the secondary heart failure.

6.1 AL amyloid

In regards to the primary disease, treatment varies substantially based on the nature of the abnormal protein that is deposited in the cardiac tissue. AL amyloid, or primary amyloid, affects the heart by depositing abnormally-folded proteins into the myocardium, rendering the ventricles concentrically thickened, thus impairing their ability to accommodate adequate filling volumes. Some studies suggest that the amyloidogenic proteins also have direct cytotoxic effects on the myocardial cells. The pathogenic proteins in AL amyloid are misfolded immunoglobulin light chains produced by a number of clonal plasma cells in the bone marrow; therefore, cytotoxic therapies against these cells have been proven to be effective. A combination of oral melphalan, dexamethasone, autologous stem cell transplantation and/or bortezomib is often utilized and tailored to each individual case based on various factors such as age, stage of disease, and patient's desire for treatment. These drug regimens are further discussed in the section on renal amyloidosis treatment.

6.2 TTR amyloid

In transthyretin amyloidosis, the protein transthyretin (TTR) loses stability, misfolds, and deposits in organs throughout the body, including the cardiac myocardium. In contrast to other types of amyloidosis, which may or may not involve the heart, TTR almost always features cardiac involvement and myocardial protein deposition. The consequences of protein deposition in the heart are essentially the same across all types of amyloidosis as the ventricles thicken and result in a restrictive type of cardiomyopathy that prevents the heart from properly filling with blood during the diastolic phase of the cardiac cycle. The restrictive cardiomyopathy leads to a clinical picture of heart failure, with symptoms that often significantly decrease the patient's quality of life. The most definitive treatment for TTR amyloidosis is liver transplantation. This is because the TTR protein is produced in the liver and eliminating the source of the protein would eliminate the pathogenic process altogether. Liver transplantation, however, may not be an option for patients who are not candidates for the procedure. This is where a recently studied drug, Tafamidis, plays a key role. Tafamidis is an agent that exhibits its therapeutic effect by stabilizing the TTR protein, thus preventing its misfolding and subsequent deposition in organs of the body. In a randomized, placebo-controlled, double blind study performed in September 2018, Tafamidis was found to improve the quality of life of amyloidosis patients by slowing the progression of the disease and reducing the functional impairment of affected nerves and systems throughout the body [58, 59]. Other drugs that also may be beneficial in TTR amyloidosis cases include an NSAID called Diflunisal, doxycycline, and an antisense therapy called ISIS-TTRrx. Both Diflunisal and doxycycline are thought to have the same mechanism of action as Tafamidis, as they stabilize the TTR protein and prevent amyloidogenesis. ISIS-TTRrx's mechanism of action differs and works by directly suppressing the gene that expresses the TTR protein. These agents are still being investigated for efficacy in experiments and clinical trials [59].

6.3 Heart failure

Heart failure secondary to cardiac amyloidosis is treated rather differently than heart failure that is organic or secondary to other causes. Agents that typically play key roles in heart failure management, such as beta blockers, ace inhibitors, and calcium channel blockers, are avoided and, sometimes, even contraindicated. These drugs are ineffective in cases of amyloid cardiomyopathy due to the pathophysiology of protein deposition rather than intrinsic cellular dysfunction of the cardiac cells. Utilization of calcium channel blockers, for example, results in an apparent amplification of the drugs' negative inotropic effects and a resultant decompensation of the amyloid cardiomyopathy [60, 61]. One class of drugs- the loop diuretics- remains the cornerstone medication utilized even in cases of heart failure due to amyloid cardiomyopathy. A loop diuretic combined with an aldosterone antagonist has been found to be the most efficacious combination of treatment for amyloid-associated heart failure [57, 62]. Along with drug therapy, other vital lifestyle changes include salt and fluid restriction, as well as regular weight measurements to monitor volume status.

7. Amyloidosis of the respiratory tract

Amyloidosis is characterized by pathological misfolding of the amyloid protein and its deposition as fibrils leading to organ dysfunction. Amyloidosis of the respiratory tract can be localized or a part of a systemic picture of dysfunction. Pulmonary amyloidosis is only symptomatic if amyloid deposits are present on the alveoli, causing impaired gas exchange. Amyloid deposition in the lung parenchyma may manifest as nodular deposits or lead to localized lymphomas.

Tissue deposits of misfolded amyloid protein in the form of fibrils characterize systemic amyloidosis. There are 15 different kinds of systemic amyloidoses, defined based on the characteristics of the deposited amyloid protein [63]. The primary kinds of amyloidosis that impact the lungs are systemic AL and localized AL consisting of monoclonal light chains, AA amyloid consisting of apolipoprotein serum amyloid A, and ATTRwt consisting of wild-type transthyretin [64]. Regardless of the type of amyloid fibril that is deposited, all fibrils have the same backbone structure that the Congo red stain binds in order to reveal an apple-green birefringence under polarized light [65]. Tissue biopsy is central to diagnosis of amyloidosis as treatment modalities vary based on the type of amyloid protein that is deposited. Less invasive procedures like abdominal fat biopsy and fine needle biopsy are indicated over more invasive procedures like transbronchial biopsy [66, 67]. Once a biopsy is obtained, it is evaluated using immunohistochemistry. The lungs are a common site of amyloid deposition, although not always symptomatic. There are three main kinds of pulmonary amyloidosis: nodular, diffuse, and tracheobronchial. Systemic amyloidosis is symptomatic, and often as a result of chronic inflammation.

7.1 Nodular pulmonary amyloidosis

Nodular amyloid deposits involving the lung are usually an incidentaloma on chest imaging and usually consist of AL light chain or mixed AL-AH light chain-heavy chain [68, 69]. Nodular amyloidosis has been associated with mucosa associated lymphoid tissue (MALT) and Sjogren disease [68]. In a study of 49 individuals with nodular AL amyloidosis, surgical resection and systemic chemotherapy were the major forms of treatment [64]. In fact, conservative excision in nodular AL amyloidosis presents with a great prognosis, although intervention is rarely required as a whole.

7.2 Diffuse alveolar amyloidosis

Presence of amyloid deposits on the alveolar walls and adjoining blood vessels signifies diffuse alveolar amyloidosis [70–72]. Since pulmonary impairment is not prominent in diffuse alveolar amyloidosis, it is often observed as a finding of post-mortem studies [73]. Positron emission tomography using radiolabeled florbetapir is one of the modalities that can help identify the diffuse alveolar variant of amyloidosis [74]. Diffuse alveolar amyloidosis has a progressive course of interstitial lung disease involving an infiltrative imaging pattern and dyspnea [75].

Diffuse alveolar amyloidosis is most commonly a manifestation of systemic AL amyloidosis, which is why treatment takes the form of targeting the underlying systemic amyloidosis. Burden reduction of free light chain is deemed to be central principle of treatment. Chemotherapy like low-dose Melphalan derived for multiple myeloma currently drives the treatment modalities used for diffuse alveolar amyloidosis [76–78]. Prednisolone is another medication used for treatment purposes. However, it is important to fashion treatment on a personalized basis based on patient needs. Pulmonary amyloidosis especially complicates the scenario when diffusion capacity reduces to less than 50%, although stem cell transplantation is an option in these cases [79]. Lung transplant is yet another option to treat isolated lung amyloidosis [80].

7.3 Laryngeal amyloidosis

Usually localized in nature, laryngeal amyloidosis is manifested by amyloid deposits superior to the glottis. The larynx is the most common location for isolated amyloid deposition in the head and neck, and symptomatically presents with stridor, dyspnea, and hoarseness [81]. Larger lesions are often surgically removed with an endoscopic excision or laryngofissure [82, 83]. Smaller lesions can be treated with carbon dioxide laser evaporation [84, 85].

7.4 Tracheobronchial amyloidosis

Tracheobronchial amyloidosis is characterized by submucosal plaques with occasional involvement of the trachea and larynx [86, 87]. Cough, dyspnea, and hemoptysis are common manifestations, with tracheal and bronchial thickening and calcifications being diagnostic markers on CT [88, 89]. Stenting is also used to prevent airway collapse in an already compromised respiratory circuit. Although treatment modalities for tracheobronchial amyloidosis are limited, systemic chemotherapy is sometimes used [89]. Tracheobronchial involvement can be symptomatically treated with debridement, bronchoscopic resection, and external beam radiation [90, 91].

7.5 A peek into the future

Agents are being developed that aim to help stabilize amyloid in their native morphology and slow down or even halt fibril deposition. Glycosaminoglycans (GAG)-like molecules inhibitors and Secreted Aspartyl Proteinase (SAP)-binding inhibitors are currently being developed. GAG binding to amyloid enhances amyloid fibril deposition, while SAP potentiates amyloidosis [92, 93]. Like mentioned earlier, it is paramount to mold each treatment plan according to the recipient to best suit the patient's needs and goals of care.

Author details

Eileen Ly, Anu Stephen, Yasmeen Alhomsy, Asal Homayouni, Joshua Fisher, Kayla Sheehan, Prashanth Venkataraman, Quinto Gesiotto, Matthew Habib and Matthew Zabel*
College of Medicine, California Northstate University, Elk Grove, CA, USA

*Address all correspondence to: matthew.zabel9352@cnsu.edu

References

[1] Nienhuis HL, Bijzet J, Hazenberg BP. The prevalence and management of systemic amyloidosis in Western countries. Kidney Diseases. 2016;**2**(1):10-19

[2] Quock TP, Yan T, Chang E, Guthrie S, Broder MS. Epidemiology of AL amyloidosis: A real-world study using US claims data. Blood Advances. 2018;**2**(10):1046-1053

[3] Kyle R, Linos A, Beard C, Linke R, Gertz M, O'Fallon W, et al. Incidence and natural history of primary systemic amyloidosis in Olmsted County, Minnesota, 1950 through 1989. Blood. 1992;**79**(7):1817-1822

[4] Pinney JH, Smith CJ, Taube JB, Lachmann HJ, Venner CP, Gibbs SD, et al. Systemic amyloidosis in England: An epidemiological study. British Journal of Haematology. 2013;**161**(4):525-532

[5] de Asúa D, Costa R, Galván JM, Filigheddu MT, Trujillo D, Cadiñanos J. Systemic AA amyloidosis: Epidemiology, diagnosis, and management. Clinical Epidemiology. 2014;**6**:369-377

[6] Hemminki K, Li X, Försti A, Sundquist J, Sundquist K. Incidence and survival in non-hereditary amyloidosis in Sweden. BMC Public Health. 2012;**12**:974

[7] El-Jawahri A, Greer JA, Pirl WF, Park ER, Jackson VA, Back AL, et al. Effects of early integrated palliative care on caregivers of patients with lung and gastrointestinal cancer: A randomized clinical trial. The Oncologist. 2017;**22**(12):1528-1534

[8] Tsukanov J, Fabbro ED. Palliative care and symptom management in amyloidosis: A review. Current Problems in Cancer. 2016;**40**(5-6):220-228

[9] Muliyala K, Varghese M. The complex relationship between depression and dementia. Annals of Indian Academy of Neurology. 2010;**13**(Suppl 2):S69-S73

[10] Rapp M, Schnaider-Beeri M, Grossman H, Sano M, Perl D, Purohit D, et al. Increased hippocampal plaques and tangles in patients with Alzheimer disease with a lifetime history of major depression. Archives of General Psychiatry. 2006;**63**(2):161-167

[11] Ganguli M. Depression, cognitive impairment and dementia: Why should clinicians care about the web of causation? Indian Journal of Psychiatry. 2009;**51**(Suppl 1):S29-S34

[12] Kim H, Kong E, Cheon E, Kim H, Koo B. Association between cerebral amyloid deposition and clinical factors including cognitive function in geriatric depression: Pilot study using amyloid. Clinical Psychopharmacology and Neuroscience. 2016;**14**(4):378-382

[13] Kantanen M, Kiuru-Enari S, Salonen O, Kaipainen M, Hokkanen L. Subtle neuropsychiatric and neurocognitive changes in hereditary gelsolin amyloidosis (AGel amyloidosis). Peer J. 2014;**2**:e493

[14] Bensamoun D, Guignard R, Furst A, Derreumaux A, Manera V, Darcourt J, et al. Associations between neuropsychiatric symptoms and cerebral amyloid deposition in cognitively impaired elderly people. Journal of Alzheimer's Disease. 2016;**49**(2):387-398

[15] Said M, Johnson H, Nonyane B, Deloria-Knoll M, O'Brien K, Andreo F, et al. Estimating the burden of pneumococcal pneumonia among adults: a systematic review and meta-analysis of diagnostic techniques. PLoS One. 2013;**8**(4):e60273

[16] Bergesio F, Ciciani A, Manganaro M, Palladini G, Santostefano M, Brugnano R, et al. Renal involvement in systemic amyloidosis: an Italian collaborative study on survival and renal outcome. Nephrology Dialysis Transplantation. 2008;**23**(3):941-51

[17] Mazdak A, Wallace W, Palma-Diaz M. Amyloid nephropathy. Clinical Kidney Journal. Apr 2014;**7**(2):97-106

[18] Seldin D, inner OB, Quillen K, Finn K. Relapse rate and long-term survival of AL amyloidosis patients treated with high-dose melphalan and autologous stem cell transplantation (HDM/SCT). Blood. 2006;**108**:3094

[19] Skinner M, Sanchorawala V, Seldin D, Dember L, Falk R, Berk J, et al. High-dose melphalan and autologous stem-cell transplantation in patients with AL amyloidosis: An 8-year study. Amyloid and Amyloidosis. 2004;**140**(2):85-93

[20] Seldin M, Shigeta R, Villoslada P, Selmi C, Tuomilehto J, Silva G, et al. European Population Substructure: Clustering of Northern and Southern Populations. PLoS Genetics. 2006; **2**(9):e143

[21] Leung N, Griffin DA, Haugen E, Gloor J, Schwab T, et al. Living donor kidney and autologous stem cell transplantation for primary systemic amyloidosis (AL) with predominant renal involvement. American Journal of Transplantation. 2005;**5**(7):1660-1670

[22] Wechalekar A, Gillmore J, Bird J, Cavenagh J, Hawkins S, Kazmi M, et al. Guidelines on the management of AL amyloidosis. British Journal of Haematology. 2015;**168**(2):186-206

[23] Palladini G, Perfetti V, Obici L, Caccialanza R, Semino A, Adami F, et al. Association of melphalan and high-dose dexamethasone is effective and well tolerated in patients with AL (primary) amyloidosis who are ineligible for stem cell transplantation. Blood. 2004;**103**(8):2936-2938

[24] Ozen S. Renal amyloidosis in familial mediterranean fever. Kidney International. 2004;**65**(3):1118-1127

[25] Elkayam O, Hawkins P, Lachmann H, Yaron M, Caspi D. Rapid and complete resolution of proteinuria due to renal amyloidosis in a patient with rheumatoid arthritis treated with infliximab. Arthritis and Rheumatism. 2002;**46**(10):2571-2573

[26] Yan DS, Zhu H, Zhu A, Golabek A, Du H, Roher A, et al. Receptor-dependent cell stress and amyloid accumulation in systemic amyloidosis. Nature Medicine. 2000;**6**(6):643-651

[27] Dember L, Hawkins P, Hazenberg B, Gorevic P, Merlini G, Butrimiene I, et al. Eprodisate for the treatment of renal disease in AA amyloidosis. NEJM. 2007;**356**(23):2349-2360

[28] Rumjon A, Coats T, Javaid M. Review of eprodisate for the treatment of renal disease in AA amyloidosis. International Journal of Nephrology and Renovascular Disease. 2012;**5**:37-43

[29] Guillaume B, N Straetmans N, Jadoul M, Cosyns J, Ferrant A. Allogeneic bone marrow transplantation for AL. Bone Marrow Transplantation. 1997;**20**:907-908

[30] Gursu M, Yelken B, Caliskan Y, Kazancioglu R, Yazici H, Kilicaslan I, et al. Outcome of patients with amyloidosis after renal transplantation: a single-center experience. International Journal of Artificial Organs. 2012; **35**(6):444-449

[31] Moreau P, Avet-Loiseau H, Facon T, Attal M, Tiab M, Hulin C, et al. Bortezomib plus dexamethasone versus reduced-dose bortezomib, thalidomide plus dexamethasone as

induction treatment prior to autologous stem cell transplantation in newly diagnosed multiple myeloma. Blood. 2011;**118**(22):5752-5758

[32] Kumar S, Dispenzieri A, Lacy M, Gertz M, Buadi F, Pandey S, et al. Continued improvement in survival in multiple myeloma: Changes in early mortality and outcomes in older patients. Leukemia. 2014;**28**(5):1122-1128

[33] Brenner H, Gondos A, Pulte D. Recent major improvement in long-term survival of younger patients with multiple myeloma. Blood. 2008;**111**(5):2521-2526

[34] Bringhen S, Milan A, Ferri C, Wäsch R, Gay F, Larocca A, et al. Cardiovascular adverse events in modern myeloma therapy–incidence and risks. A review from the European myeloma network (EMN) and Italian Society of Arterial Hypertension. Haematologica. 2018;**103**(9):1422-1432

[35] Niesvizky R, Flinn I, Rifkin R, Gabrail N, Charu V, Clowney B, et al. Community-based phase IIIB trial of three UPFRONT bortezomib-based myeloma regimens. Journal of Clinical Oncology. 2015;**33**(33):3921-3929

[36] Cerrato C, Raimondo DF, Paoli DL, Spada S, Patriarca F, Crippa C, et al. Maintenance in myeloma patients achieving complete response after upfront therapy: A pooled analysis. Journal of Cancer Research and Clinical Oncology. 2018;**144**(7):1357-1366

[37] Madan S, Dispenzieri A, Lacy M, Buadi F, Hayman S, Zeldenrust S, et al. Clinical features and treatment response of light chain (AL) amyloidosis diagnosed in patients with previous diagnosis of multiple myeloma. Mayo Clinic Proceedings. 2010;**85**(3):232-238

[38] Kastritis E, Anagnostopoulos A, Roussou M, Toumanidis S, Pamboukas C, et al. Treatment of light chain (AL) amyloidosis with the combination of bortezomib and dexamethasone. Haematologica. 2007;**92**(10):1351-1358

[39] Chaulagain C, Comenzo R. How we treat systemic light-chain amyloidosis. Clinical Advances in Hematology & Oncology. 2015;**13**(5):315-324

[40] Reece D, Hegenbart U, Sanchorawala V, Merlini G, Paladini G, Blade J, et al. Long-term follow-up from a phase 1/2 study of single-agent bortezomib in relapsed systemic AL amyloidosis. Blood. 2014;**124**(16):2498-2506

[41] Reece D, Hegenbart U, Sanchorawala V, Merlini G, Paladini G, Blade J, et al. Efficacy and safety of once-weekly and twice-weekly bortezomib in patients with relapsed systemic AL amyloidosis: Results of a phase 1/2 study. Blood. 2011;**118**(4):865-873

[42] Kastritis E, Leleu X, Arnulf B, Zamagni E, Cibeira M, et al. A randomized phase III trial of melphalan and dexamethasone (MDex) versus bortezomib, melphalan and dexamethasone (BMDex) for untreated patients. Blood. 2016;**128**:646

[43] Lasek-Bal A, Holecki M, Czapska A, Karuga A, Dulawa J. Primary clinical manifestation of systemic amyloidosis in the central nervous system. Polskie Archiwum Medycyny Wewnętrznej. 2014;**124**(3):138-139

[44] Adav S, Gallart-Palau X, Tan K, Lim S, Tam J, et al. Dementia-linked amyloidosis is associated with brain protein deamidation as revealed by proteomic profiling of human brain tissues. Molecular Brain. 2016;**9**(20):1-10

[45] Banerjee G, Carare R, Cardonnier C, Greenberg S, Schneider J, et al. The increasing impact of cerebral amyloid angiopathy: Essential new insights for

clinical practice. Journal of Neurology, Neurosurgery, and Psychiatry. 2017;**88**(11):982-994

[46] Shin SC, Robinson-Papp J. Amyloid neuropathies. Mount Sinai Journal of Medicine: A Journal of Translational and Personalized Medicine. 2012;**79**(6):733-748

[47] Bard F, Cannon C, Barbour R, Burke R, medicine GD. Peripherally administered antibodies against amyloid β-peptide enter the central nervous system and reduce pathology in a mouse model of alzheimer disease. Nature. 2000;**6**:916-919

[48] Van Dyck C. Anti-amyloid-β monoclonal antibodies for Alzheimer's disease: Pitfalls and promise. Biological Psychiatry. 2018;**83**(4):311-319

[49] Coelho T, Adams D, Silva A, Lozeron P, Hawkins P, Mant T, et al. Safety and efficacy of RNAi therapy for transthyretin amyloidosis. NEJM. 2013;**369**:819-829

[50] Sekijima Y, Yazaki M, Oguchi K, Ezawa N, Yoshinaga T, Yamada M, et al. Cerebral amyloid angiopathy in posttransplant patients with hereditary ATTR amyloidosis. Neurology. 2016;**87**:1-9

[51] Suhr OB, Herlenius G, Friman S, Ericzon B. Liver transplantation for hereditary transthyretin amyloidosis. Liver Transplantation. 2000;**6**(3):263-276

[52] Merlini G, Ascari E, Amboldi N, Bellotti V, Arbustini E, Perfetti V, et al. Interaction of the anthracycline 4′-iodo-4′-deoxydoxorubicin with amyloid fibrils: Inhibition of amyloidogenesis. PNAS. 1995;**92**(7):2959-2963

[53] Cardoso I, Saraiva M. Doxycycline disrupts transthyretin amyloid: Evidence from studies in a FAP transgenic mice model. The FASEB Journal. 2006;**20**(2):234-239

[54] Obici L, Cortese A, Lozza A, Lucchetti J, Amyloid GM. Doxycycline plus tauroursodeoxycholic acid for transthyretin amyloidosis: a phase II Study. Amyloid: the international journal of experimental and clinical investigation. 2012;**19**(1):34-36

[55] Adams D, Gonzalez-Duarte A, O'Riordan WD, Yang C-C, Ueda M, Kristen AV, et al. Patisiran, an RNAi therapeutic, for hereditary transthyretin amyloidosis. New England Journal of Medicine. 2018;**379**(1):11-21

[56] Benson MD, Waddington-Cruz M, Berk JL, Polydefkis M, Dyck PJ, Wang AK, et al. Inotersen treatment for patients with hereditary transthyretin amyloidosis. New England Journal of Medicine. 2018;**379**(1):22-31

[57] Donnelly JP, Hanna M. Cardiac amyloidosis: An update on diagnosis and treatment. Cleveland Clinic Journal of Medicine. 2017;**84**(12 Suppl 3):12-26

[58] Maurer MS, Schwartz JH, Gundapaneni B, Elliott PM, Merlini G, Waddington-Cruz M, et al. Tafamidis treatment for patients with transthyretin amyloid cardiomyopathy. New England Journal of Medicine. 2018;**379**(11):1007-1016

[59] Mesquita E, Jorge A, Junior C, de Andrade T. Cardiac amyloidosis and its new clinical phenotype: Heart failure with preserved ejection fraction. Arquivos Brasileiros de Cardiologia. 2017;**109**(1):71-80

[60] Gertz MA, Falk RH, Skinner M, Cohen AS, Kyle RA. Worsening of congestive heart failure in amyloid heart disease treated by calcium channel-blocking agents. The American Journal of Cardiology. 1985;**55**(13):1645

[61] Pollak A, Falk RH. Left ventricular systolic dysfunction precipitated by verapamil in cardiac amyloidosis. Chest. 1993;**104**(2):618-620

[62] Patel K, Hawkins P. Cardiac amyloidosis: Where are we today? Journal of Internal Medicine. 2015;**278**(2):126-144

[63] Sipe JD, Benson MD, Buxbaum JN, Ikeda S, Merlini G, Saraiva MJ, et al. Amyloid fibril proteins and amyloidosis: Chemical identification and clinical classification International Society of Amyloidosis 2016 nomenclature guidelines. Amyloid. 2016;**4**:1-5

[64] Milani P, Basset M, Russo F, Foli A, Palladini G, Merlini G. The lung in amyloidosis. European Respiratory Review. 2017;**26**(145):170046

[65] Riek R, Eisenberg DS. The activities of amyloids from a structural perspective. Nature. 2016;**539**(7628):227-235

[66] Foli A, Palladini G, Caporali R, Verga L, Morbini P, Obici L, et al. The role of minor salivary gland patients. Amyloid. 2011;**18**(sup1):80-82

[67] de Larrea C, Verga L, Morbini P, Klersy C, Lavatelli F, Foli A, et al. A practical approach to the diagnosis of systemic amyloidoses. Blood. 2015;**125**(14):2239-2244

[68] Grogg KL, Aubry M-C, Vrana JA, Theis JD, Dogan A. Nodular pulmonary amyloidosis is characterized by localized immunoglobulin deposition and is frequently associated with an indolent B-cell lymphoproliferative disorder. The American Journal of Surgical Pathology. 2013;**37**(3):406

[69] Kaplan B, Martin BM, Boykov O, Gal R, Pras M, Shechtman I, et al. Co-deposition of amyloidogenic immunoglobulin light and heavy chains in localized pulmonary amyloidosis. Virchows Archiv. 2005;**447**(4):756-761

[70] Hui A, Koss M, Hochholzer L, Wehunt W. Amyloidosis presenting in the lower respiratory tract. Clinicopathologic, radiologic, immunohistochemical, and histochemical studies on 48 cases. Archives of Pathology & Laboratory Medicine. 1986;**110**(3):212-218

[71] Nivas R, Singh N, Gupta K, Gupta D. Pulmonary amyloidosis in Sjogren's syndrome: A case report and systematic review of the literature. Respirology. 2010;**15**(5):860-866

[72] BoydKing A, Sharma O, Stevenson K. Localized interstitial pulmonary amyloid: A case report and review of the literature. Current Opinion in Pulmonary Medicine. 2009;**15**(5):517

[73] Smith R, Hutchins GM, Moore GW, Humphrey RL. Type and distribution of pulmonary parenchymal and vascular amyloid correlation with cardiac amyloidosis. The American Journal of Medicine. 1979;**66**(1):96-104

[74] Park M-A, Padera RF, Belanger A, Dubey S, Hwang DH, Veeranna V, et al. 18F-Florbetapir binds specifically to myocardial light chain and transthyretin amyloid deposits. Circulation. Cardiovascular Imaging. 2018;**8**(8):e002954

[75] Ohdama S, Akagawa S, Matsubara O, Yoshizawa Y. Primary diffuse alveolar septal amyloidosis with multiple cysts and calcification. European Respiratory Journal. 1996;**9**(7):1569-1571

[76] Kyle RA, Gertz MA, Greipp PR, Witzig TE, Lust JA, Lacy MQ, et al. A trial of three regimens for primary amyloidosis: Colchicine alone, melphalan and prednisone, and melphalan, prednisone, and colchicine. New England Journal of Medicine. 1997;**336**(17):1202-1207

[77] Comenzo R, Vosburgh E, Falk R, Sanchorawala V, Reisinger J, Dubrey S, et al. Dose-intensive melphalan with blood stem-cell support for

the treatment of AL (amyloid light-chain) amyloidosis: Survival and responses in 25 patients. Blood. 1998;**91**(10):3662-3670

[78] Gillmore JD, Davies J, Iqbal A, Madhoo S, Russell NH, Hawkins PN. Allogeneic bone marrow transplantation for systemic AL amyloidosis. British Journal of Haematology. 1998;**100**(1):226-228

[79] Gertz M, Lacy M, Dispenzieri A, Kumar S, Dingli D, Leung N, et al. Refinement in patient selection to reduce treatment-related mortality from autologous stem cell transplantation in amyloidosis. Bone Marrow Transplantation. 2013;**48**(4):557

[80] Ware L, Keith F, Gordon R, Ries C, Seitz R, Gold W, et al. Lung transplantation for pulmonary amyloidosis: A case report. The Journal of Heart and Lung Transplantation. 1998;**17**(11):1129-1132

[81] Lewis JE, Olsen KD, Kurtin PJ, Kyle RA. Laryngeal amyloidosis: A clinicopathologic and Immunohistochemical review. Otolaryngology–Head and Neck Surgery. 1991;**106**(4):372-377

[82] Darcy F. Localized amyloidosis of the larynx. The Journal of Laryngology & Otology. 1972;**86**(9):929-931

[83] Walker PA, Courey MS, Ossoff RH. Staged endoscopic treatment of laryngeal amyloidosis. Otolaryngology–Head and Neck Surgery. 1996;**114**(6):801-805

[84] Finn DG, Farmer JC. Management of amyloidosis of the larynx and trachea. Archives of Otolaryngology. 1982;**108**(1):54-56

[85] Mcilwain J, Shepperd H. Laser treatment of primary amyloidosis of the larynx. The Journal of Laryngology & Otology. 1986;**100**(9):1079-1080

[86] Utz J, Swensen S, Gertz M. Pulmonary amyloidosis. The Mayo clinic experience from 1980 to 1993. Annals of Internal Medicine. 1996;**124**(4):407-413

[87] Graham C, Stern E, Finkbeiner W, Webb W. High-resolution CT appearance of diffuse alveolar septal amyloidosis. AJR American Journal of Roentgenology. 1992;**158**(2):265-267

[88] Crestani B, Monnier A, Kambouchner M, Battesti J, Reynaud P, Valeyre D. Tracheobronchial amyloidosis with hilar lymphadenopathy associated with a serum monoclonal immunoglobulin. The European Respiratory Journal. 1993;**6**(10):1569-1571

[89] O'Regan A, Fenlon HM, Beamis JF, Steele MP, Skinner M, Berk JL. Tracheobronchial amyloidosis: The Boston University experience from 1984 to 1999. Medicine. 2000;**79**(2):69

[90] Monroe AT, Walia R, Zlotecki RA, Jantz MA. Tracheobronchial amyloidosis a case report of successful treatment with external beam radiation therapy. Chest. 2004;**125**(2):784-789

[91] Neben-Wittich MA, Foote RL, Kalra S. External beam radiation therapy for tracheobronchial amyloidosis. Chest. 2007;**132**(1):262-267

[92] Botto M, Hawkins PN, Bickerstaff M, Herbert J, Bygrave AE, Mcbride A, et al. Amyloid deposition is delayed in mice with targeted deletion of the serum amyloid P component gene. Nature Medicine. 1997;**3**(8):nm0897-nm0855

[93] Kisilevsky R, Lemieux LJ, Fraser PE, Kong X, Hultin PG, Szarek WA. Arresting amyloidosis in vivo using small-molecule anionic sulphonates or sulphates: Implications for Alzheimer's disease. Nature Medicine. 1995;**1**(2):143

Chapter 3

The Role of Inflammation in Amyloid Diseases

Estefania P. Azevedo and Debora Foguel

Abstract

Amyloid diseases are characterized by the abnormal accumulation of proteinaceous aggregates (amyloid fibrils or plaques) in tissues and organs. This class of diseases is also characterized by the presence of inflammation. Amyloid fibrils arise from the partial denaturing and unfolding of native proteins. The accumulation of amyloid fibrils causes tissue damage and elicits local and nonlocal immune cell infiltration into tissue and proinflammatory cytokine production. Moreover, these conditions fuel a vicious cycle that can increase amyloid production and create an environment of chronic inflammation. A chronically inflamed tissue rapidly deteriorates and loses its function. In this chapter, we will discuss important data gathered over the years describing the role of inflammation in amyloid diseases. We will describe how inflammation begins and how it affects disease progression for major amyloid diseases, such as Alzheimer's disease (AD) and hereditary TTR amyloidosis (hATTR). Lastly, we will discuss the recent advancements in treatments for amyloid diseases and how they address inflammation in affected patients.

Keywords: amyloid diseases, neutrophils, proteases, fibrils, inflammation

1. Introduction

In 1849, the term "amyloid" was first introduced by Matthias Schleiden to describe a starch-like material identified by an iodine-sulfuric acid staining of plant tissues [1]. Later in 1854, Rudolph Virchow observed similar deposits in human nervous tissue that reacted in an analogous manner as the deposits in plants after the addition of Schleiden's iodine-sulfuric acid stain [1]. With the advance in technological power and the advent of microscopy, researchers found that the starch-like deposits found in the diseased tissues of humans were made of proteinaceous structures that were organized as fibrils (termed "amyloid fibrils") and coated with carbohydrates, hence the reaction to iodine-sulfuric acid stains [1]. More than 40 pathologies are part of the family of diseases characterized as "Amyloid Diseases" [2]. The criteria that allow such characterization rely on the fact that these pathologies contain a very specific hallmark: the accumulation of amyloid fibrils in cells, tissues and/or organs. Fibrils are formed after native proteins partly unfold and aggregate into oligomers or amorphous aggregates that later organize themselves into mature, β-sheet-rich fibrillar structures [2]. On a molecular level, amyloid fibrils extracted from different patients can be indistinguishable from each other [2]. These structures can be formed outside the cell or inside the cell [2], and when they accumulate, they cause cellular damage or mechanical damage (if accumulating in between or on top of tissues).

IntechOpen

For decades, scientists believed that amyloid fibrils were stable and inert, and the end result of a nontoxic natural pathway that serves to scavenge and store highly reactive and toxic oligomeric intermediates formed during the process of protein folding [3–5]. The reactive hydrophobic residues found exposed in oligomeric intermediates are hidden in mature amyloid fibrils, thus unable to react with important cellular components [6]. Although the latter is true about amyloid fibrils, research in the last two decades shows that these structures are neither inert nor nontoxic [5, 7]. When extracellular, amyloid fibrils are readily identified by the host immune system, mainly by macrophages or neutrophils [8–10]. These immune cells have receptors that recognize and bind to the amyloid fibrils and intermediates, activating a signaling cascade that results in the production of proinflammatory molecules [8–10]. In this chapter, we will review the inflammatory component of some clinically important amyloid diseases, such as Alzheimer's disease (AD) and familial amyloid pathologies, such as hereditary TTR amyloidosis (hATTR or familial amyloid polyneuropathy—FAP). We will also discuss how inflammatory cells contribute to disease progression by causing bystander damage to tissues or by enhancing protein aggregation, in the case of AA amyloidosis. Finally, we will provide the recent therapeutic approaches based on immune regulatory strategies for these diseases.

2. Inflammation in amyloid diseases

Inflammation is the term given to a form of immune defense that is widespread and requires a complex network of immune effector mechanisms to address tissue dysfunction or injury. The notion that inflammation is involved in amyloid pathogenesis was first suggested in the 1970s in two reports on serum amyloid A (SAA) [11, 12]. Nowadays, it is known that this particular amyloidogenic protein expression is regulated by IL-6, an inflammatory cytokine, which results in increased levels of SAA [13]. Hyperexpression of SAA for long periods of time results in amyloid formation and deposition in tissue, characterizing amyloid A (AA) amyloidosis [13]. This particular type of amyloidosis occurs in chronic inflammation conditions, such as autoimmune diseases or cancer [13]. With the exception of inflammation-induced amyloidosis, such as AA amyloidosis, the role of inflammation in most amyloid diseases is a more recent concept that emerged in the late 1980s with the observation of microglia, a brain immune cell, found near amyloid plaques in postmortem brain tissue from Alzheimer's disease (AD) patients [14–16]. After these first observations, more evidence on the involvement of inflammatory mechanism in amyloid pathogenesis has emerged.

2.1 Alzheimer's disease (AD)

Alzheimer's disease (AD) is known as the most common neurodegenerative disease worldwide. It afflicts over 40 million people in the world, and because aging is the major risk factor for developing AD, its incidence will likely increase in the future as medical advances lead to increasing life span [17]. Although there is no definite known causative agent, most scientists agree that amyloid-β peptide (Aβ) is an important factor leading to AD [18]. Aβ is highly amyloidogenic, meaning that it has great potential to aggregate in solution [18]. Aβ is a small peptide ranging from 25 to 42 amino acids [18]. Extracellular aggregates of Aβ are the main protein present in amyloid plaques, a hallmark of AD [18]. Moreover, a small fraction of AD patients is diagnosed with familial AD, which is known to be the result of an infrequently inherited autosomal dominant mutation in one of the three genes involved with the production of Aβ: the amyloid precursor protein (APP) gene, presenilin 1 (PSEN1), and presenilin 2 (PSEN2) [19]. The first findings pointing to a possible involvement of inflammatory mechanisms emerged around 1980 when scientists reported reactive microglia and astrocytes surrounding amyloid plaques of AD patients [14–16]. Nowadays, after years of research, inflammation is known to be implicated in AD by having a role in neuronal damage [20], Aβ generation [21], increased hyperphosphorylation of tau protein [22] (another hallmark of AD), and cognitive impairment [23]. In this part of the chapter, we will be focusing on summarizing the role of microglia in the progression of AD.

2.1.1 Role of microglia in AD

Microglia are the immune cells of the brain. They derive from myeloid precursors which migrate into the brain during early embryonic development and play a major role in maintaining a healthy environment in the brain [24, 25]. Microglia use their surface receptors to constantly scan the central nervous system (CNS) for microbes or other damaging molecules [26]. When activated by a stimulus, microglia mediate innate and adaptive immune responses or perform various functions in response to CNS disease or injury [26]. Microglia are of great importance for brain homeostasis, but uncontrolled or overactivated microglia can also contribute to brain diseases, such as AD.

Years of research is allowing deeper understanding of how microglia contribute to AD. Microglia produce inflammatory mediators, such as TNF-α [26], that can have a detrimental role when overproduced for long periods of time. Microglia are able to produce large quantities of TNF-α upon exposure to fibrillar and oligomeric Aβ [23, 27]. TNF-α is increased in the serum and CSF of AD patients and has additionally been detected in amyloid plaques [28–32]. Inhibiting TNF-α production with the use of unspecific anti-inflammatory compounds, such as minocycline, or a specific neutralizing TNF-α antibody, (infliximab) results in downregulated inflammatory pathways (e.g., MAPK, AKT, and NF-κB) and abrogates cognitive deficits in mice [23, 33]. It has been shown that fibrillar and oligomeric Aβ can induce production of not only TNF-α but also other important inflammatory cytokines in microglia by binding and activating several receptors [23, 34]. This suggests the existence of a universal epitope found in aggregated material and a nonspecific response to amyloids. Also supporting this idea is the fact that two generic, widely used, conformation-specific antibodies have been generated (A11 and OC antibodies) that recognize mutually exclusive structural epitopes in a range of amyloid-forming proteins, including Aβ, independently of any primary amino acid sequence similarities. A11 antibodies recognize anti-parallel β-sheet structures found in intermediate states, and OC antibodies detect parallel β-sheets found in mature amyloid fibrils [35]. Inflammation is a downstream consequence of aggregated Aβ binding to receptors such as TLR-4 (toll-like receptor 4), RAGE (receptor for advanced glycation end products), CD36 [23, 36, 37], etc. It is important to note that some of these receptors are also able to recognize other aggregated non-Aβ materials [38]. Interestingly, these receptors are not only present in microglia, but some are also present in endothelial cells and neurons [39]. This suggests that the role of Aβ in AD is very complex.

Some receptors that primarily bind monomeric Aβ are not involved in pathological, inflammatory processes. Receptors such as LRP1 (low-density lipoprotein receptor-related protein 1), PrPc (cellular prion protein), and PICALM (phosphatidylinositol-binding clathrin assembly protein) are able to bind monomeric Aβ and are thought to be involved in Aβ clearance, decreasing the Aβ burden and plaque formation in the brain [40]. Moreover, mutations in PICALM, which is a gene that encodes a clathrin assembly protein and thus is involved in endocytosis, have been shown to be a risk factor for developing late-onset AD [41]. More convincing evidence of the significant role of neuroinflammation in AD is found in recent genome-wide association studies (GWAS). These studies have identified more than 20 gene variants as risk factors for developing late-onset AD. These disease-modifying genes include genes involved in both innate and adaptive immune system responses: *CR1*, *CLU*, *CD33*, *MS4A*, *ABCA7 EPHA1*, *TREM2*, and *HLA-DRB5/HLA-DRB1* [41, 42]. It is interesting to note that all of these genes are present in microglia cells as well [41]. It is thought that these genes can change microglia function and increase the risk of AD.

2.1.2 Role of peripheral inflammation in AD

An emerging concept based on recent work is that peripheral inflammation, in addition to local, brain inflammation, also affects AD pathogenesis. Studies suggest that myeloid cells, such as neutrophils, can enter the brain and may also involve in Aβ clearance [10, 43]. Neutrophils can recognize fibrillar Aβ and produce *in vitro* and *in vivo* extracellular traps (NETs; a defense mechanism that results in neutrophil cell death) [10, 43]. Extracellular traps are protein and DNA-made meshes that can immobilize Aβ particles, degrade fibrillar amyloids, but are known to modulate other immune system effector mechanisms as well [44].

Acute systemic inflammation, caused by bacterial infection, exacerbates AD pathology [45], and chronic systemic inflammation, occurring in diseases such as rheumatoid arthritis (RA), depression, and obesity, has also been reported to modify the amyloid phenotype of AD mice and is considered common co-morbid states of AD patients. In autoimmune disease, chronic inflammation can increase the risk of developing AD. Patients with the autoimmune disease Sjögren's syndrome (SS) are twice as likely to develop AD [46]. In RA, it has been shown that anti-TNF-α therapy has a protective effect on dementia [47]. In the case of depression, Aβ accumulation in AD mouse models induces depressive-like behavior, which is dependent on inflammation [23]. Inflammatory cytokine production reduces serotonin levels and contributes to behavioral changes in mice with AD [23]. Again, this can be prevented by anti-TNF-α therapy [23]. Obesity is a known comorbidity of AD and a low-grade chronic inflammatory disease. In humans and AD mouse models, cafeteria diet consumption and a higher BMI are known to accelerate AD pathology [48, 49]. For example, in humans, for every 1.0 increase in BMI at age 70 years, AD risk increased by 36% in female patients [49].

In an attempt to cure AD, active immunization against Aβ was performed in mice and humans [50, 51]. Studies reported that immunization had a therapeutic effect on mouse models of AD [50–52]. Unfortunately, clinical Aβ vaccination trials have been interrupted due to the development of meningoencephalitis in 6% of the patients, likely involving the appearance of pro-inflammatory macrophages, CD4+ and CD8+ T cells [50]. As well as myeloid cells, T cells can enter the brain. There are myriads of T-cell subtypes surveilling the CSF and the meningeal membranes [53], and they can enter the brain parenchyma upon cell injury [53]. It is not only brain-local T cells that react to Aβ but also blood T cells have been shown to have hyperreactivity to the Aβ peptide [54], specifically to epitopes within the residues 15–42 [54]. This evidence together suggests that the immune system and inflammation play significant roles in AD: not only helping with homeostatic Aβ clearance and preventing AD plaque formation but also by contributing to cell injury. Unfortunately, to date, tackling the immune system to prevent AD has yet to prove clinically effective.

2.2 Hereditary ATTR (hATTR) amyloidosis

Transthyretin (TTR) is a 55-kDa tetrameric protein expressed and secreted mainly not only by the liver, but also by the choroid plexus in the brain [55]. This protein received this specific name due to its function: once in the plasma or in the cerebrospinal fluid, TTR acts as a retinol-binding protein and thyroxine transporter across the body [55]. More than 100 point mutations in the TTR gene have been described worldwide and most of them culminate in the production of abnormal protein with a high thermodynamic instability compared to its wild-type counterpart [55]. Only a handful of mutations are not pathogenic, such as the T119M mutation [56]. The pathogenic V30M variant is the most common mutation affecting a large population of people worldwide and results in the accumulation of TTR in various tissues, such as cardiac and nervous tissue [57]. Most TTR mutations have a high propensity to aggregate under denaturing and even physiological conditions [58], forming amyloid fibrils that deposit in various tissues and organs [58]. For decades, most physicians and pathologists still regard hATTR amyloidosis as a disease without an inflammatory component, since most biopsies and *ex vivo* analysis showed no leukocyte infiltration [59]. However, with the appearance of new data in the last decade, hATTR amyloidosis is now being recognized as a disease with an important inflammatory component. Moreover, TTR amyloid fibrils are similar in structure to other amyloid fibrils and thus should induce similar inflammatory responses. One of the most common types of hATTR amyloidosis is known as familial amyloid polyneuropathy (FAP). FAP is an autosomal dominant hereditary disease characterized by the accumulation of amyloid fibrils in peripheral nerves, the gastrointestinal tract, and the heart [59]. This disease has three discernable stages: FAP 1 = unimpaired ambulation; mostly mild sensory, motor, and autonomic neuropathy in the lower limbs; FAP 2 = assistance with ambulation required; mostly moderate impairment progression to the lower limbs, upper limbs, and trunk; FAP 3 = wheelchair-bound or bedridden; severe sensory, motor, and autonomic involvement of all limbs. This disease, as most amyloidosis, is incurable and results in death [59].

The diagnosis of FAP is challenging, often relying on genetic screening to identify TTR mutations as well as on the identification of Congo red-positive amyloid deposits in biopsies. These biopsies are generally invasive, and tissue is usually taken from the sural nerve, abdominal fat, or salivary glands [59]. The main *go-to* treatment for FAP is liver transplantation (LT), since the liver is the major organ of TTR production. Unfortunately, LT presents mortality risks, and it is not available to all patients [60]. More recently, two new drug-based treatments have been FDA approved. One of these treatments use a new drug (Tafamidis) that works by stabilizing the TTR protein that is available in several countries showing effective results in controlling disease progression [61]. The other, just recently approved by the FDA, uses antisense oligonucleotides (ASOs) to target TTR production in the liver directly, decreasing the amount of TTR in the plasma, thus reducing protein aggregation [62].

Since the first study in 2001, the new concept that inflammation may play a role in the pathogenesis of FAP has emerged. Sousa and colleagues showed the presence of proinflammatory markers such as TNF-α and IL-1β in biopsies of FAP patients [63, 64]. Interestingly, the levels of proinflammatory and oxidative markers in *ex vivo* tissue positively correlate with the scoring stage proposed by Coutinho and colleagues in FAP patients, which is an index used to discriminate disease progression [65]. In addition, their study also showed the participation of the receptor RAGE, which can also bind Aβ fibrils, in the recognition of TTR amyloid fibrils [63]. In this first study, the authors suggest that Schwann cells, which are cells that myelinate peripheral nerves, were responsible for the cytokine production observed in the neural tissue. A few years later, the presence of neutrophil-derived proteins in TTR amyloid deposits was described [66]. Proteins such as lipocalin and metalloproteinases were found together with TTR deposits in FAP patients [66]. The authors suggest that the sural nerve itself is the possible tissue producing these proteins for extracellular matrix remodeling and might be an effort to degrade amyloid fibrils deposited around them. Interestingly, a forgotten report in 1986 already reported the presence of neutrophil-derived proteins in amyloid-containing tissue [67]. The report in 1986 describes the presence of elastase, a neutrophil's granule enzyme, in amyloid-containing tissue from patients diagnosed with AA amyloidosis, primary amyloidosis caused by immunoglobulin light-chain aggregation and hATTR amyloidosis [67]. Notably, intact neutrophils were not found, which confirms the most pathologist reports of FAP tissues not having leukocyte infiltration. But how intracellular components from neutrophils appeared in amyloid-containing tissue? Azevedo and colleagues reported in 2012 that a common epitope found in amyloid fibrils arising from different proteins, one of them being TTR, are able to activate neutrophils and induce elastase secretion in the form of extracellular traps [10]. These structures, called neutrophil extracellular traps (NETs), represent an important strategy to immobilize and kill invading microorganisms or in this case, aggregated proteins. The NET scaffold consists of DNA fibers associated with various granule proteins, one of them being elastase [10]. These elastase and DNA-traps accumulate in amyloid tissue and thus could explain why elastase and neutrophil-derived proteins are found around amyloid tissues in FAP patients [10]. This immune response could also be an effort to eliminate amyloid fibrils or oligomers from the affected tissue. In 2012, another important report by Buxbaum and colleagues used an animal model of FAP to study the disease progression in mice [68]. The study showed the increased levels of inflammation-related transcripts in both liver and heart of transgenic mice, strengthening the concept that inflammation might play an important role in FAP progression [68]. Additionally, Kurian and colleagues have observed sex-specific changes in blood cell gene expression in FAP patients, suggesting that inflammatory gene markers in circulating blood cells might be influenced by sexual dimorphisms [69]. More recently, new evidence shows the presence of elevated levels of IL-6 in FAP carriers that may be produced by myeloid cells and T cells [70].

These studies altogether suggest that inflammation in FAP consists of two different phases. One phase in which inflammation possibly begins at the moment of TTR production in the liver. The synthesis and abnormal folding process of the mutated and unstable TTR in the liver requires a high energetic state and thus, may cause endoplasmic reticulum (ER) stress and the activation of the liver unfolding protein response (UPR). ER stress and the activation of UPR in liver were shown to cause pro-inflammatory cytokines production, such as IL-6 [71, 72]. IL-6 is known to increase the production of other proinflammatory intermediates and could enhance inflammation levels locally in the liver by activating liver-associated macrophages as seen in other nonamyloid diseases [73, 74]. It is ultimately important to understand whether the liver plays an important role in the inflammation observed in FAP patients due to the fact that most of these patients undergo domino liver transplant. In this procedure, a liver failure patient receives a liver from a FAP patient. However, a five-year study described that 35% of patients that underwent domino liver transplantation presented FAP symptoms earlier than donor FAP patients [75]. These data indicate that FAP patients may have altered liver capacity and a low-grade chronic inflammation, decreasing the success of liver transplants. The second phase occurs after unstable TTR reaches the bloodstream and aggregation starts. TTR oligomers have been found in blood from FAP patients [76] and could elicit the production of various inflammatory cascades in circulating leukocytes and T cells. Amyloid oligomers are formed before fibril deposition and have been shown to be toxic to cells [77] and elicit inflammation when presented to immune cells [23]. Small, toxic oligomers can also be produced in situ after the cleavage of mature fibrils through the action of local proteases, such as elastase and metalloproteinase-9 [10, 66].

So far, in FAP patients and hATTR mouse models as well as in vitro, TTR fibrils are able to elicit inflammation and activate a myriad of cell types. In a broader clinical context, the underlying inflammation that begins in asymptomatic patients and continues chronically might be important for the development of FAP-associated symptoms. Patients with FAP present symptoms other than neuropathy, such as gastrointestinal symptoms, cachexia, malnutrition, diarrhea, and others [59]. Inflammatory molecules are known to change neuroendocrine pathways leading to anorexia and thus cachexia in FAP patients. These new data point to an explanation for a lot of unknowns concerning the pathogenesis of FAP. Additionally, understanding the role of inflammation in hATTR will help improve the quality of life and disease management in affected patients. There are currently no studies showing if inflammation can increase the risk of developing hATTR. However, it is possible that an inflammatory environment could decrease liver function and predispose an individual for the production of misfolded proteins, such as TTR.

2.3 Other amyloid diseases

Although recent papers have confirmed that amyloid fibrils present polymorphisms in topology, amyloids still possess an unchangeable structural fingerprint that is shared across species [78]. A lot of different proteins are able to form amyloid fibrils and not all amyloids are pathogenic. Various hormones are present in amyloid form in the pituitary gland [79], and melanocytes possess amyloids, which contribute to melanin formation [80], etc. What makes an amyloid pathogenic or not is still unclear. However, amyloids also possess another universal characteristic: they are able to activate the immune system and induce inflammation. This suggests that inflammation may be an important component of many other amyloid diseases. Indeed, inflammation has been described in many other amyloid diseases. In Parkinson's disease (PD), the involvement of inflammation in the disease process is supported by data showing the infiltration of activated microglia and T cells in post-mortem PD brains [81, 82] Additionally, there is accumulation of proinflammatory cytokines such as TNF-α, IFN-γ, and IL-6 IL-1β in the brain and cerebrospinal fluid of PD patients [83, 84]. The PD culprit protein, α-synuclein, is able to bind to several immune receptors and elicits *in vitro* and *in vivo* inflammatory response [85]. Local inflammation has been thoroughly reported for PD patients, mainly derived from activated microglia [82, 85]. Protein aggregation in PD extends well beyond the CNS and also affects peripheral autonomic neuronal circuits, such as the enteric nervous system [86]. Gut inflammation has been recently reported in PD and is thought to be an important component of the disease [86].

Prion disease is another widely studied amyloid disease and is also known as Creutzfeldt-Jakob disease, fatal insomnia, spongiform encephalopathy, and Kuru. Prion diseases are rare, progressive neurodegenerative disorders that affect both humans and animals [87]. They are caused by the aggregation of PrPc (cellular prion protein) into transmissible, pathogenic prions [87]. These diseases are accompanied by long incubation periods and brain changes associated with neuronal loss [87]. Identifying a role of inflammation in these diseases is rather recent and begun with studies showing that the pathological hallmarks of the prion diseases are associated with the presence of activated astrocytes and microglia [88]. CD8+ T cells are also present in prion-affected brains and usually are found near activated microglia and prion amyloid plaques [89]. As inflammation progresses, inflammatory cytokines are also detected in prion-containing brains [88], and these are thought to play an important role in behavioral changes and neuronal loss observed in affected mice. And this is yet another example of inflammation being widely present and contributing to pathogenesis in an amyloid disease which was first thought to not have an inflammatory component.

3. What is in store for the future: Therapies for amyloid diseases

Most amyloid diseases are still incurable. However, most of them can be managed using palliative care and drugs to decrease symptoms and extend the patients' lives. In AD, efforts are concentrated in decreasing symptoms such as cognitive deficits [90]. Currently, there are five FDA-approved drugs to treat cognitive symptoms associated with AD. These drugs are basically acting on two different neurotransmitter systems in the brain: the cholinergic system and the glutamatergic system [90]. They act by blocking glutamate receptors and inhibiting cholinesterase activity, thus these drugs, when combined, can decrease excitotoxicity induced by an overload of glutamate in the synapse and making acetylcholine more available for a healthy synaptic transmission [90]. While in theory, and as seen in mouse models of AD, these drugs seem effective, in humans they work to certain extent decreasing the symptoms. Although these drugs can temporarily decrease symptoms, they are not able to stop the progression of AD, as they do not address amyloid accumulation [90]. Although great results were seen in mouse models, in AD patients, clinical trial using nonsteroidal anti-inflammatory drugs (NSAID) were unsuccessful to prevent or treat the disease, but these drugs only account for a small part of inflammatory pathways dependent on cyclooxygenases (COX) and have diverse side effects. For PD, treatment using drugs is aimed at enhancing cholinergic and dopaminergic transmissions and hence decreasing motor and gut-related symptoms, such as tremors and constipation [91]. Deep-brain stimulation is a surgical treatment available for PD and can also decrease motor symptoms [91]. Most treatments, as the ones described above, are aimed at treating the consequence of amyloid accumulation rather than treating the amyloid accumulation itself or the inflammatory components of these many amyloid diseases.

For the hATTR diseases, two FDA-approved drugs have been developed to prevent amyloid accumulation in patients: tafamidis, a drug that stabilizes TTR and decreases TTR aggregation and antisense oligonucleotides against TTR, a drug that aims in reducing TTR production in the liver [61, 62]. In structure, tafamidis resembles most NSAID, and hence, it does not have any NSAID activity [92]. Notably, many other NSAID drugs also bind to TTR, stabilizing it [93]. However, many have not been to clinical trials at all or have not been successful in clinical trials because chronic use of NSAIDs is not indicated for patients with liver, renal, and heart problems [94], which are part of the symptoms affecting FAP patients. NSAIDs have also been used for treating other amyloid diseases, such as AD and PD, but again without success [95, 96]. Indeed, many AD and PD patients are older individuals that also possess additional conditions that exclude them from the chronic use of NSAIDs. The use of immunotherapies, especially for AD, has been thought to be an effective approach to treating the disease, but clinical trials have shown that autoimmune meningoencephalitis develops in a significant number of patients undergoing immunotherapy [50]. Usually these treatments aim to use antibodies to neutralize the culprit of the disease, in the case of AD, the Aβ peptide [50]. Unfortunately, the autoimmune response, consisting of hyperreactive T cells, of patients has prevented the clinical trials from continuing further. Researchers are still investigating immunotherapies as a way to treat AD and managing the T cell response.

The use of antisense nucleotides (ASOs) for successfully decreasing the amount of native protein in the body remains the most effective therapy and maybe the path to cure amyloid diseases. ASOs have already been shown to be effective in hATTR disease [62], without eliciting any further autoimmune inflammatory response in patients receiving the therapy. There is growing interest in using ASOs in AD and PD, since many proteins that cause amyloid diseases have unknown or redundant physiological function [2]. This suggests that decreasing the levels of native, healthy protein in individuals may not cause problems for most bodily functions. By reducing the levels of native protein, ASOs ultimately decrease amyloid formation and accumulation and finally, all the immune responses that might come with unstable protein synthesis, aggregation, and amyloid deposition in tissue.

4. Conclusion

Amyloid diseases have been described in humans and animals since the 1800s. This family of diseases has one defining characteristic: the presence of extracellular proteinaceous aggregates (amyloid fibrils or plaques) in tissues and organs. These amyloid fibrils arise from the unfolding of native protein, which vary according to the disease (for example, Aβ peptide in AD). Another common characteristic of amyloid diseases is the installment of inflammation during and after amyloid formation. Amyloid fibrils and tissue damage elicit local and nonlocal immune cell infiltration into tissue and proinflammatory cytokine production. Together, these fuel a vicious cycle that can increase amyloid production, as seen in AA amyloidosis, and create an environment of chronic inflammation. A chronically inflamed tissue, as seen in autoimmune diseases, rapidly loose function and deteriorates. This is especially true for the nervous system, a delicate tissue in which self-repair is almost impossible. As most amyloid diseases affect the CNS, and inflammation is a fundamental component of amyloid disease, studying inflammation in the CNS is imperative to our understanding of how to treat amyloid disease. Many current treatments focus on the consequences of amyloid accumulation and fail to address the basic underlying causes. The use of ASOs brings promise of improvements in amyloid disease therapeutics and fortunately is growing as an important tool used in disease therapy. Recognizing that inflammation plays a significant role in amyloid disease is essential to understand the pathogenesis of amyloidosis and important for developing new targeted treatments in an era of growing demand.

Acknowledgements

I would like to thank Dr. Kristina Hedbacker for careful proof reading of this chapter.

Conflict of interest

We report no conflict of interest.

Author details

Estefania P. Azevedo[1]* and Debora Foguel[2]

1 Laboratory of Molecular Genetics, The Rockefeller University, New York, NY, USA

2 Universidade Federal do Rio de Janeiro, Rio de Janeiro, RJ, Brazil

*Address all correspondence to: eazevedo@rockefeller.edu

References

[1] Puchtler H, Sweat F. A review of early concepts of amyloid in context with contemporary chemical literature from 1839 to 1859. The Journal of Histochemistry and Cytochemistry. 1966;**2**:123-134. DOI: doi.org/10.1177/14.2.123

[2] Chiti F, Dobson CM. Protein misfolding, amyloid formation, and human disease: A summary of progress over the last decade. Annual Review of Biochemistry. 2017;**20**(86):27-68. DOI: 10.1146/annurev-biochem-061516-045115

[3] Kayed R, Head E, Thompson JL, Mcintire TM, Milton SC, Cotman CW, et al. Common structure of soluble amyloid oligomers implies common mechanism of pathogenesis. Science. 2003;**5618**:486-489. DOI: 10.1126/science.1079469

[4] Knowles TP, Fitzpatrick AW, Meehan S, Mott HR, Vendruscolo M, Dobson CM, et al. Role of intermolecular forces in defining material properties of protein nanofibrils. Science. 2007;**318**(5858):1900-1903. DOI: 10.1126/science.1150057

[5] Tipping KW, van Oosten-Hawle P, Hewitt EW, Radford SE. Amyloid fibres: Inert end-stage aggregates or key players in disease? Trends in Biochemical Sciences. 2015;(12):719-727. DOI: 10.1016/j.tibs.2015.10.002

[6] Smaoui MR, Poitevin F, Delarue M, Koehl P, Orland H, Waldispühl J. Computational assembly of polymorphic amyloid fibrils reveals stable aggregates. Biophysical Journal. 2013;(3):683-693. DOI: 10.1016/j.bpj.2012.12.037

[7] Balchin D, Hayer-Hartl M, Hartl FU. In vivo aspects of protein folding and quality control. Science. 2016;**353**:aac4354. DOI: 10.1126/science.aac4354

[8] Gustot A, Gallea JI, Sarroukh R, Celej MS, Ruysschaert JM, Raussens V. Amyloid fibrils are the molecular trigger of inflammation in Parkinson's disease. The Biochemical Journal. 2015;(3):323-333. DOI: 10.1042/BJ20150617

[9] Gustot A, Raussens V, Dehousse M, Dumoulin M, Bryant CE, Ruysschaert JM, et al. Activation of innate immunity by lysozyme fibrils is critically dependent on cross-β sheet structure. Cellular and Molecular Life Sciences. 2013;(16):2999-3012. DOI: 10.1007/s00018-012-1245-5

[10] Azevedo EP, Guimarães-Costa AB, Torezani GS, Braga CA, Palhano FL, Kelly JW, et al. Amyloid fibrils trigger the release of neutrophil extracellular traps (NETs), causing fibril fragmentation by NET-associated elastase. The Journal of Biological Chemistry. 2012;(44):37206-37218. DOI: 10.1074/jbc.M112.369942

[11] Benditt EP, Eriksen N. Chemical similarity among amyloid substances associated with long standing inflammation. Laboratory Investigation. 1972;**6**:615-625

[12] Schumacher HR Jr. Multiple myeloma with synovial amyloid deposition. Rheumatology and Physical Medicine. 1972;**7**:349-353

[13] Sack GH Jr. Serum amyloid a - A review. Molecular Medicine. 2018;**1**:46. DOI: 10.1186/s10020-018-0047-0

[14] Itagaki S, McGeer PL, Akiyama H, Zhu S, Selkoe D. Relationship of microglia and astrocytes to amyloid deposits of Alzheimer disease. Journal of Neuroimmunology. 1989;(3):173-182

[15] Vostrikov VM. Electron-cytochemical study of microglia in Alzheimer's disease and senile dementia.

Zhurnal Nevropatologii i Psikhiatrii Imeni S.S. Korsakova. 1985;7:974-976

[16] Rozemuller JM, Eikelenboom P, Stam FC. Role of microglia in plaque formation in senile dementia of the Alzheimer type. An immunohistochemical study. Virchows Archiv. B, Cell Pathology Including Molecular Pathology. 1986;**51**:247-254

[17] Dos Santos Picanco LC, Ozela PF, de Fatima de Brito Brito M, Pinheiro AA, Padilha EC, Braga FS, et al. Alzheimer's disease: A review from the pathophysiology to diagnosis, new perspectives for pharmacological treatment. Current Medicinal Chemistry. 2018;(26):3141-3159. DOI: 10.2174/0929867323666161213101126

[18] Barage SH, Sonawane KD. Amyloid cascade hypothesis: Pathogenesis and therapeutic strategies in Alzheimer's disease. Neuropeptides. 2015;**52**:1-18. DOI: 10.1016/j.npep.2015.06.008

[19] Karch CM, Cruchaga C, Goate AM. Alzheimer's disease genetics: From the bench to the clinic. Neuron. 2014;(1):11-26. DOI: 10.1016/j.neuron.2014.05.041

[20] Ill-Raga G, Ramos-Fernández E, Guix FX, Tajes M, Bosch-Morató M, Palomer E, et al. Amyloid-β peptide fibrils induce nitro-oxidative stress in neuronal cells. Journal of Alzheimer's Disease. 2010;**2**:641-652. DOI: 10.3233/JAD-2010-100474

[21] Joshi P, Turola E, Ruiz A, Bergami A, Libera DD, Benussi L, et al. Microglia convert aggregated amyloid-β into neurotoxic forms through the shedding of microvesicles. Cell Death and Differentiation. 2014;(4):582-593. DOI: 10.1038/cdd.2013.180

[22] Maphis N, Xu G, Kokiko-Cochran ON, Jiang S, Cardona A, Ransohoff RM, et al. Reactive microglia drive tau pathology and contribute to the spreading of pathological tau in the brain. Brain. 2015;**6**:1738-1755. DOI: 10.1093/brain/awv081

[23] Ledo JH, Azevedo EP, Clarke JR, Ribeiro FC, Figueiredo CP, Foguel D, et al. Amyloid-β oligomers link depressive-like behavior and cognitive deficits in mice. Molecular Psychiatry. 2013;**10**:1053-1054. DOI: 10.1038/mp.2012.168

[24] Ginhoux F, Greter M, Leboeuf M, Nandi S, See P, Gokhan S, et al. Fate mapping analysis reveals that adult microglia derive from primitive macrophages. Science. 2010;(6005):841-845. DOI: 10.1126/science.1194637

[25] Prinz M, Mildner A. Microglia in the CNS: Immigrants from another world. Glia. 2011;(2):177-187. DOI: 10.1002/glia.21104

[26] Tambuyzer BR, Ponsaerts P, Nouwen EJ. Microglia: Gatekeepers of central nervous system immunology. Journal of Leukocyte Biology. 2009;(3):352-370. DOI: 10.1189/jlb.0608385

[27] Jana M, Palencia CA, Pahan K. Fibrillar amyloid-beta peptides activate microglia via TLR2: Implications for Alzheimer's disease. Journal of Immunology. 2008;(10):7254-7262

[28] Fillit H, Ding WH, Buee L, Kalman J, Altstiel L, Lawlor B, et al. Elevated circulating tumor necrosis factor levels in Alzheimer's disease. Neuroscience Letters. 1991;(2):318-320

[29] Dickson DW. Neuropathological diagnosis of Alzheimer's disease: A perspective from longitudinal clinicopathological studies. Neurobiology of Aging. 1997;**18**:21-26

[30] Janelsins MC, Mastrangelo MA, Oddo S, LaFerla FM, Federoff HJ, Bowers WJ. Early correlation of

microglial activation with enhanced tumor necrosis factor-alpha and monocyte chemoattractant protein-1 expression specifically within the entorhinal cortex of triple transgenic Alzheimer's disease mice. Journal of Neuroinflammation. 2005;**2**:23

[31] Galimberti D, Fenoglio C, Scarpini E. Inflammation in neurodegenerative disorders: Friend or foe? Current Aging Science. 2008;**1**:30-41

[32] Montgomery SL, Bowers WJ. Tumor necrosis factor-alpha and the roles it plays in homeostatic and degenerative processes within the central nervous system. Journal of Neuroimmune Pharmacology. 2012;(1):42-59. DOI: 10.1007/s11481-011-9287-2

[33] Kim DH, Choi SM, Jho J, Park MS, Kang J, Park SJ, et al. Infliximab ameliorates AD-associated object recognition memory impairment. Behavioural Brain Research. 2016;**311**:384-391. DOI: 10.1016/j.bbr.2016.06.001

[34] Lotz M, Ebert S, Esselmann H, Iliev AI, Prinz M, Wiazewicz N, et al. Amyloid beta peptide 1-40 enhances the action of toll-like receptor-2 and -4 agonists but antagonizes toll-like receptor-9-induced inflammation in primary mouse microglial cell cultures. Journal of Neurochemistry. 2005;**2**:289-298

[35] Kayed R, Head E, Sarsoza F, Saing T, Cotman CW, Necula M, et al. Fibril specific, conformation dependent antibodies recognize a generic epitope common to amyloid fibrils and fibrillar oligomers that is absent in prefibrillar oligomers. Molecular Neurodegeneration. 2007;**2**:18

[36] Lee JJ, Wang PW, Yang IH, Wu CL, Chuang JH. Amyloid-beta mediates the receptor of advanced glycation end product-induced pro-inflammatory response via toll-like receptor 4 signaling pathway in retinal ganglion cell line RGC-5. The International Journal of Biochemistry & Cell Biology. 2015;**64**:1-10. DOI: 10.1016/j.biocel.2015.03.002

[37] Moore KJ, El Khoury J, Medeiros LA, Terada K, Geula C, Luster AD, et al. A CD36-initiated signaling cascade mediates inflammatory effects of beta-amyloid. The Journal of Biological Chemistry. 2002;(49):47373-47379

[38] Salahuddin P, Rabbani G, Khan RH. The role of advanced glycation end products in various types of neurodegenerative disease: A therapeutic approach. Cellular & Molecular Biology Letters. 2014;(3):407-437. DOI: 10.2478/s11658-014-0205-5

[39] Gasparotto J, Ribeiro CT, da Rosa-Silva HT, Bortolin RC, Rabelo TK, Peixoto DO, et al. Systemic inflammation changes the site of RAGE expression from endothelial cells to neurons in different brain areas. Molecular Neurobiology. 2018. DOI: 10.1007/s12035-018-1291-6

[40] Jarosz-Griffiths HH, Noble E, Rushworth JV, Hooper NM. Amyloid-β receptors: The good, the bad, and the prion protein. The Journal of Biological Chemistry. 2016;(7):3174-3183. DOI: 10.1074/jbc.R115.702704

[41] Hansen DV, Hanson JE, Sheng M. Microglia in Alzheimer's disease. The Journal of Cell Biology. 2018;(2): 459-472. DOI: 10.1083/jcb.201709069

[42] Harold D, Abraham R, Hollingworth P, Sims R, Gerrish A, Hamshere ML, et al. Genome-wide association study identifies variants at CLU and PICALM associated with Alzheimer's disease. Nature Genetics. 2009;(10):1088-1093. DOI: 10.1038/ng.440

[43] Zenaro E, Pietronigro E, Della Bianca V, Piacentino G, Marongiu L, Budui S, et al. Neutrophils promote Alzheimer's disease-like pathology and cognitive decline via LFA-1 integrin. Nature Medicine. 2015;(8):880-886. DOI: 10.1038/nm.3913

[44] Guimarães-Costa AB, Rochael NC, Oliveira F, Echevarria-Lima J, Saraiva EM. Neutrophil extracellular traps reprogram IL-4/GM-CSF-induced monocyte differentiation to anti-inflammatory macrophages. Frontiers in Immunology. 2017;**8**:523. DOI: 10.3389/fimmu.2017.00523

[45] O'Banion MK. Does peripheral inflammation contribute to Alzheimer disease? Evidence from animal models. Neurology. 2014;**83**:480-481. DOI: 10.1212/WNL.0000000000000663

[46] Liliang PC, Liang CL, Lu K, Yang SN, Hsieh MT, Tai YC, et al. Population-based study suggests an increased risk of Alzheimer'sdisease in Sjögren's syndrome. Clinical Rheumatology. 2018;**37**:935-941. DOI: 10.1007/s10067-017-3940-y

[47] Judge A, Garriga C, Arden NK, Lovestone S, Prieto-Alhambra D, Cooper C, et al. Protective effect of antirheumatic drugs on dementia in rheumatoid arthritis patients. Alzheimers Dement (N Y). 2017;(4):612-621. DOI: 10.1016/j.trci.2017.10.002

[48] Luchsinger JA, Cheng D, Tang MX, Schupf N, Mayeux R. Central obesity in the elderly is related to late-onset Alzheimer disease. Alzheimer Disease and Associated Disorders. 2012;(2):101-105. DOI: 10.1097/WAD.0b013e318222f0d4

[49] Gustafson D, Rothenberg E, Blennow K, Steen B, Skoog I. An 18-year follow-up of overweight and risk of Alzheimer disease. Archives of Internal Medicine. 2003;(13):1524-1528

[50] Sterner RM, Takahashi PY, Yu Ballard AC. Active vaccines for alzheimer disease treatment. Journal of the American Medical Directors Association. 2016;(9):862.e11-862.e15. DOI: 10.1016/j.jamda.2016.06.009

[51] Zhang HY, Zhu K, Meng Y, Ding L, Wang JC, Yin WC, et al. Reduction of amyloid beta by Aβ3-10-KLH vaccine also decreases tau pathology in 3×Tg-AD mice. Brain Research Bulletin. 2018;**142**:233-240. DOI: 10.1016/j.brainresbull.2018.07.019

[52] Panza F, Frisardi V, Solfrizzi V, Imbimbo BP, Logroscino G, Santamato A, et al. Immunotherapy for Alzheimer's disease: From anti-β-amyloid to tau-based immunization strategies. Immunotherapy. 2012;**2**:213-238. DOI: 10.2217/imt.11.170

[53] Rua R, McGavern DB. Advances in meningeal immunity. Trends in Molecular Medicine. 2018;(6):542-559. DOI: 10.1016/j.molmed.2018.04.003

[54] Monsonego A, Zota V, Karni A, Krieger JI, Bar-Or A, Bitan G, et al. Increased T cell reactivity to amyloid beta protein in older humans and patients with Alzheimer disease. The Journal of Clinical Investigation. 2003;(3):415-422

[55] Vieira M, Saraiva MJ. Transthyretin: A multifaceted protein. Biomolecular Concepts. 2014;**1**:45-54. DOI: 10.1515/bmc-2013-0038

[56] Almeida MR, Alves IL, Terazaki H, Ando Y, Saraiva MJ. Comparative studies of two transthyretin variants with protective effects on familial amyloidotic polyneuropathy: TTR R104H and TTR T119M. Biochemical and Biophysical Research Communications. 2000;**270**:1024-1028

[57] Soares ML, Coelho T, Sousa A, Batalov S, Conceição I, Sales-Luís ML, et al. Susceptibility and modifier genes

in Portuguese transthyretin V30M amyloid polyneuropathy: Complexity in a single-gene disease. Human Molecular Genetics. 2005;(4):543-553

[58] Hurshman Babbes AR, Powers ET, Kelly JW. Quantification of the thermodynamically linked quaternary and tertiary structural stabilities of transthyretin and its disease-associated variants: The relationship between stability and amyloidosis. Biochemistry. 2008;**47**:6969-6984. DOI: 10.1021/bi800636q

[59] Planté-Bordeneuve V, Said G. Familial amyloid polyneuropathy. Lancet Neurology. 2011;**10**:1086-1097

[60] Benson MD. Liver transplantation and transthyretin amyloidosis. Muscle & Nerve. 2013;**47**:157-162

[61] Coelho T, Maia LF, da Silva AM, Cruz MW, Planté-Bordeneuve V, Suhr OB, et al. Long-term effects of tafamidis for the treatment of transthyretin familial amyloid polyneuropathy. Journal of Neurology. 2013;**260**:2802-2814

[62] Benson MD, Waddington-Cruz M, Berk JL, Polydefkis M, Dyck PJ, Wang AK, et al. Inotersen treatment for patients with hereditary transthyretin amyloidosis. The New England Journal of Medicine. 2018;**379**:22-31. DOI: 10.1056/NEJMoa1716793

[63] Sousa MM, Du Yan S, Fernandes R, Guimaraes A, Stern D, Saraiva MJ. Familial amyloid polyneuropathy: Receptor for advanced glycation end products-dependent triggering of neuronal inflammatory and apoptotic pathways. The Journal of Neuroscience. 2001;**21**:7576-7586

[64] Gonçalves NP, Vieira P, Saraiva MJ. Interleukin-1 signaling pathway as a therapeutic target in transthyretin amyloidosis. Amyloid. 2014;**21**:175-184

[65] Coutinho P, Martins da Silva A, Lopes Lima J, Resende Barbosa A. In: Glenner GG, Pinho e Costa P, Falcao de Freitas A, editors. Amyloid and Amyloidosis. Amsterdam: Excerpta Medica; 1980. Forty years of experience with type I amyloid neuropathy. Review of 483 cases. pp. 88-98

[66] Sousa MM, do Amaral JB, Guimarães A, Saraiva MJ. Up-regulation of the extracellular matrix remodeling genes, biglycan, neutrophil gelatinase-associated lipocalin, and matrix metalloproteinase-9 in familial amyloid polyneuropathy. The FASEB Journal. 2005;**19**:124-126

[67] Stone PJ, Campistol JM, Abraham CR, Rodgers O, Shirahama T, Skinner M. Neutrophil proteases associated with amyloid fibrils. Biochemical and Biophysical Research Communications. 1993;**197**:130-136

[68] Buxbaum JN, Tagoe C, Gallo G, Walker JR, Kurian S, Salomon DR. Why are some amyloidoses systemic? Does hepatic "chaperoning at a distance" prevent cardiac deposition in a transgenic model of human senile systemic (transthyretin) amyloidosis? The FASEB Journal. 2012;**26**:2283-2293

[69] Kurian SM, Novais M, Whisenant T, Gelbart T, Buxbaum JN, Kelly JW, et al. Peripheral blood cell gene expression diagnostic for identifying symptomatic transthyretin amyloidosis patients: Male and female specific signatures. Theranostics. 2016;**6**:1792-1809

[70] Suenaga G, Ikeda T, Masuda T, Motokawa H, Yamashita T, Takamatsu K, et al. Inflammatory state exists in familial amyloid polyneuropathy that may be triggered by mutated transthyretin. Scientific Reports. 2017;**7**:1579

[71] Scheller J, Chalaris A, Schmidt-Arras D, Rose-John S. The pro- and anti-inflammatory properties of the cytokine

interleukin-6. Biochimica et Biophysica Acta. 2011;**1813**:878-888

[72] Urano F, Wang X, Bertolotti A, Zhang Y, Chung P, Harding HP, et al. Coupling of stress in the ER to activation of JNK protein kinases by transmembrane protein kinase IRE1. Science. 2000;**287**:664-666

[73] Liaskou E, Wilson DV, Oo YH. Innate immune cells in liver inflammation. Mediators of Inflammation. 2012;**2012**:949157

[74] Helk E, Bernin H, Ernst T, Ittrich H, Jacobs T, Heeren J, et al. TNFα-mediated liver destruction by kupffer cells and Ly6Chi monocytes during entamoeba histolytica infection. PLoS Pathogens. 2013;**9**:e1003096

[75] Lladó L, Baliellas C, Casasnovas C, Ferrer I, Fabregat J, Ramos E, et al. Risk of transmission of systemic transthyretin amyloidosis after domino liver transplantation. Liver Transplantation. 2010;**16**:1386-1392

[76] Schonhoft JD, Monteiro C, Plate L, Eisele YS, Kelly JM, Boland D, et al. Peptide probes detect misfolded transthyretin oligomers in plasma of hereditary amyloidosis patients. Science Translational Medicine. 2017;**9**(407). DOI: 10.1126/scitranslmed.aam7621

[77] Reixach N, Deechongkit S, Jiang X, Kelly JW, Buxbaum JN. Tissue damage in the amyloidoses: Transthyretin monomers and nonnative oligomers are the major cytotoxic species in tissue culture. Proceedings of the National Academy of Sciences of the United States of America. 2004;**101**:2817-2822

[78] Assenza S, Adamcik J, Mezzenga R, De Los Rios P. Universal behavior in the mesoscale properties of amyloid fibrils. Physical Review Letters. 2014;**113**:268103

[79] Maji SK, Perrin MH, Sawaya MR, Jessberger S, Vadodaria K, Rissman RA, et al. Functional amyloids as natural storage of peptide hormones in pituitary secretory granules. Science. 2009;**5938**:328-332

[80] Fowler DM, Koulov AV, Balch WE, Kelly JW. Functional amyloid -from bacteria to humans. Trends in Biochemical Sciences. 2007;**32**:217-224

[81] Brochard V, Combadière B, Prigent A, Laouar Y, Perrin A, Beray-Berthat V, et al. Infiltration of CD4+ lymphocytes into the brain contributes to neurodegeneration in a mouse model of Parkinson disease. The Journal of Clinical Investigation. 2009;**119**: 182-192. DOI: 10.1172/JCI36470

[82] McGeer PL, Itagaki S, Boyes BE, McGeer EG. Reactive microglia are positive for HLA-DR in the substantia nigra of Parkinson's and Alzheimer's disease brains. Neurology. 1988;**38**:1285-1291

[83] Blum-Degen D, Müller T, Kuhn W, Gerlach M, Przuntek H, Riederer P. Interleukin-1 beta and interleukin-6 are elevated in the cerebrospinal fluid of Alzheimer's and de novo Parkinson's disease patients. Neuroscience Letters. 1995;**202**:17-20

[84] Reale M, Iarlori C, Thomas A, Gambi D, Perfetti B, Di Nicola M, et al. Peripheral cytokines profile in Parkinson's disease. Brain, Behavior, and Immunity. 2009;**23**:55-63. DOI: 10.1016/j.bbi.2008.07.003

[85] Joshi N, Singh S. Updates on immunity and inflammation in Parkinson disease pathology. Journal of Neuroscience Research. 2018;**96**: 379-390. DOI: 10.1002/jnr.24185

[86] Caputi V, Giron MC. Microbiome-gut-brain axis and toll-like receptors in Parkinson's disease. International Journal of Molecular Sciences. 2018;**19**(6). DOI: 10.3390/ijms19061689

[87] Geschwind MD. Prion diseases. Continuum (Minneap Minn). 2015;**6**:1612-1638. DOI: 10.1212/CON.0000000000000251

[88] Brown DR, Kretzschmar HA. Microglia and prion disease: A review. Histology and Histopathology. 1997;**12**:883-892

[89] Douet JY, Lacroux C, Litaise C, Lugan S, Corbière F, Arnold M, et al. Mononucleated blood cell populations display different abilities to transmit prion disease by the transfusion route. Journal of Virology. 2016;**90**:3439-3445. DOI: 10.1128/JVI.02783-15

[90] Hung SY, Fu WM. Drug candidates in clinical trials for Alzheimer's disease. Journal of Biomedical Science. 2017;**24**:47. DOI: 10.1186/s12929-017-0355-7

[91] Muthuraman M, Koirala N, Ciolac D, Pintea B, Glaser M, Groppa S, et al. Deep brain stimulation and L-DOPA therapy: Concepts of action and clinical applications in Parkinson's disease. Frontiers in Neurology. 2018;**9**:711. DOI: 10.3389/fneur.2018.00711

[92] Bulawa CE, Connelly S, Devit M, Wang L, Weigel C, Fleming JA, et al. Tafamidis, a potent and selective transthyretin kinetic stabilizer that inhibits the amyloid cascade. Proceedings of the National Academy of Sciences of the United States of America. 2012;**109**:9629-9634. DOI: 10.1073/pnas.1121005109

[93] Adams D, Cauquil C, Labeyrie C, Beaudonnet G, Algalarrondo V, Théaudin M. TTR kinetic stabilizers and TTR gene silencing: A new era in therapy for familial amyloidotic polyneuropathies. Expert Opinion on Pharmacotherapy. 2016;(6):791-802. DOI: 10.1517/14656566.2016.1145664

[94] Murphy EJ. Acute pain management pharmacology for the patient with concurrent renal or hepatic disease. Anaesthesia and Intensive Care. 2005;**33**:311-322

[95] Miguel-Álvarez M, Santos-Lozano A, Sanchis-Gomar F, Fiuza-Luces C, Pareja-Galeano H, Garatachea N, et al. Non-steroidal anti-inflammatory drugs as a treatment for Alzheimer's disease: A systematic review and meta-analysis of treatment effect. Drugs & Aging. 2015;**32**:139-147. DOI: 10.1007/s40266-015-0239-z

[96] Samii A, Etminan M, Wiens MO, Jafari S. NSAID use and the risk of Parkinson's disease: Systematic review and meta-analysis of observational studies. Drugs & Aging. 2009;**26**:769-779. DOI: 10.2165/11316780-000000000-00000

Chapter 4

Pathologic Findings of Amyloidosis: Recent Advances

Moon Joo Kim, Donghwa Baek, Luan Truong and Jae Y. Ro

Abstract

Amyloids are aggregations of misfolded protein, which creates fibrillary structures. Unlike normally folded proteins, misfolded fibrils are insoluble and deposited extracellularly or intracellularly. The pathologic mechanism is still unclear, but resultant toxic oligomers within the tissue are known to damage the tissue via aberrant protein interactions. This condition has been known as amyloidosis. Different kinds of amyloid protein may cause similar or different clinical signs and symptoms, largely depending on the target organ it is deposited. However, because treatments and prognoses of each type are different drastically, it is critical to distinguish them and determine the specific type of amyloidosis. The confirmation and typing of amyloid heavily depend on pathologic examination of tissue. The gold standard method for the former is a Congo red staining and birefringence under polarized microscopy. The conventional way for the latter is immunohistochemistry (IHC), where most of the amyloid types can be classified. However, electron microscopy, mass spectrometry, or other molecular methods are required for typing some amyloids that are difficult to identify through IHC. In this chapter, we will describe basic concepts of amyloidosis and pathologic findings of amyloid deposition, including atypical structural deposition. Furthermore, we will review methodologies for amyloid typing briefly.

Keywords: amyloid, amyloidosis, immunohistochemistry, molecular diagnosis, immunoelectron microscopy, atypical amyloid feature

1. Introduction

Amyloids are an aggregation of misfolded protein that creates fibrillary structures for various causes including hereditary or de novo mutations of the proteins and errors in the normal folding processes. This abnormally misfolded protein can aggregate into insoluble polymers or develop resistance against proteolysis. As a result, amyloid is deposited extracellularly or intracellularly within the tissue, causing tissue damage. This condition is called amyloidosis.

More than 90% of amyloid deposition is composed of protein fibrils, and the remainder of the deposition is proteoglycans, glycoproteins, or serum amyloid P components. Because more than 30 previously described species of amyloid protein share the same fibril structure, they may look similar when they are deposited within an organ. The structure of amyloid is observed by electron microscopy showing fibrils with a diameter of approximately 7.5–10 nm. Furthermore, β-pleated sheet structures within the fibrils were shown by X-ray crystallography and infrared spectroscopy.

IntechOpen

Depending on the chemical nature and the origin of the amyloid, each amyloid type has a tendency to be deposited in certain tissue or organ. However, the clinical signs and symptoms of different types can be remarkably similar when those types of amyloid are deposited within the same organ. Moreover, the deposited amyloid will show the same bright pink homogeneous amorphous materials when the affected organ is examined microscopically. This can be confirmed by apple-green birefringence on Congo red stain with polarization and fluorescence microscopy. Even if they have a similar morphologic appearance and similar clinical pictures, the treatment and prognosis vary significantly according to the type of amyloid. Thus, distinguishing the amyloid type is essential.

2. Molecular pathogenesis

The mechanisms of amyloidogenesis of each protein are quite variable and involve different overlapping mechanisms and environmental factors. The four recurring themes include intrinsic amyloidogenic tendency, increased concentration, altered proteolytic cleavage, and genetic mutation.

Several indigenous proteins have an innate tendency to fold into amyloid structure. Such proteins include transthyretin (TTR) and atrial natriuretic peptide (ANF). The former can deposit in the heart, joint, and other organs in the elderly, even without genetic mutations, and cause **wild-type TTR amyloidosis (wtATTR)** (formerly, **senile systemic amyloidosis**). In contrary to transthyretin, which is deposited in both the atria and ventricle, ANF deposits selectively in the atria and causes **isolated atrial amyloidosis (IAA)**. This condition is also more common among the elderly and associated with atrial fibrillation. Other intrinsically prone proteins include apolipoproteins A-I, A-IV, and E and serum amyloid protein (SAP), which are incorporated in other forms of amyloid plaques nonspecifically.

Interestingly, exogenous proteins that have an amyloidogenic property can also cause amyloidosis. Two peptide drugs, insulin and enfuvirtide, have recently been described to cause localized amyloidosis [1]. Both drugs are injected subcutaneously, and the drug polypeptides may aggregate into amyloid fibril forming a localized amyloidoma. The amyloid fibrils are composed of the drug peptides themselves, which was confirmed by mass spectrometry. This **pharmaceutical amyloidosis** is an important differential diagnosis in a patient who presents with abdominal nodules and has been on insulin or enfuvirtide therapy.

Another contributing factor is persistently high concentrations of amyloidogenic proteins. Such elevated concentrations make it easier for the proteins to deposit and form a nidus for fibril extension and stabilization. These high levels can be achieved by either overproduction or undersecretion. For instance, SAP expression is greatly increased under inflammatory conditions, where the protein can aggregate to cause **AA amyloidosis**. Another example is **dialysis-associated amyloidosis (Aβ2M)**, where β-2 microglobulin (β2M) level is increased in patients with end-stage renal disease due to ineffective elimination.

Amyloidosis caused by altered proteolytic cleavage is classically exemplified by **Alzheimer's disease**, in which amyloid-β precursor protein (AβPP) forms neuritic plaques. When AβPP is cleaved by β- and γ-secretases rather than normal α- and γ-secretases, a highly amyloidogenic and neurotoxic oligomer Aβ is produced. The Aβ is believed to cause cellular dysfunction and neurodegeneration in **Alzheimer's disease**.

Lastly, genetic mutations of proteins can form amyloid fibrils by one or more mechanisms previously mentioned. These alterations may involve either gene overexpression or structural changes. The former promotes amyloidogenesis by increased concentrations and the latter by either conferring amyloidogenic instability to the protein or making the protein subject to amyloidogenic proteolytic cleavage. One important example is duplication or triplication of the *SNCA* gene, which results in increased production of the gene product α-synuclein. It aggregates into toxic oligomer and amyloid plaques (Lewy body) and causes familial **Parkinson's disease**. In **hereditary transthyretin amyloidosis (hereditary ATTR)**, more than 130 mutations in *TTR* gene induce further instability to intrinsically unstable transthyretin and result in amyloid deposition in the heart, kidney, and peripheral nerves. Another interesting kind of mutation that can potentially produce amyloid by altered proteolytic cleavage involves gelsolin protein. Several mutations of gelsolin make the protein vulnerable to cleavage by furin, a ubiquitous protein convertase, producing amyloidogenic fragment C68 and causing **hereditary familial amyloidosis of Finnish type**.

Although different mechanisms are shown to be involved in amyloidogenesis, how some amyloid fibrils are deposited selectively in certain organs is not well known. In localized amyloidosis, the location of amyloid deposition may be related to the tissue where the amyloid protein is originated. For instance, islet amyloid polypeptide (IAPP or amylin) is an amyloidogenic peptide with physiologic roles in glucose regulation and secreted along with insulin by Langerhans islet cells. In **type 2 diabetes** and **insulinoma**, IAPP is deposited only in the islet of Langerhans, not exocrine pancreas. Other factors that may explain organotropism of amyloid fibrils include physiochemical environment and extracellular matrix. In **dialysis-associated amyloidosis**, β2m deposition in joint and bone tissue may be explained by the affinity of β2m for collagen, enhanced fibril extension by glycosaminoglycans such as heparan sulfate and bone resorption and nidus formation by proinflammatory cytokines and acidosis.

Another unsettled issue is how amyloid formation can damage the target tissue. Extracellular deposition of amyloid fibrils itself may disrupt the organ integrity as in **cerebral amyloid angiopathy (CAA)**, where Aβ is deposited in the walls of meningeal or cortical vessels, weakens the vessel, and leads to lobar hemorrhage. However, available evidence indicates that the primary mechanism of tissue damage in the majority of amyloidosis involves toxic oligomers rather than mature amyloid fibrils themselves. Despite various cellular defensive mechanisms to prevent proteins from misfolding like molecular chaperones and cochaperones, ubiquitin-protease pathway, and autophagy, such "proteostasis" machineries can be overwhelmed by mechanisms mentioned above. The resultant misfolded oligomers may exhibit hydrophobic residues that are normally buried inside the normal quaternary structure of the protein, and they seem to induce aberrant interactions with other proteins, triggering unfolded protein response, cell death, inflammation, and other pathways of cell injury. Moreover, these toxic oligomers seem to "spread" to the surrounding tissue in a prion-like manner, further propagating cell injury.

3. Major types of amyloidosis

The most recent classification of amyloidosis has been published by the Nomenclature Committee of the International Society of Amyloidosis (ISA) in 2016. The classification listed 36 different extracellular fibril proteins seen in humans and animals, whose sequence is identified unequivocally (**Table 1**). According to this scheme, amyloid proteins can be broadly divided into systemic or localized in relation to the extent of organ involved by the condition. Systemic forms of amyloidosis are common and may result in serious clinical consequences, while localized forms tend to be less common and clinically indolent unless they involve critical organs such as CNS. Therefore, the distinction between the two is important.

Fibril protein	Precursor protein	Associated disease
Systemic		
AL	Immunoglobulin light chain	Plasma cell disorders
AH	Immunoglobulin heavy chain	Plasma cell disorders
AA	(Apo) Serum amyloid A	Inflammation-associated amyloidosis, familial Mediterranean fever
ATTR	Transthyretin	Familial amyloidosis, senile cardiac amyloidosis
Aβ2M	β2-Microglobulin	Dialysis-associated amyloidosis
AApoAI	Apolipoprotein A I, variants	Familial systemic amyloidosis
AApoAII	Apolipoprotein A II, variants	Familial systemic amyloidosis
AApoAIV	Apolipoprotein A IV, wild type	
AApoCII	Apolipoprotein C II, variants	
AApoCIII	Apolipoprotein C III, variants	
AGel	Gelsolin, variants	Familial amyloidosis (Finnish)
ALys	Lysozyme, variants	Familial systemic amyloidosis
ALECT2	Leukocyte chemotactic factor-2	
AFib	Fibrinogen α, variants	Familial systemic amyloidosis
ACys	Cystatin C, variants	Hereditary cerebral hemorrhage with amyloidosis (Icelandic)
Abri	ABriPP, variants	Familial dementia (British)
Localized		
Adan	ADanPP, variants	Familial dementia (Danish)
Aβ	Aβ protein precursor	Alzheimer disease, Down syndrome, hereditary cerebral hemorrhage with amyloidosis (Dutch)
AαSyn	α-Synuclein	Alzheimer disease
ATau	Tau	Alzheimer disease
APrP	Prion protein	Creutzfeldt-Jakob disease, Gerstmann-Stäussler-Scheinker disease, fatal familial insomnia, kuru
ACal	(Pro)calcitonin	Medullary thyroid carcinoma
AIAPP	Islet amyloid polypeptide	Insulinoma, type 2 diabetes
AANF	Atrial natriuretic factor	Isolated atrial amyloidosis
APro	Prolactin	Pituitary amyloidoma
AIns	Insulin	
ASPC	Lung surfactant protein	
AGal7	Galectin 7	
ACor	Corneodesmosin	
AMed	Lactadherin	Aortic amyloidosis in elderly people
Aker	Kerato-epithelin	Familial corneal amyloidosis
ALac	Lactoferrin	Familial corneal amyloidosis
AOAAP	Odontogenic ameloblast-associated protein	
ASem1	Semenogelin 1	
AEnf	Enfurvitide	
ACas*	A-S2C casein	

* ACas has been identified in Animal.

Table 1.
Amyloid fibril protein classification and associated disease.

Exhaustive review of every subtype is beyond the scope of this chapter. The more common and clinically important types of amyloid protein are described below.

3.1 Amyloid light chain (AL) protein

AL type amyloid is the most common amyloid in the United States. The AL chain is a clonal immunoglobulin light chain or light chain fragment, which is produced by the uncontrolled productions of antibodies by plasma cells. Lambda (λ) type (ALλ) is more common than kappa (κ) type (ALκ) light chain. This type of amyloidosis is related to monoclonal plasma cell disorders, especially multiple myeloma or other B-lymphocyte-related disorders. If we cannot determine AL type amyloidosis to a certain disease, it is categorized as primary amyloidosis. Even if we cannot demonstrate a specific disease to AL type amyloidosis, we still see monoclonal plasma cell proliferation in these patients. In either case, we can find immunoglobulin or light chain within the serum or urine. The most commonly affected organ is the kidney. The heart, peripheral nervous system, gastrointestinal tract, and respiratory tract can also be affected. A localized form of AL type amyloid can be seen in the gastrointestinal tract [2]. Amyloid heavy chain (AH) is rarely reported but also associated with monoclonal plasma cell disorder [3].

3.2 Amyloid-associated type (AA) protein

AA type amyloidosis is the most common amyloid worldwide. AA type amyloid is an acute phase protein derived from SAP by proteolysis. AA type amyloid is made in the liver, bounds to high-density lipoprotein (HDL), and is associated with chronic inflammatory disorder. In the past, the primary cause was predominantly of infections such as tuberculosis and chronic osteomyelitis. Nowadays, with the development of antibiotics, the most common source of AA type amyloid has become noninfectious inflammatory conditions, such as rheumatoid arthritis or inflammatory bowel diseases including Crohn's disease and ulcerative colitis. Typical organs of AA type amyloid deposition are the kidney, liver, and spleen. AA type amyloidosis is also related to hereditary amyloidosis, caused by familial Mediterranean fever inherited as an autosomal recessive pattern. This is an auto-inflammatory disorder characterized by frequent fever and serosal inflammation. The main affected organ is the kidney, but other organs such as the heart, spleen, and gastrointestinal tract can be affected [4].

3.3 Transthyretin amyloid (ATTR) protein

TTR is a transport protein made in the liver and choroid plexus. TTR transfers thyroxin and retinol in the blood and cerebrospinal fluid. TTR proteins can be differentiated into wild type and mutant type. TTR wild-type amyloid is associated with systemic senile amyloidosis and mostly affects heart ventricles in elderly patients. In this population, a prevalence of monoclonal gammopathy of undetermined significance (MGUS) has been reported [5]. TTR mutant type protein is related to hereditary amyloidosis. TTR mutant type protein can affect commonly peripheral nerves and other organs including the heart and gastrointestinal tract. This is inherited as an autosomal dominant pattern. The clinical course of TTR mutant type is relatively faster than TTR wild type in terms of onset and progression. Also, treatment and prognosis of two types are different. Therefore, distinguishing two types in early stage is important.

3.4 Dialysis-related amyloidosis (Aβ2M)

β2M is a light chain component of the major histocompatibility complex (MHC) class I molecules. It is found in patients on dialysis and is rarely seen in renal failure patients who have not undergone dialysis. Since β2M is catabolized in the kidney, this protein may accumulate in renal failure patients. Conventional dialysis membranes do not remove this protein, thus dialysis-related β2M deposits occur in dialysis patients. Deposits occur mostly in the carpal ligaments, synovium, and bone. Other organs such as the heart, gastrointestinal tract, liver, lungs, prostate, adrenal glands, and tongue can be affected. These days, we use polyamide high-flux membranes to remove β2M, resulting in a lower incidence of this type of amyloid.

3.5 Amyloid β (Aβ) protein

Aβ protein comes from the proteolysis of an amyloid precursor protein known as transmembrane glycoprotein and accumulates as plaque in the cerebral cortex and in the blood vessel. Deposits within the blood vessels cause CAA, which induces progressive cognitive decline and lobar hemorrhage. The most well-known disease related to Aβ is Alzheimer's disease. Rarely, familial Alzheimer's disease, which occurs in an autosomal dominant pattern, is seen. In addition, by about age 50, Down syndrome patients present with amyloid deposits in the brain similar to those of patients with Alzheimer's disease. Furthermore, a very rare form of hereditary cerebral hemorrhage with amyloidosis occurring in an autosomal dominant pattern has been reported.

Clinical symptoms are mostly nonspecific and may include headache, general weakness, edema, and weight change. Symptoms may also depend on the location and amount of amyloid deposition. Amyloid deposition in the heart causes arrhythmia, heart failure, or abnormal electric rhythm. Amyloid in the kidney eventually induces renal failure with proteinuria and uremia. If amyloid deposits within the blood vessels, it creates ischemic or hemorrhagic condition for the organ. Amyloid deposition also mimics arthritis and peripheral neuropathy. Within the brain, it causes cognitive and memory disorders seen in Alzheimer's disease or prion diseases. Localized deposition in the gastrointestinal tract has nonspecific gastrointestinal symptoms, such as dyspepsia or diarrhea. Since clinical symptoms are nonspecific, and most of the amyloid types can cause similar clinical features in the same organ; the clinical approach to amyloidosis is very limited. Therefore, a pathologic diagnosis of amyloidosis is critical.

4. Pathologic findings

Amyloid deposition is seen in the same manner within the same tissue no matter what protein it contains, except in a few cases. Grossly, amyloidosis deposition can appear as nodules and organomegaly, and sometimes it can show a pale gray to waxy color change with firm consistency. Microscopically, bright pink amorphous material deposition in extracellular space is most commonly observed under conventional hematoxylin–eosin stain. Peculiar intracellular and spheroid type amyloid depositions may be seen, but they are rare.

Since the adventitious discovery by Hans Hermann Bennhold in 1922, Congo red stain has been the gold standard of confirming the presence of amyloid protein. When properly stained, the amyloid imparts red, orange, or salmon pink color. The subsequent demonstration of apple-green birefringence confirms the diagnosis of amyloidosis. However, this two-step method still suffers low sensitivity, specificity and reproducibility and heavily depends on the interpretation of highly experienced pathologists. For instance, aside from the inherent sampling error, negative birefringence on positive Congo red stain may result in a false-negative result, even if the stained material actually contains amyloid. This "polarization shadow" can be overcome by rotating the slide table, which may detect additional small amount of amyloid protein. The intensity of the stain is also significantly affected by the washing process in the staining protocol, resulting in low reproducibility and mandating the use of positive control tissue. In addition, Congo red also stains collagen, elastin, or even non-fibrillary materials such as eosinophils, further complicating the interpretation.

To overcome such limitations of Congo red stain, additional filters such as a fluorescein isothiocyanate (FITC) or Texas red filter can be used [6]. These filters can augment the weak signal from Congo red into red fluorescence, greatly improving the detection sensitivity. Additional fluorochrome dyes, such as thioflavin T, can also be recruited. The stain becomes highly fluorogenic only when they are bound to amyloid, which imparts a yellow-green fluorescence when it is examined under fluorescence microscopy. Because both fluorescence filters and dyes are not entirely specific for amyloid, they should be used as adjunct in the context of Congo red stain. In conclusion, the light microscopic diagnosis of amyloidosis pertains not only to the on–off signal but also to staining techniques, specimen alignment under polarized light, fluorescence microscopy, and experience of the pathologist.

Generally, histological features are similar throughout the organ, but there are still specific features for specific organs, as will be discussed below.

4.1 Heart

Heart amyloidosis is induced by various types of amyloid. AL type is the most common amyloid found in the heart, while wtATTR, which causes systemic senile amyloidosis, is the second most common amyloid in the heart. Mostly, gross features will be normal unless it is late-stage amyloidosis. Minimal to mild enlargement of the heart, along with pale and waxy changes on the external surface, can be seen. Within the heart, ventricular wall concentric thickening, including that of the septum, is seen. The epicardium, endocardium, and valves can show nodular deposits. Histologically, there is no definite pattern of amyloid deposition based on the type of amyloid, and it normally shows blight pink amorphous deposition, showing an infiltrative pattern within the interstitium. Expanding to the myocardium can cause atrophy of myocardial muscle. Also, arteriolar deposition can be seen in AL amyloidosis. Depending on the site of deposition and amount of deposition, it can cause conduction abnormality inducing arrhythmia, restrictive cardiomyopathy, and heart failure.

4.2 Kidney

The kidney is the most common organ where amyloid deposits. Various types of amyloid deposits can occur, but AA and AL type amyloids are the most common amyloid types seen in the kidney. Grossly, the kidney is firm, pale, and waxy. The size can vary between normal, enlarged, or small; if amyloid deposits within the arteries or arterioles and causes ischemia, the kidney becomes small. Histologically, there is no type-specific pattern. Amorphous bright pink deposits are mostly seen in the mesangium and capillary wall (**Figures 1** and **2**). In addition, interstitial peritubular tissue, arteries, and arterioles can be affected. Capillary wall thickening and mesangial expansion are seen. Sometimes, amyloid deposits protrude to the basement membrane of glomerular capillaries, showing discontinuity of the membrane. Expansion of amyloid within the mesangium eventually causes capillary obstruction and renal failure. Proteinuria is a very common finding among patients with kidney amyloidosis.

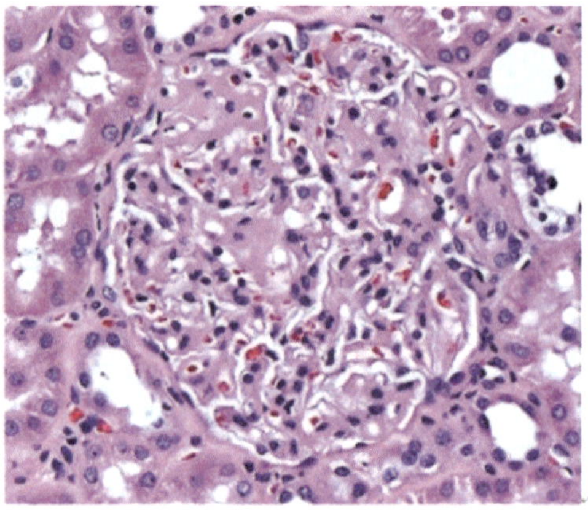

Figure 1.
Mesangium depositions of homogeneously bright pink material in kidney, H&E stain.

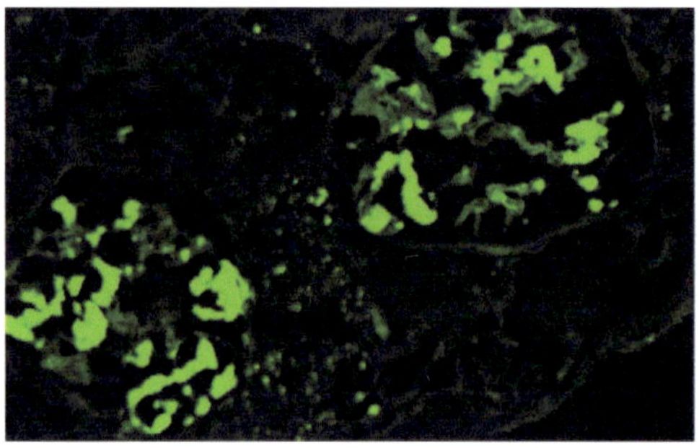

Figure 2.
Mesangium deposition of amyloid in kidney, ALλ type in immunofluorescence.

4.3 Liver

The most common amyloid type in the liver is AL and leukocyte-derived chemotaxin 2 (LECT2) type [7]. LECT 2 type amyloid (ALECT2) deposition was relatively recently found within the kidney and first reported in 2008 [8]. LECT 2 is synthesized in the liver and is a chemotaxin that attracts neutrophils. Grossly, appearance ranges from normal to moderate and massive hepatomegaly. Histologically, we can see bright pink amorphous deposition within the sinusoidal space and vessel in the portal tract. AL type tends to have a sinusoidal pattern and a vascular pattern in the portal tract, but AA type shows a vascular pattern within the portal tract [9] (**Figures 3** and **4**). A globular pattern in sinusoids has been reported in LECT 2 hepatic amyloidosis [10]. Even if there are more specific patterns depending on the type, they are not accurate, and sometimes there are overlapping patterns. Thus, confirmation with a specific stain is important. Kupffer cells and Multinucleated giant cells can be seen near the amyloid deposition. If amyloid expands, it induces hepatocyte atrophy and replaces normal hepatic tissue, causing liver failure.

4.4 Spleen

The spleen is mostly affected by AL type with plasmacytoid lymphovascular proliferation. The spleen shows two distinct gross patterns which are sago spleen and lardaceous spleen. Sago spleen has a gray, waxy, nodular appearance and is mild to moderately enlarged, and histologically, white pulp (follicles) is affected.

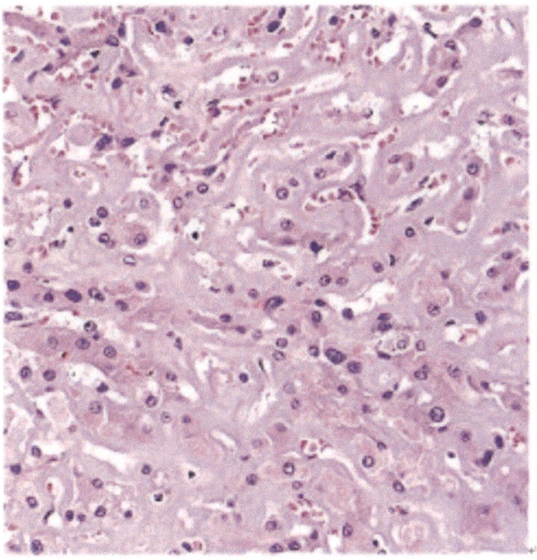

Figure 3.
Sinusoidal depositions of homogeneously bright pink material in liver, H&E stain.

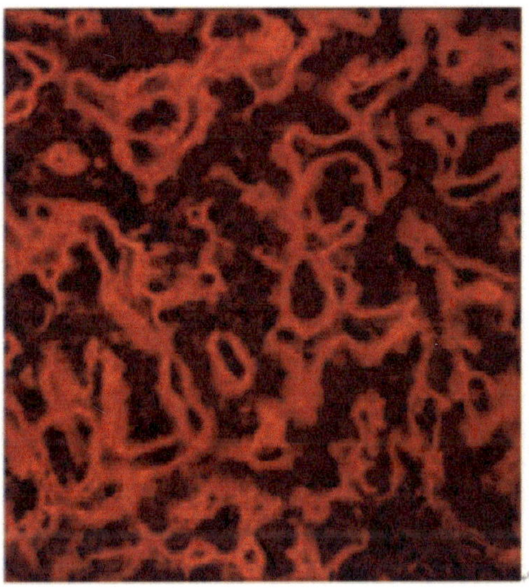

Figure 4.
Sinusoidal deposition of amyloid in liver, Congo red stain under Texas red filter.

If amyloid deposits grow, they replace the white pulp. Lardaceous spleen shows a diffuse waxy appearance and moderate to marked enlargement. Histologically, amyloid deposition is seen within the splenic sinuses and blood vessels.

4.5 Brain

The most common amyloid we see in the brain is β-amyloid. β-amyloid accumulates diffusely in the extracellular space of the cerebral cortex and is most commonly related to Alzheimer's disease. Characteristically, we can appreciate numerous extracellular depositions of amyloid plaques within the cortex (**Figure 5**). Amyloid plaques show filamentous appearance and can be demonstrated with a Congo red and a silver stain and β-amyloid IHC. Some dense amyloid plaques are surrounded by dystrophic neurites, reactive astrocytes, and microglia. Additionally, β-amyloid

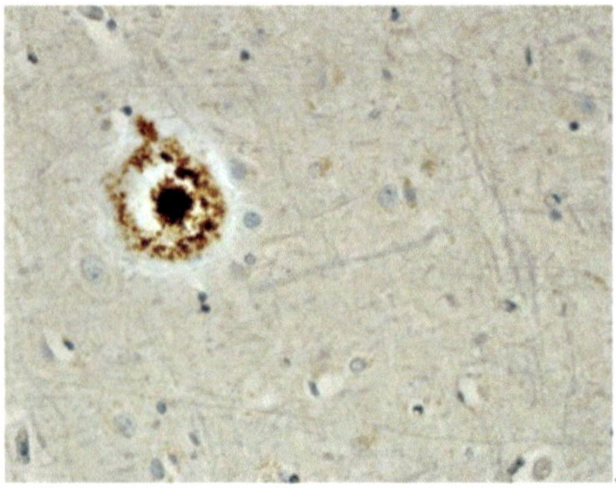

Figure 5.
Amyloid plaque seen in Alzheimer disease, β amyloid antibody in IHC.

can deposit within small-to-medium-sized arteries in the superficial cortex and leptomeningeal space and causes cerebral amyloid angiopathy. Cerebral amyloid angiopathy causes recurrent lobar hemorrhage. Furthermore, most Alzheimer's-affected brains show cerebral amyloid angiopathy as well.

4.6 Other organs

In the tongue, nodular deposition is seen, causing macroglossia. Gastrointestinal tract deposition of amyloid is common with polyps or ulcerative lesions. In the late stage, the cut surface shows yellow and waxy mural thickening. Clinically, it can cause motility disorders or stricture. Not uncommonly, vessels in the gastrointestinal tract can have amyloid deposition. In the respiratory tract, grossly nodular appearance is seen, and histologically, such depositions can be divided into four patterns including tracheobronchial, nodular parenchymal, diffuse alveolar septal, and lymphatic [11]. Skin depositions vary in size and shape, from papules to nodules and plaque. As an endocrine organ, the thyroid can present with goiter and is associated with medullary carcinoma. Localized nodular deposition in the bone causes amyloidoma. Inflammation including giant cell, lymphocyte, and spheroid structure has been reported [12]. Joint depositions are seen mimicking rheumatoid arthritis, but less synovial inflammation is seen. Bone marrow deposition is commonly seen in multiple myeloma patients. For patients on chronic dialysis, amyloid-related carpal tunnel has been seen.

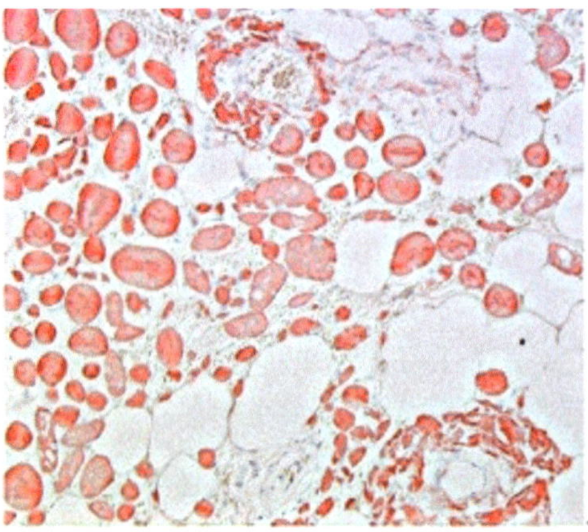

Figure 6.
Spheroid type amyloid deposition in colonic submucosa, Congo red stain.

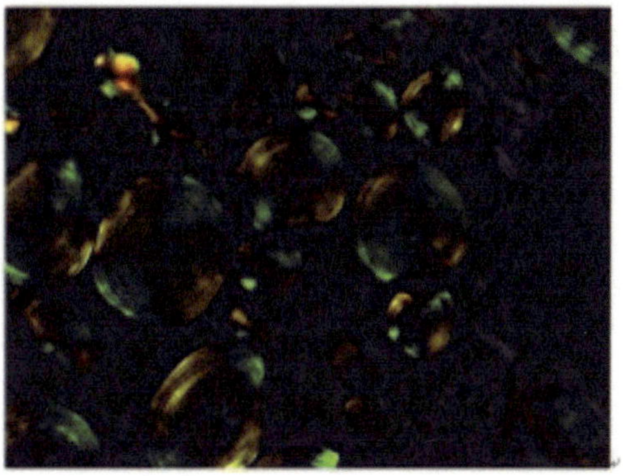

Figure 7.
Spheroid type amyloid deposition in colonic submucosa, Congo red stain under polarizer filter.

4.7 Atypical amyloid findings

Cases of intracellular amyloid deposition have been reported in few organs including cardiomyocytes, plasma cells, as well as the histiocytes and β cells of the pancreas [12–14]. Spheroid type (corpora amylacea-like) amyloid deposition is reported in pituitary adenoma, squamous cell carcinoma of the uterine cervix, and amyloidoma of the bone, jejunum, and colon [15–18]. One case of spheroid type amyloid deposition from our group in association with colon adenocarcinoma is identified [2] (**Figures 6** and **7**). Current hypothesis regarding spheroid type amyloid deposition is that during the process of amyloid removal by macrophages, amyloid is packed inside the macrophage, making spheroid formations that are extracted into the surrounding tissue [18].

5. Immunohistochemistry and immunoelectron microscopy

While the Congo red stain positivity and birefringence are the gold standard of confirming amyloidosis, they do not tell what type of amyloid is deposited. Considering managements and clinical outcomes vary drastically according to the types, further studies to identify the causative protein are critical. Clinicopathologic correlation cannot substitute for amyloid typing.

Immunohistochemistry (IHC) is the most commonly utilized method for subtyping amyloidosis. IHC takes advantage of relatively specific binding properties of antibodies against different types of amyloid fibrils to illuminate the amyloid protein in tissue. A panel of antibodies for more common types can subtype the majority of amyloidosis cases. Such antibodies include those against ALλ, ALκ, AHγ, ATTR, Aβ2M, and AFib (fibrinogen). The method has been widely used due to low cost, ease of use, rapid turnaround time, and formalin-fixed paraffin-embedded (FFPE) section compatibility.

However, there is one important pitfall in IHC. Because of heterogeneity of amyloid fibrils, nonspecific staining is common, and this potentially complicates the interpretation. For instance, the antibody against Aλ is notorious for nonspecific staining of amyloid other than Aλ. This diagnostic pitfall mandates the use of multiple comparative IHC stains to separate the true diagnostic positivity from the nonspecific reaction. In comparative IHC, subtyping of amyloid is determined by the specific amyloid with the strongest immunohistochemical reactivity.

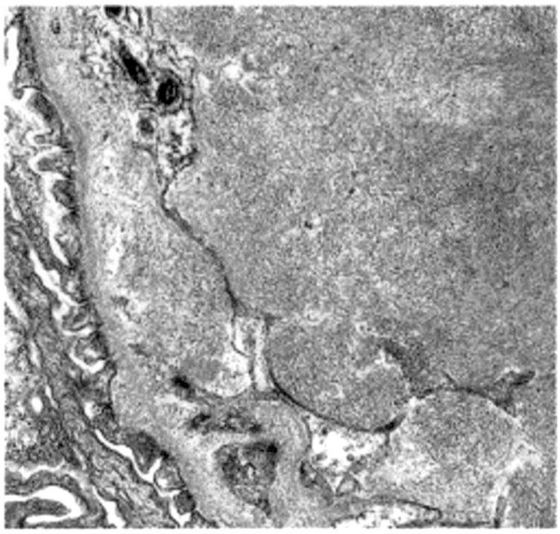

Figure 8.
Amyloid fibrils diameter of approximately 7.5–10 nm non branched fibers in kidney, EM.

Although not as commonly utilized as IHC, electron microscopy (EM) is a preferred method over Congo red birefringence or IHC in some institutions due to ambiguity of these stains in the interpretation. EM can confirm or rule out amyloidosis by visualizing amyloid fibrils in tissue as non-branching fibers with an average diameter of 7.5–10 nm. Because these fibers are considerably thicker than collagen fibers in EM, this technique can avoid diagnosing collagen fibers as amyloid fibrils, which is common in Congo red stain due to birefringence of collagen fibers in abdominal fat biopsy.

Morphologic patterns of EM have been described in amyloidosis affecting certain organs. Selective deposition in mesangial matrix and basement membrane and subepithelial "spikes" or "spicules" under podocyte foot processes are seen in glomerular amyloidosis (**Figure 8**). Amyloid deposition in tubular basement membrane, interstitial space, and vascular wall are observed in extraglomerular amyloid. However, such differences in distribution are not specific enough to indicate certain subtypes of amyloidosis.

Some authors may further utilize immunoelectron microscopy (IEM), in which immunogold stains—antibody probes conjugated with gold particles—for ALλ, ALκ, AA, and ATTR are used to subtype the amyloid fibril. These stains "decorate" the target amyloid fibers and can be seen as "beads" in the fibrillary matrix of amyloid. IEM can detect even small amounts of amyloid fibrils, at earlier stages of the disease. However, the processing deals with a very small piece of tissue and leads to a false-negative result due to the limited sampling, especially in cases where the amyloid deposits are focal. Another barrier is fixation, where architectural details are preserved by cross-linking, but at the same time loss of antigenicity may result from dehydration and embedding procedures. Therefore, alternative fixatives such as modified Karnovsky's solution rather than conventional glutaraldehyde with different protocols are used for IEM examination.

6. Molecular diagnosis

Recent advances in MS-based proteomic analysis have revolutionized detecting and subtyping of amyloidosis. The analytic method has made it possible to detect and identify new kinds of amyloid fibrils as well as previously known ones in a given specimen without direct sequencing. One such example is ALECT2. As mentioned above, LECT2 is synthesized by the liver and released into the circulation and has uncertain physiologic roles in the cartilage and liver. It has been shown that ALECT2 is one of the major causes of kidney and liver amyloidosis after AL and AA amyloidosis, especially among Hispanics. This major amyloidosis may have been unrecognized due to a relatively indolent clinical course and limited ethnic distribution. Because serum LECT2 levels are not elevated, and no mutations are found in LECT2 gene so far, ALECT2 might have been misdiagnosed as AL or AA amyloidosis and treated as such without MS-based analysis.

The MS-based proteomic analysis utilizes techniques like laser microdissection (LMD), high-performance liquid chromatography (HPLC), and a variety of computational database tools. Although earlier HPLC- and MS-based analysis suffered from lack of specificity due to heterogeneous nature of the specimen, LMD largely overcame such diagnostic inaccuracy. LMD deals with microscopic examination of the specimen, selection of a field of interest, and microdissection of the field using laser in an attempt to achieve pure amyloid plaques. The dissected specimen can be submitted for histochemistry, IHC, or MS analysis. For FFPE specimens, an extra step for protein release similar to antigen retrieval used in IHC is applied. The released proteins are treated with a proteolytic enzyme (most commonly trypsin), and the resultant digested peptide fragments are separated by HPLC and analyzed with MS. This analytic method is based on an assumption that each human protein has their unique tryptic fragmentation patterns, which serves as a "fingerprint" of the protein. The analysis involves a previously curated database on human proteins and a number of computational algorithms to predict the amino acid sequences of the proteins that are contained in a given specimen.

Although the LMD- and MS-based proteomic analysis has demonstrated great sensitivity and specificity, they have one major pitfall. Because MS-based proteomic analysis heavily depends on human protein databases available in public, new polymorphisms or mutations may not be listed in the databases and, thus, cannot be identified using the technique. In such situations, a separate workflow to compare the newly identified mutations against previously known variants is utilized.

7. Conclusion

Amyloidosis is characterized morphologically by amorphous deposition of amyloid within tissue. The deposition is caused by aggregation of misfolded protein. Any disruptive processes in protein homeostasis (proteinostasis) can cause such misfolding and aggregation. Although different species of amyloid protein have different organotropisms and physiochemical properties, they appear remarkably similar when deposited within the target tissue. Clinical signs and symptoms of different types are largely affected by the organ where the amyloid is deposited. However, different treatment modalities and clinical courses according to the type mandate the exact subtyping of amyloid.

The confirmation and subtyping of amyloidosis heavily depend on pathologic examination of abdominal fat, minor salivary gland, or target organs. The gold standard for confirmation of amyloidosis is Congophilia and birefringence. Additional modalities such as IHC, EM, and MS can help further subclassify the type of amyloidosis.

Lately, new types of amyloidosis have been identified by MS. Atypical structure of amyloid continues to be found in various organs. Contrary to the conventional definition of amyloid, such as extracellular amorphous deposition, intracellular and spherical structure amyloids have been discovered. In addition, novel mutations of the same protein have been shown to confer totally different clinical implications.

The accumulation of new histologic findings and molecular studies will be an important key to understanding the disease mechanisms and, further on, the treatment of amyloid-associated diseases.

Author details

Moon Joo Kim, Donghwa Baek, Luan Truong and Jae Y. Ro*
Department of Pathology and Genomic Medicine, Houston Methodist Hospital, Weill Medical College of Cornell University, Houston, Texas, USA

*Address all correspondence to: jaero@houstonmethodist.orf

References

[1] D'Souza A, Theis JD, Vrana JA, Dogan A. Pharmaceutical amyloidosis associated with subcutaneous insulin and enfuvirtide administration. Amyloid. 2014;**21**(2):71-75

[2] Kim MJ, McCroskey Z, Piao Y, Belcheva A, Truong L, Kurtin PJ, et al. Spheroid-type of AL amyloid deposition associated with colonic adenocarcinoma: A case report with literature review. Pathology International. 2018;**68**(2):123-127

[3] Miyazaki D, Yazaki M, Gono T, Kametani F, Tsuchiya A, Matsuda M, et al. AH amyloidosis associated with an immunoglobulin heavy chain variable region (VH1) fragment: A case report. Amyloid. 2008;**15**(2):125-128

[4] Livneh A, Langevitz P. Diagnostic and treatment concerns in familial Mediterranean fever. Baillière's Best Practice & Research. Clinical Rheumatology. 2000;**14**(3):477-498

[5] Phull P, Sanchorawala V, Connors LH, Doros G, Ruberg FL, Berk JL, et al. Monoclonal gammopathy of undetermined significance in systemic transthyretin amyloidosis (ATTR). Amyloid. 2018;**25**(1):62-67

[6] Clement CG, Truong LD. An evaluation of Congo red fluorescence for the diagnosis of amyloidosis. Human Pathology. 2014;**45**(8):1766-1772

[7] Mereuta OM, Theis JD, Vrana JA, Law ME, Grogg KL, Dasari S, et al. Leukocyte cell-derived chemotaxin 2 (LECT2)-associated amyloidosis is a frequent cause of hepatic amyloidosis in the United States. Blood. 2014;**123**(10):1479-1482

[8] Benson MD, James S, Scott K, Liepnieks JJ, Kluve-Beckerman B. Leukocyte chemotactic factor 2: A novel renal amyloid protein. Kidney International. 2008;**74**(2):218-222

[9] Buck FS, Koss MN. Hepatic amyloidosis: Morphologic differences between systemic AL and AA types. Human Pathology. 1991;**22**(9):904-907

[10] Chandan VS, Shah SS, Lam-Himlin DM, Petris GD, Mereuta OM, Dogan A, et al. Globular hepatic amyloid is highly sensitive and specific for LECT2 amyloidosis. The American Journal of Surgical Pathology. 2015;**39**(4):558-564

[11] Almeida RR, Zanetti G, Pereira E Silva JL, Neto CA, Gomes AC, Meirelles GS, et al. Respiratory tract amyloidosis. State-of-the-art review with a focus on pulmonary involvement. Lung. 2015;**193**(6):875-883

[12] Otto M, Hansen T, Kriegsmann J. Images in cardiology: Intracellular cardiac amyloidosis in familiar amyloid polyneuropathy of the Portuguese type. Heart. 2002;**88**(1):90

[13] Kjeldsberg CR, Eyre HJ, Totzke H. Evidence for intracellular amyloid formation in myeloma. Blood. 1977;**50**(3):493-504

[14] O'Brien TD, Butler AE, Roche PC, Johnson KH, Butler PC. Islet amyloid polypeptide in human insulinomas. Evidence for intracellular amyloidogenesis. Diabetes. 1994;**43**(2):329-336

[15] Landolt AM, Kleihues P, Heitz PU. A myloid deposits in pituitary adenomas. Differentiation of two types. Archives of Pathology & Laboratory Medicine. 1987;**111**(5):453-458

[16] Val-Bernal JF. Localized amyloidosis of the uterine cervix with spheroid type of amyloid. International Journal of Gynecological Pathology. 1999;**18**(2):188

[17] Pambuccian SE, Horyd ID, Cawte T, Huvos AG. Amyloidoma of bone, a

plasma cell/plasmacytoid neoplasm. Report of three cases and review of the literature. The American Journal of Surgical Pathology. 1997;**21**(2):179-186

[18] Acebo E, Mayorga M, Fernando Val-Bernal J. Primary amyloid tumor (amyloidoma) of the jejunum with spheroid type of amyloid. Pathology. 1999;**31**(1):8-11

Section 2

Amyloidosis: Specific Cases

Chapter 5

Renal Amyloidosis

Elena Zakharova

Abstract

Modern amyloid nomenclature, based on the amyloid fibril proteins, includes 31 types of amyloidosis. Renal involvement is commonly seen in AA, AL, and several other hereditary and acquired amyloidoses. AA amyloidosis, constituting up to 45% of all systemic amyloidosis cases, is associated with wide variety of chronic inflammatory conditions. The precursor protein of the fibrils in AA amyloidosis is an apolipoprotein, called serum amyloid A, and produced in the liver in response to proinflammatory cytokines. AL amyloidosis is actually known to be the most common form of systemic amyloidosis in the Western countries. In this type of amyloidosis the precursor proteins are monoclonal immunoglobulin light chains, produced by plasma cell clone. Clinical diagnosis of AA and AL systemic amyloidosis is based on the presence of proteinuria or nephrotic syndrome and impaired kidney function in patients with extrarenal manifestations. Kidney biopsy is crucial for the diagnostics, and while Congo red staining with examination of Congo-positive material in the polarized light is confirmative for amyloidosis as such, immune staining, helpful to distinguish AA and AL types, guides treatment strategies. In cases when neither AA nor AL amyloidosis are confirmed, one should consider rare types of amyloidosis—ALECT2, AapolA, AFib or ALys.

Keywords: light chains, serum amyloid A, nephrotic syndrome, kidney function, kidney biopsy

1. Introduction

Modern amyloid nomenclature, based on the amyloid fibril proteins, includes 31 types of amyloidosis [1]. Renal involvement is commonly seen in AL, AH, AA, ALECT2, and several other hereditary and acquired amyloidoses [1–4], main features are summarized in **Table 1**.

We describe below two most common types of amyloidosis, damaging kidneys—AA amyloidosis and AL amyloidosis.

2. AA amyloidosis

The precursor protein of the fibrils in AA amyloidosis is an apolipoprotein, called serum amyloid A, and produced in the liver in response to proinflammatory cytokines. AA amyloidosis, constituting up to 45% of all systemic amyloidosis cases, is associated with wide variety of chronic inflammatory conditions [5–7], summarized in the **Table 2**.

Protein precursor	Fibril protein	Clinical setting	Kidney damage	Other target organs
Immunoglobulin light chain	AL	"Primary" amyloidosis, LPD	70%	All organs
Immunoglobulin heavy chain	AH	LPD	—	All organs
Serum amyloid A	AA	Chronic inflammation	90%	All organs except CNS
Leucocyte chemotactic factor-2	ALECT2	Not defined as acquired or hereditary	Primarily	Liver
Transthyretin	ATTR	Hereditary and acquired	Common	Heart, Eye, PNS, ANS, ligaments, tendon synovium, leptomeninges
Apolipoprotein A I	AapoAI	Hereditary	Common	Heart, liver, PNS, testis, larynx, skin
Apolipoprotein A II	AapoAII	Hereditary	Primarily	Many organs
Apolipoprotein A IV	AapoAIV	Acquired	Primarily	—
Fibrinogen α	AFib	Hereditary	Primarily	—
Lysozyme	ALys	Hereditary	Primarily	Liver

LPD, lymphoproliferative disorders; CNS, central nervous system; PNS, peripheral nervous system; ANS, autonomous nervous system.

Table 1.
Amyloidoses with renal involvement.

Kidneys are the main site of involvement in AA amyloidosis, renal damage (**Figure 1**) occurs in 90% of cases, presenting with proteinuria, nephrotic syndrome (NS) and impaired kidney function [3, 6].

Rheumatoid arthritis, if poorly controlled, still remains one of the most common inflammatory diseases, associated with AA amyloidosis (**Figure 2**).

However, many other conditions, listed in **Table 2**, may be causative for AA amyloidosis. Frequency of the diseases, associated with AA amyloidosis in the patients, followed in our unit, is shown in **Table 3**.

Worthy to note, that beyond traditional causes, several rare conditions, such as sarcoidosis, cystic fibrosis and Castleman's disease, complicated by AA amyloidosis, might be seen in the real practice (**Figures 3** and **4**).

Moreover, we recently described a patient with sclerosing angiomatoid nodular transformation of the spleen and AA amyloidosis [8], association previously unreported (**Figures 5** and **6**).

Presence of NS or proteinuria in patients with the history of any kind of chronic inflammatory conditions, indicates a high "suspicion index' with AA amyloidosis. The diagnosis demands pathology confirmation with kidney biopsy, demonstrating not only positive Congo red staining of the material, infiltrating kidney tissue (see **Figure 1**), but also apple-green birefringence in polarized light (**Figure 7**) and serum amyloid A expression (**Figure 8**).

Treatment goal in patients with AA amyloidosis is a complete control of the inflammatory process [6]. Due to the various characters of the underlying diseases, treatment may include surgery, antibiotics, anti-TNF agents, colchicine and several novel drugs. Kidney transplantation for the patients with the end stage of renal disease (ESRD) is an important option and may be considered if a stable control of the underlying disease has been achieved.

Infectious conditions with persistent inflammation	**Chronic non-infectious diseases with persistent inflammation**
Conditions predisposing to chronic infections	*Arthritis*
• Cystic fibrosis	• Rheumatoid arthritis
• Epidermolysis bullosa	• Ankylosing spondylitis
• Paraplegia	• Adult Still disease
• Jejunoileal bypass	• Juvenile idiopathic arthritis
• Intravenous drugs use	• Psoriatic arthritis
	• Gout
Immunodeficiency's predisposing to chronic infections	*Bowel diseases*
• Common variable immunodeficiency	• Crohn's disease
• Hypogammaglobulinemia	• Ulcerative colitis
• X-linked agammaglobulinemia	*Systemic vasculitis*
• Cyclic neutropenia	• Behcet's disease
• HIV/AIDS	• Polyarteritis nodosa
• Other immunodeficiencies	• Giant cell vasculitis
	• Takayasu's arteritis
	• Polymyalgia rheumatica
Chronic infections	*Other diseases*
• Bronchiectasis	• Sarcoidosis
• Osteomyelitis	• SAPHO syndrome
• Tuberculosis	• Schnitzler syndrome
• Leprosy	• Rosai-Dorfman disease
• Chronic pyelonephritis	• Recurrent idiopathic pericarditis
• Whipple's disease	
• Chronic cutaneous ulcers	
Neoplastic diseases	**Hereditary autoinflammatory syndromes**
Blood malignancies	*Classic*
• Castleman's disease	• Familial Mediterranean fever
• Hodgkin's lymphoma	*Rare*
• Waldenstrom macroglobulinemia	• TRAPS
• Hairy cell leukemia	• Muckle-Wells syndrome
Solid tumors	• NOMID/CINCA syndrome
• Hepatic adenoma	• Hyper-IgD syndrome
• Renal cell carcinoma	• Other monogenic autoinflammatory syndromes
• Adenocarcinoma of the lung	
• Adenocarcinoma of the gut	
• Mesothelioma	

HIV, human immunodeficiency virus; AIDS, acquired immunodeficiency syndrome; SAPHO, synovitis, acne, pustules, hyperostosis, osteitis; TRAPS, TNF receptor associated periodic syndrome; NOMID, neonatal multisystem inflammatory disease; CINCA, chronic infantile neurological cutaneous and articular syndrome.

Table 2.
Diseases, associated with AA amyloidosis.

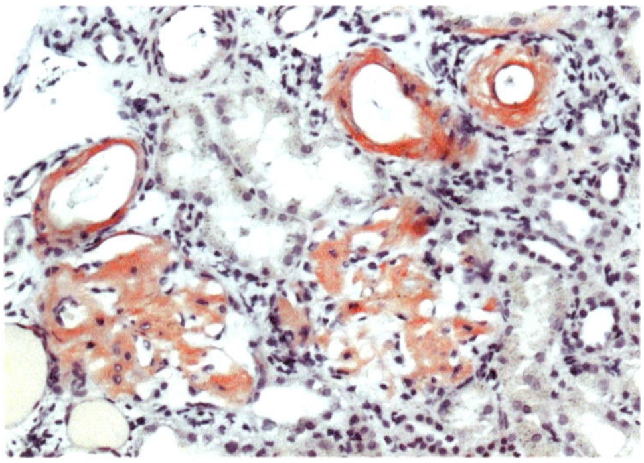

Figure 1.
Renal AA amyloidosis, Congo red 100×.

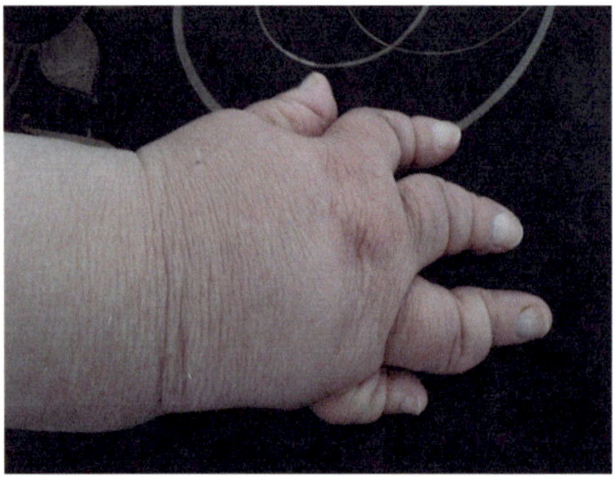

Figure 2.
Rheumatoid arthritis, complicated by renal AA amyloidosis with nephrotic syndrome.

Associated disease	Patients (N)	%
Rheumatoid arthritis	64	44.1
Ankylosing spondylitis	16	11.0
Psoriatic arthritis	7	4.8
Crohn's disease/ulcerative colitis	3	2.0
Sarcoidosis	1	0.7
Mediterranean fever	14	9.6
Hyper-IgD syndrome	1	0.7
Bronchiectasis	10	6.8
Osteomyelitis	7	4.8
Paraplegia	6	4.1
Tuberculosis	4	2.7
Chronic cutaneous ulcers	3	2.0
Cystic fibrosis	1	0.7
Lung tumors	3	2.0
Hodgkin's lymphoma	2	1.4
Castleman's disease	2	1.4
Sclerosing angiomatoid nodular transformation of the spleen	1	0.7
Total	145	100

Table 3.
Spectrum of the diseases, associated with AA amyloidosis, personal data, unpublished.

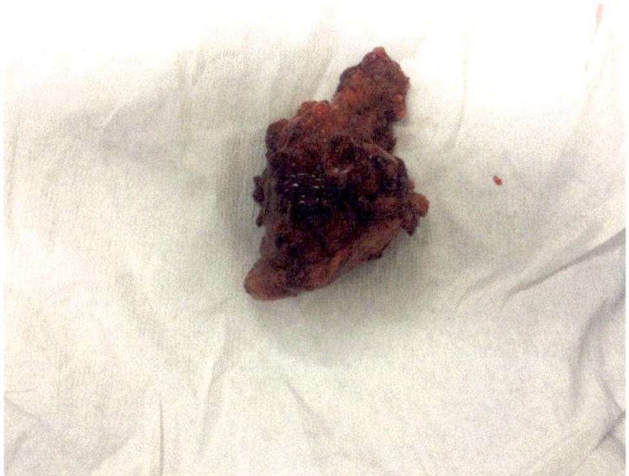

Figure 3.
Castleman's disease, unfixed gross specimen.

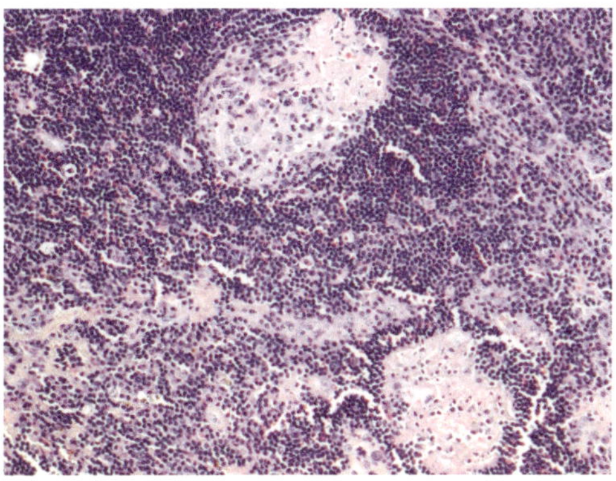

Figure 4.
Castleman's disease, atypical lymphoid tissue, hematoxylin & eosin 100×.

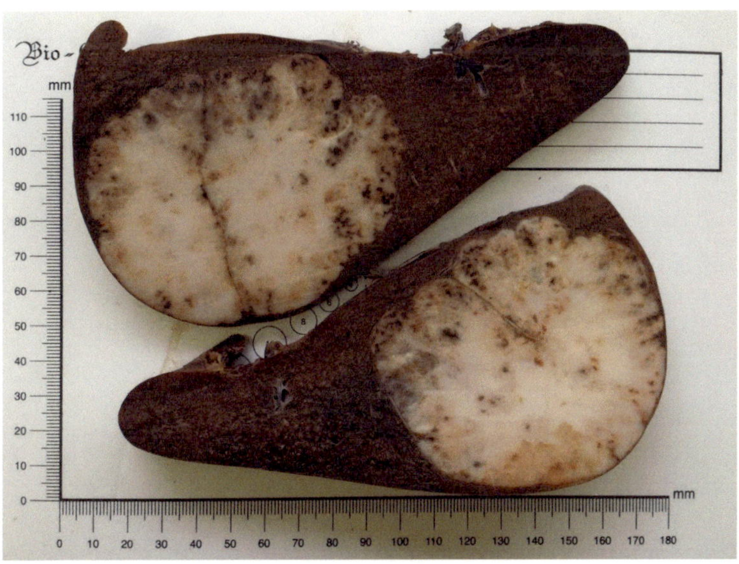

Figure 5.
Sclerosing angiomatoid nodular transformation of the spleen. Formalin-fixed gross specimen.

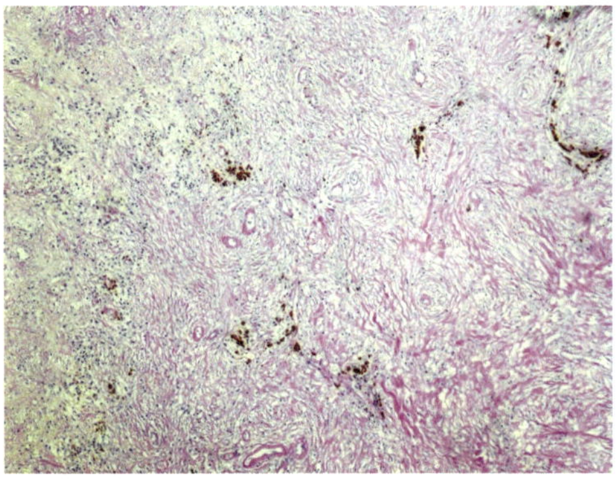

Figure 6.
Sclerosing angiomatoid nodular transformation of the spleen. PAS 100×.

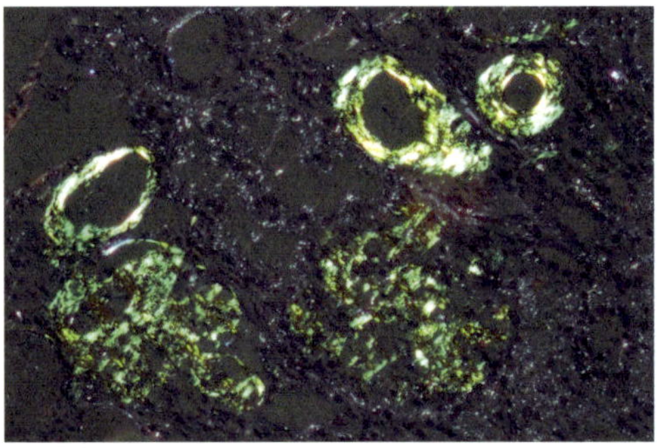

Figure 7.
Renal AA amyloidosis, Congo red 100×, polarized light.

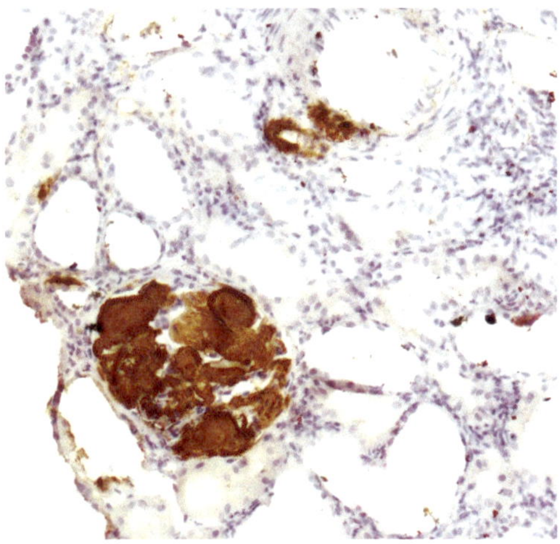

Figure 8.
Renal AA amyloidosis, serum amyloid A, immunoperoxidase 100×.

3. AL amyloidosis

The precursor proteins of the fibrils in AL amyloidosis are monoclonal immunoglobulin light chains, produced by plasma cell clone. AL amyloidosis, which is the most prevalent type of systemic amyloidosis in the Western countries, sometimes is associated with B cell lymphoproliferative disorders—multiple myeloma, Waldenström macroglobulinemia and non-Hodgkin lymphomas [9–14]. However usually AL amyloidosis is associated with low-grade plasma cell clone and do not meet the criteria for multiple myeloma or lymphoplasmacytic lymphoma, therefore formerly it was known as "primary" [15–18].

In the real practice, among 128 patients with biopsy-proven AL amyloidosis, followed in our unit, 25 were diagnosed with multiple myeloma, 1—with Waldenström macroglobulinemia, and 102—with AL amyloidosis ("primary").

Kidneys and heart are the main sites of involvement in AL amyloidosis with the occurrence up to 70% of cases. Renal involvement typically presents with proteinuria or NS, which is manifested in more than 50% of patients at the time of diagnosis, and impaired kidney function progressing towards ESRD in about 20% of cases over time [19–21].

AL amyloidosis is diagnosed by demonstration of monoclonal deposits in the sites of amyloid deposition in the kidney (**Figures 9–11**).

Kidney biopsy is usually indicated for significant proteinuria and/or renal insufficiency in patients with signs and symptoms of heart, liver, tongue, intestine, peripheral and autonomous nervous system and soft tissues damage (**Figures 12–17**).

Monoclonal protein studies should be performed to match the monoclonal protein in circulation with the monoclonal deposits in the kidney (**Figure 18**).

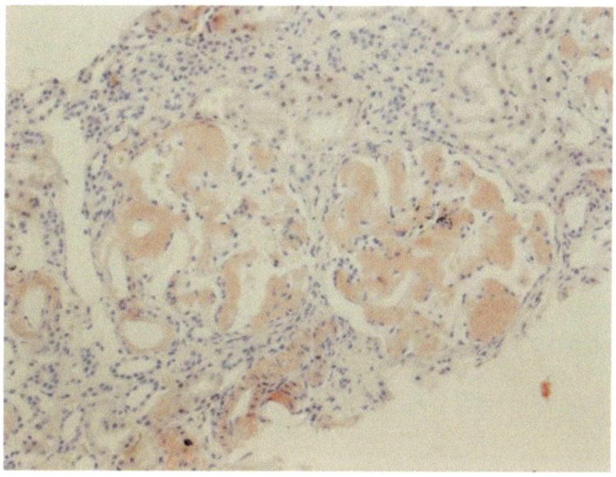

Figure 9.
Renal AL amyloidosis, Congo red 100×.

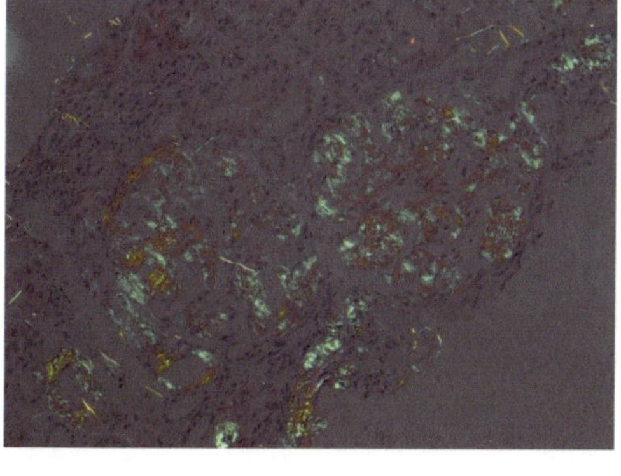

Figure 10.
Renal AL amyloidosis, Congo red 100×, polarized light.

Different treatment regimens had been used since 1997, when melphalan was introduced—melphalan and prednisone (MP), melphalan and dexamethasone (MD), and high dose melphalan with autologous stem cell transplantation (ASCT).

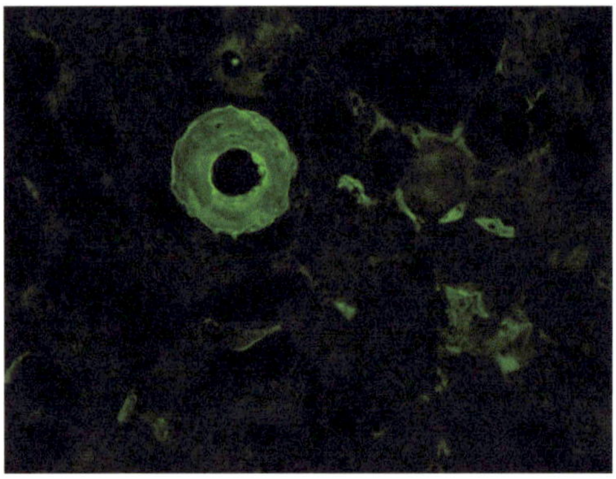

Figure 11.
Renal AL amyloidosis, light chain lambda, immunofluorescence 100×.

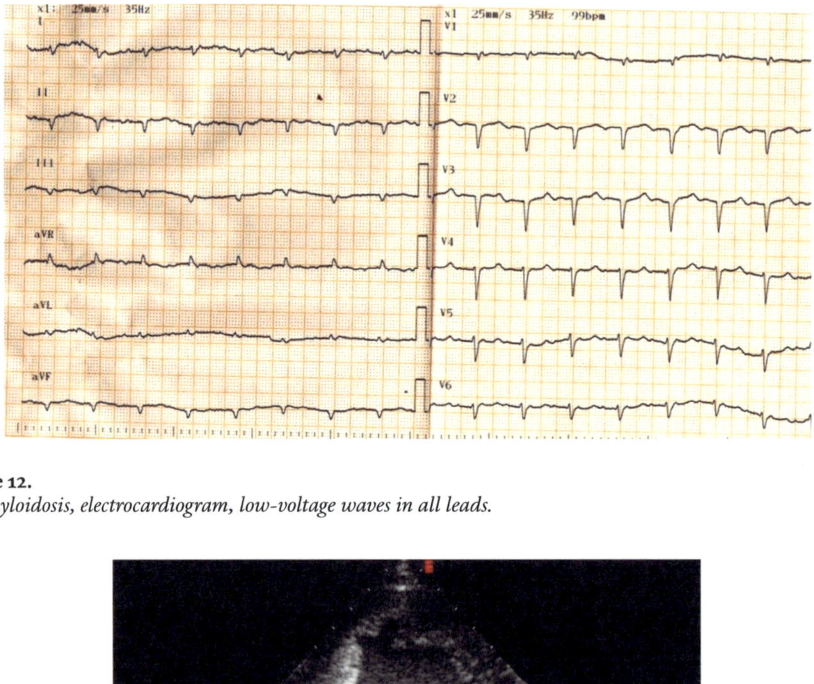

Figure 12.
AL amyloidosis, electrocardiogram, low-voltage waves in all leads.

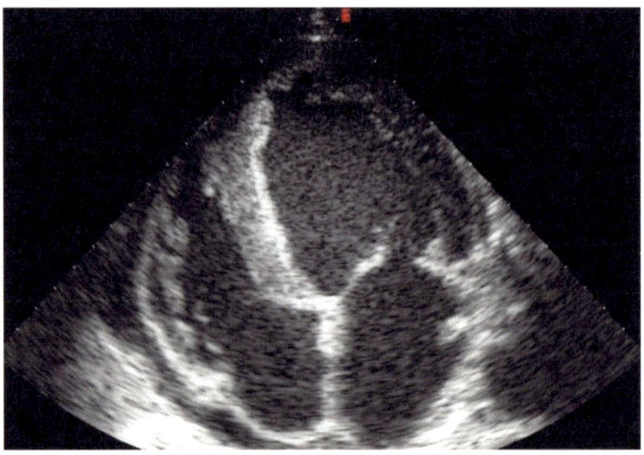

Figure 13.
AL amyloidosis, echocardiogram, myocardial mirror-like appearance.

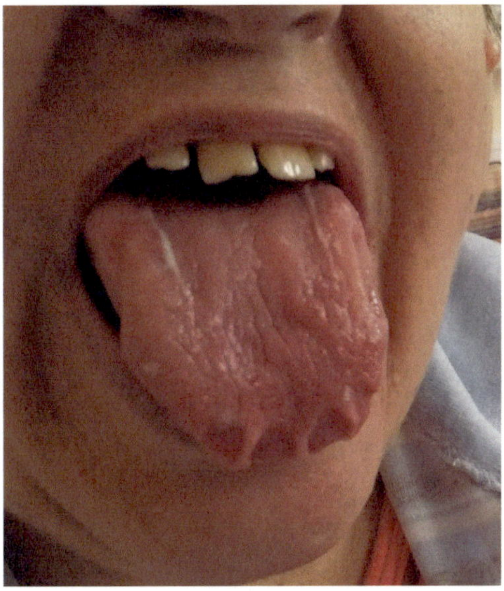

Figure 14.
AL amyloidosis, macroglossia.

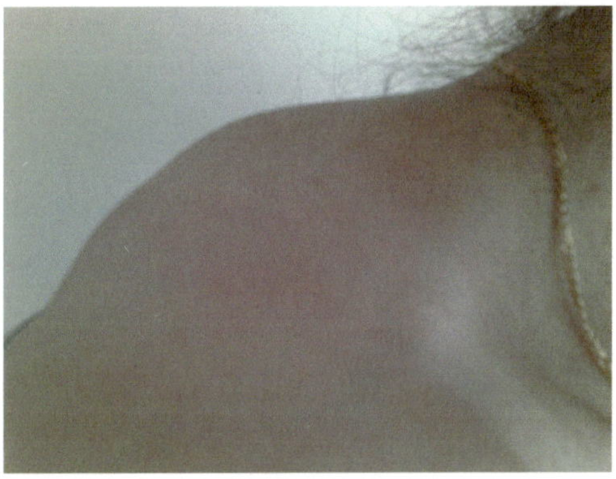

Figure 15.
AL amyloidosis, "shoulder pad" symptom.

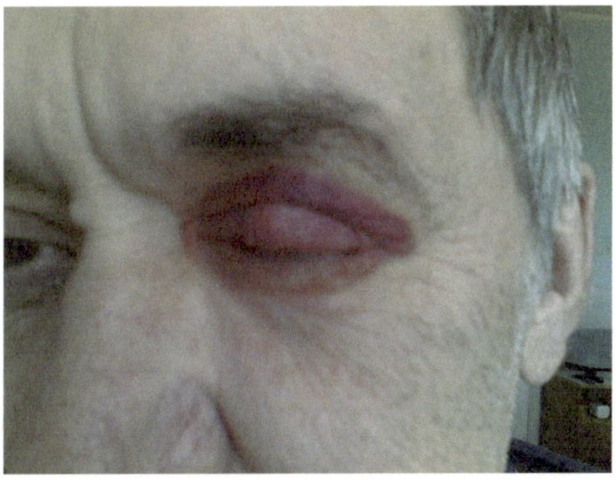

Figure 16.
AL amyloidosis, "racoon eye" symptom.

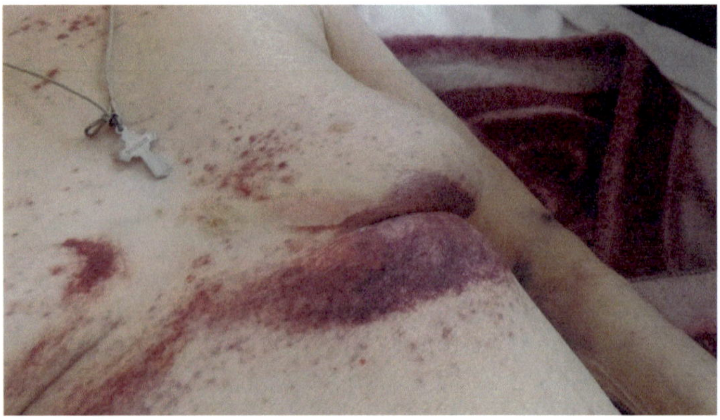

Figure 17.
AL amyloidosis, spontaneous subcutaneous hemorrhages.

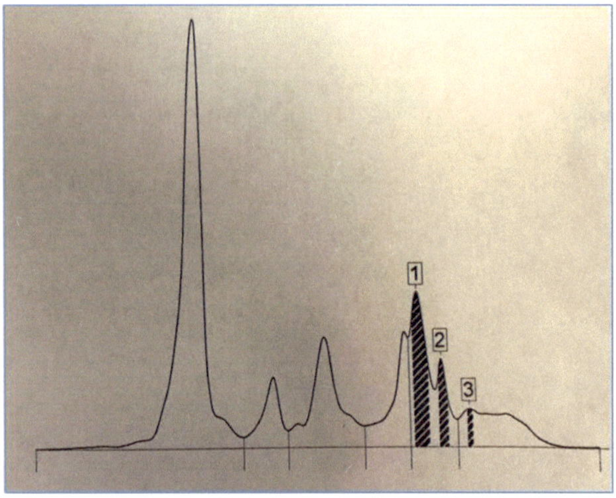

Figure 18.
Serum electrophoresis, M-spike.

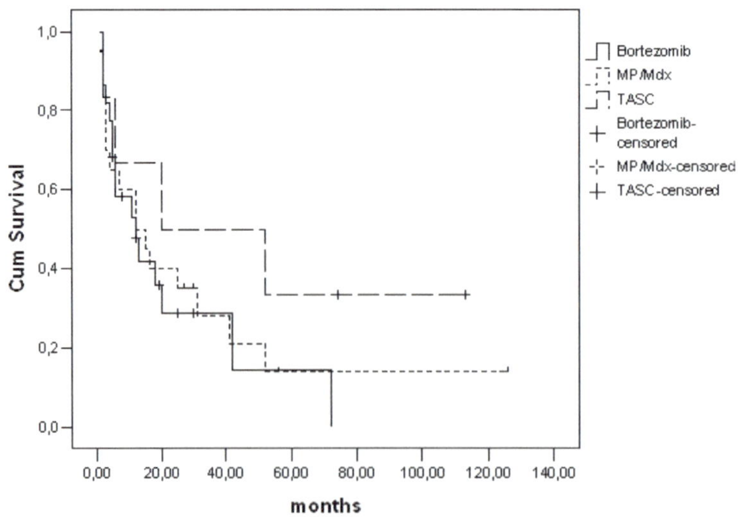

Figure 19.
Treatment results in 49 patients with AL amyloidosis, personal data [23].

Currently recommended treatment for AL amyloidosis, including cyclophosphamide-thalidomide-dexamethasone (CTD), bortezomib-dexamethasone (BD), cyclophosphamide-bortezomib-dexamethasone(CBD) regimens with relatively fast hematological response were adopted from multiple myeloma treatment protocols [22]. In our experience of treatment of systemic "primary" AL amyloidosis with kidney involvement using different regimens over almost three decades, cumulative survival did not differ statistically between melphalan-based and bortezomib-based regimens (**Figure 19**) [23].

4. Conclusions

Clinical diagnosis of AA and AL systemic amyloidosis, most often affecting kidneys, is based on the presence of proteinuria or nephrotic syndrome and impaired kidney function in patients with extrarenal manifestations. Kidney biopsy is crucial for the diagnostics, and while Congo red staining with examination of Congo-positive material in the polarized light is confirmative for amyloidosis as such, immunofluorescence and immunohistochemistry technics are helpful to distinguish AA and AL types. Differential diagnostics of AA and AL types guides the treatment strategies. In cases when neither AA nor AL amyloidosis are confirmed, one should consider rare types of amyloidosis, based on the presence of renal involvement—ALECT2, AapolA I, II and IV, AFib or ALys amyloidosis.

Acknowledgements

Author thanks doctors Olga Vorobova, Ekaterina Stolyarevich, Vladimir Bedin, Mikhail Tavobilov, Evgeny Shutov, Eugene Nikitin, Marina Rybakova and Igor Miloserdov for their help in diagnostics and treatment of the patients.

Conflict of interest

Author declares no conflict of interests.

Author details

Elena Zakharova
City Clinical Hospital n.a. S.P. Botkin, Russian Medical Academy of Continuous Postgraduate Education, Moscow, Russian Federation

*Address all correspondence to: helena.zakharova@gmail.com

References

[1] Sipe JD, Benson MD, Buxbaum JN, Ikeda S, Merlini G, Saraiva MJ, et al. Nomenclature 2014: Amyloid fibril proteins and clinical classification of the amyloidosis. Amyloid. 2014;**21**(4):221-224. DOI: 10.3109/13506129.2014.964858

[2] Said SM, Sethi S, Valeri AM, Leung N, Cornell LD, Fidler ME, et al. Renal amyloidosis: Origin and clinicopathologic correlations of 474 recent cases. Clinical Journal of the American Society of Nephrology. 2013;**8**:1515-1523

[3] Picken MM, Dogan A. Amyloidosis of the kidney, the lower urinary and genital tract (male and female) and the breast. In Picken MM, Herrera GA, Dogan A, editors. Amyloid and Related Disorders. Totowa, NJ, USA: Humana Press (Springer) 2015. p. 369-390

[4] Benson MD. The hereditary amyloidoses. In: Picken MM, Herrera GA, Dogan A, editors. Amyloid and Related Disorders. Totowa, NJ, USA: Humana Press (Springer); 2015. pp. 65-80

[5] Lachmann HJ, Goodman HJB, Gilbertson AJ, Gallimore JR, Sabin SA, Gillmore JD, et al. Natural history and outcome in systemic AA amyloidosis. The New England Journal of Medicine. 2007;**356**:2361-2371

[6] Obici L, Merlini G. AA amyloidosis: Basic knowledge, unmet needs and future treatments. Swiss Medical Weekly. 2012;**31**:142. DOI: 10.4414/smw.2012.13580

[7] Ombrello AK, Aksentijevich IAA. Amyloidosis. In: Picken MM, Herrera GA, Dogan A, editors. Amyloid and Related Disorders. Totowa, NJ, USA: Humana Press (Springer); 2015. pp. 31-54

[8] Zakharova EV, Shutov EV, Vorobyova OA, Nikitin EA. AA amyloidosis in a patient with essential thrombocythemia and sclerosing angiomatoid nodular transformation of the spleen. Journal of Onco-Nephrology. 2017;**1**(3):13-17. DOI: 10.5301/jo-n.5000028

[9] Kyle RA, Linos A, Beard SM, Linke RP, Gertz MA, O'Fallon WM, et al. Incidence and natural history of primary systemic amyloidosis in Olmsted County, Minnesota, 1950 through 1989. Blood. 1992;**79**:1817-1822

[10] Pinney JH, Smyth CJ, Taube JB, Lachmann HJ, Venner CP, Gibbs SD. Systemic amyloidosis in England: An epidemiological study. British Journal of Haematology. 2013;**161**:523-532

[11] Herrera G, Picken M. Renal diseases associated with plasma cell dyscrasias, amyloidosis, Waldenstrom macroglobulinemia and cryoglobulinemic nephropathies. In: Jennette J, Olson J, Silva F, D'Agati V, editors. Heptinstall's Pathology of the Kidney. 7th ed. Philadelphia, PA: Lippincott Williams & Wilkins; 2014. pp. 951-114

[12] Blade J, Fernandez-Llama P, Bosch F, Montoliu J, Lens XM, Montoto S. Renal failure in multiple myeloma: Presenting features and predictors of outcome in 94 patients from a single institution. Archives of Internal Medicine. 1998;**158**(17):1889-1893

[13] Cohen AH, Zhou P, Xiao Q, Fleisher M, Kalakonda N, Akhurst T, et al. Systemic AL amyloidosis due to non-Hodgkin's lymphoma: An unusual clinicopathologic association. British Journal of Haematology. 2004;**124**:309-314

[14] Ikee R, Kobayashi S, Hemmi N, Suzuki S, Miura S. Amyloidosis associated with chronic lymphocytic leukemia. Amyloid. 2005;**12**:131-134

[15] Gertz M, Kyle R. The plasma cell labelling index: A valuable tool in

primary systemic amyloidosis. Blood. 1989;**74**:1008-1011

[16] Gertz M, Kyle R, Noel P. Primary systemic amyloidosis: A rare complication of immunoglobulin M monoclonal gammopathies and Waldenstrom's macroglobulinemia. Journal of Clinical Oncology. 1993;**11**:914-920

[17] Merlini G, Stone MJ. Dangerous small B-cell clones. Blood. 2006;**108**(8):2520-2530

[18] Said S, Sethi S, Valeri A, Leung N, Cornell L, Fidler ME, et al. Renal amyloidosis: Origin and clinicopathologic correlations of 474 recent cases. Clinical Journal of the American Society of Nephrology. 2013;**8**:1515-1523

[19] Gertz M, Lacy M, Dispenzieri A. Immunoglobulin light chain amyloidosis and the kidney. Kidney International. 2002;**61**:1-9

[20] Gertz M, Leung N, Lacy MQ, Dispenzieri A, Zeldenrust SR, Haymann SR, et al. Clinical outcomes in immunoglobulin light chain amyloidosis affecting kidney. Nephrology Dialysis Transplantation. 2009;**24**:3132-3137

[21] Falk R, Comenzo R, Skinner M. The systemic amyloidosis. The New England Journal of Medicine. 1997;**337**:898-909

[22] Fermand J-P, Bridoux F, Kyle RA, Kastritis E, Weiss BM, Cook MA, et al. On behalf of the international kidney and monoclonal Gammopathy research group. How I treat monoclonal gammopathy of renal significance (MGRS). Blood. 2013;**122**(22):3583-3590

[23] Zakharova EV, Stolyarevich ES. Chemotherapy for renal AL amyloidosis: Treatment results and outcomes in 49 patients from a single center. Clinical Practice. 2016;**13**(1):11-18

Chapter 6

Neurological Manifestations of Transthyretin-Related Amyloidosis

Kourosh Rezania and Laleh Saadat

Abstract

Transthyretin related amyloidosis (ATTR) results from the tissue deposition of misfolded mutant or wild-type transthyretin (TTR). Involvement of nervous system often heralds the onset of ATTR. Familial ATTR is because of mutations in the TTR gene which lead to destabilization of the tetrameric structure of TTR and generation of amyloidogenic monomers, tissue deposition of which causes end organ injury specially neuropathy and cardiomyopathy. Peripheral neuropathy is typically axonal with early involvement of the autonomic nerves. Wild-type TTR (ATTRwt), is a common cause of cardiomyopathy in the elderly and may play a role in the pathogenesis of carpal tunnel syndrome and spinal stenosis in that age group. Diagnosis of ATTR is made by demonstrating tissue amyloid deposits, then proving that the amyloid deposits consist of mutant or wild-type TTR, which necessitates assessment of TTR gene sequencing. Disease modifying treatments have become available for ATTR through liver transplantation, stabilization of the TTR molecule (diflunisal and tafamidis) and suppressing the gene expression of TTR (inotersen and patisiran).

Keywords: TTR, ATTR, transthyretin amyloidosis, ATTRwt, tafamidis, diflunisal, inotersen, patisiran

1. Introduction

Systemic amyloidosis comprises a group of diseases characterized by deposition of misfolded proteins which express abnormal β-sheet conformation usually in the extracellular spaces in different tissues [1]. At least 36 amyloid precursor proteins are recognized so far in the humans [2]. There are several general pathogenetic pathways that proteins become misfolded and create amyloid fibrils [3]: (1) presence of abnormal protein such as amyloid light chain (AL) or those caused by a mutation (such as familial ATTR and amyloidosis related to gelsolin mutations), (2) prolonged exposure to a normal protein such as systemic reactive (AA) and dialysis related amyloidosis; and (3) age related amyloidosis such as senile systemic amyloidosis. This book chapter will discuss the neurological manifestations of familial and wild-type ATTR, their diagnosis and treatment. Although neuropathy related to familial ATTR is uncommon, it is underdiagnosed and causes profound disability and mortality, largely as a result of concomitant cardiomyopathy. Timely diagnosis and treatment improves the outcome as new disease modifying treatments have become available.

IntechOpen

2. Transthyretin (TTR)

TTR is a 127 amino acid protein, is encoded by 7 kb of DNA spanning exons 1–4 of a single gene on chromosome 18 [4]. TTR is a carrier molecule of thyroxine and vitamin A. Serum TTR is synthesized and excreted by the liver as a tetrameric structure. Other sources of local TTR synthesis include epithelial cells of the choroid plexus and the retinal pigment epithelium. TTR is however dispensable for thyroid hormone homeostasis; TTR knockout mice are euthyroid and have a normal phenotype [5, 6]. The presence of point mutations in TTR results in destabilization of the tetramere, and dissociation into amyloidogenic monomers, which misfold and self-aggregate into insoluble amyloid fibrils (**Figure 1**). Two distinct types of amyloid fibrils have been described in TTR amyloid deposits: type A, consists of C-terminal TTR fragments and full-length TTR, and type B, which only consists of full-length TTR [7]. Type A fibrils often target the heart and type B fibrils occur predominantly with neurological symptoms [8]. Every organ of an individual patient contains the same (either type A or type B) fibrils, and the composition is unchanged over time. The presence of C-terminal TTR fragments has an impact on the affinity for various tracers used for intensity of tissue Congo red staining and of noninvasive imaging of amyloid depositions using 99 m-technetium-diphosphono-propanodicarboxylic acid scintigraphy [7].

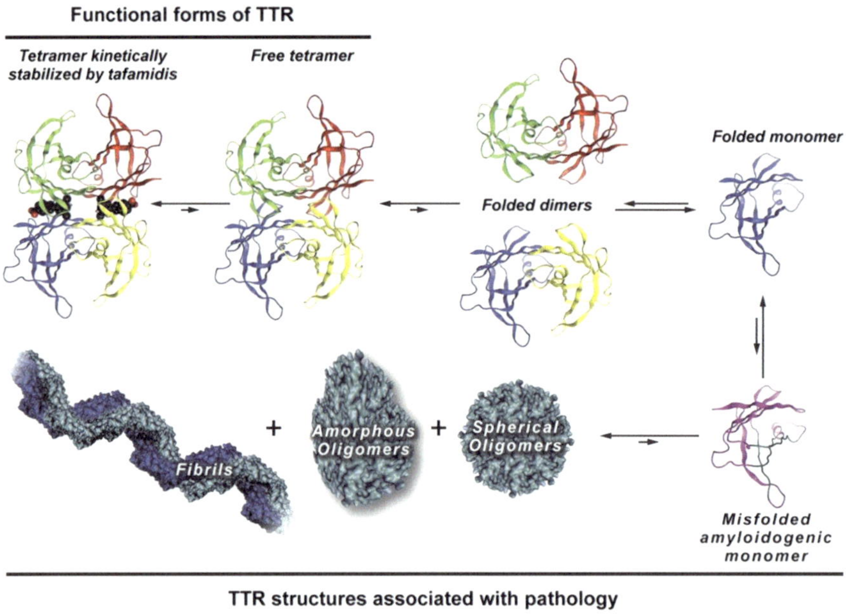

Figure 1.
Amyloid formation by TTR requires rate-limiting tetramer dissociation to a pair of folded dimers, which then quickly dissociate into folded monomers. Partial unfolding of the monomers yields the aggregation-prone amyloidogenic intermediate. The amyloidogenic intermediate can misassemble to form a variety of aggregate morphologies, including spherical oligomers, amorphous aggregates, and fibrils. Tafamidis binding to the TTR tetramer (upper left, see text below) dramatically slows dissociation, thereby efficiently inhibiting aggregation [from [63], with permission].

3. Familial transthyretin related amyloidosis (fATTR)

fATTR is a multisystem disease involving the heart (cardiomyopathy, conduction disturbances), gastrointestinal tract, kidneys, thyroid, salivary glands, eyes, peripheral and central nervous system. More than 130 pathological mutations have been associated with fATTR [9, 10].

3.1 Epidemiology

There is a marked variation in the prevalence and age of onset of ATTR in different countries, partly as a result of variation in the type of pathogenic mutation. fATTR is endemic in northern Portugal, Sweden and Japan, but sporadically occurs everywhere in the globe, with estimated number of about 5–10,000 patients worldwide [11]. The global prevalence is estimated at 0.87–1.1 per million; prevalence in Europe and Japan are estimated at 1/100,000 and 1 per million individuals respectively [12, 13]. The age of onset has a wide range, between 10s and 90s [10]. In Japan, the age of onset is bimodal, with early (30–40 year old) and late (60s) onset peaks [10]; on the other hand, the age of onset is more likely to be early (25–35 years old) in Portugal and late in Sweden [14, 15]. The most common mutation associated with familial amyloid polyneuropathy (FAP) is Val30Met mutation (replacement of valine with methionine at position 30), with endemic spots in northern Portugal (where its prevalence is estimated at 1/538), Sweden, Japan, and Brazil. On the other hand, the most common mutation in the US metropolitan areas is Val122Ile (isoleucine is substituted for valine at position 122); this mutation almost exclusively occurs in patients of African descent and has he allele prevalence of 0.0173; i.e. 3.43% of African Americans carry at least one copy of the mutant gene [16]. Val122Ile related fATTR generally has a cardiac phenotype. In the UK population the majority of patients have the T60A missense mutation where tyrosine is replaced by adenine at position 60. This has been traced to a single founder mutation from north-west Ireland [17].

3.2 Neurological manifestations

Depending on the mutation in TTR, the phenotype can be cardiologic, neurologic, or mixed. Neurological manifestations, particularly polyneuropathy are the most common manifestations of some of the mutations.

3.2.1 Familial amyloid polyneuropathy (FAP)

FAP is the most common neurological manifestation of fATTR. It is autosomal dominant, but the penetrance is variable and dependent on the type of mutation. If untreated, patients will have progressive neuropathy and disability resulting in death 10–15 years after disease onset [18]. The Val30Met mutation is the most common mutation associated with FAP, with a variable disease phenotype. Early onset disease (age < 50), which is more common in endemic regions of Japan and Portugal has a high penetrance and presents with a progressive polyneuropathy predominantly involving the small fiber nerves, which is typically manifested by loss of distal pain and temperature sensation, and progressive autonomic dysfunction; the latter includes orthostatic hypotension, neurogenic bladder, erectile dysfunction and impaired bowel function (malabsorption, diarrhea and constipation), and the presence of cardiac conduction blocks often necessitate pacemaker placement [10, 19]. On the other hand, late onset (>50 year old) phenotype, which occurs in non-endemic regions of Portugal, Sweden and Japan and sporadic cases in other parts of the world, is characterized by a low penetrance rate, male sex predominance. Late onset cases may not have significant clinical dysautonomia, and often present with a progressive distal neuropathy involving large and small fiber modalities, presenting with motor weakness and loss of vibratory and position sense early on, often with significant neuropathic pain. Autonomic dysfunction was the initial manifestation of 48% of early onset and 10% of late onset FAP in a previous study [20]. Late onset FAP is often misdiagnosed for more common entities in that age group such as idiopathic neuropathy or chronic inflammatory demyelinating polyneuropathy (CIDP) partly because of lack of positive family history and autonomic symptoms [9, 19, 21]. Other reasons for misdiagnosis include presence of demyelinating features in the nerve conduction study, elevated cerebrospinal fluid (CSF) protein level [22, 23], and negative abdominal fat pad a nerve biopsy for Congo-red amyloid staining [9]. In a previous study on patients with familial amyloid cardiomyopathy, abdominal fat pad and bone marrow biopsy showed amyloid deposits in 67 and 41% of the patients respectively, while a sural nerve biopsy was positive in 83% of the patients who had that procedure [27]. It is therefore very important to do an amyloidosis workup, including echocardiography, nuclear imaging studies, and nerve biopsy on CIDP patients who do not respond to immunomodulatory treatment [9, 22, 23]. Val122Ile is the most common fATTR mutation in the USA, and usually has a cardiac phenotype, rather similar to ATTRwt (see below) [24, 25]; but carpal tunnel syndrome is rather common and neuropathy has also been reported in Val122Ile ATTR [26]. Unusual neuropathy phenotypes of FAP include upper extremity onset, ataxic and motor predominant [13]. For example, FAP associated with T60A mutation (which one of the more common mutations in UK) is characterized by a non-length dependent sensory loss and motor deficits, often rapidly progressive disease, and lack of positive sensory symptoms [17]. There is a diagnostic delay of up to 4 years for FAP diagnosis, especially when the autonomic symptoms are lacking [9, 21, 27]; As effective treatments are now available for FAP, it is very important to diagnose it in early stages, and before the cardiovascular and neurological disability are not severe. Presence of "red-flag" symptomatology have been emphasized to expedite the diagnosis, these include positive family history for neuropathy, unexplained heart disease including but not limited to atrial fibrillation, cardiac hypertrophy on echocardiography, carpal tunnel syndrome, gastrointestinal symptoms (anorexia, constipation, diarrhea, nausea, vomiting and unexplained weight loss, alternating constipation and diarrhea), renal involvement (proteinuria and renal failure) and ocular disease. The presence of >1 of the aforementioned features should prompt genetic testing for fATTR, as well as neurological and cardiovascular workup directed at the detection of amyloidosis [10, 28]. Gene sequencing has become increasingly affordable, and currently can be done free of charge for some patients in the USA (www.invitae.com/en/alnylam-act-hattr-amyloidosis; www.ambrygen.com/partners/hattr-compass/healthcare-provider). Another rather common diagnostic challenge is differentiating ATTR from primary (AL) amyloidosis. Monoclonal gammopathy of unclear significance (MGUS) has been reported in ~20–50% of patients with ATTR cardiomyopathy [29, 30]. Very high (>5.0) or low (<0.2) kappa/lambda ratio usually imply AL amyloidosis whereas normal ratio (0.7–1.2) suggests ATTR [31]. Sometimes, however, the result of kappa/lambda ratio is inconclusive. Immunohistochemistry (IHC), i.e. staining of amyloid deposits with antibodies to kappa and lambda light chains as well as TTR can be used to make the differentiation between AL amyloidosis and ATTR, however, amyloid subtype cannot be determined in 20–25% of cases with IHC alone [32]. Laser capture microdissection of amyloid deposits (microdissection done on Congo red stained tissue materials) followed by mass spectroscopy has increased the sensitivity and specificity of amyloid subtyping to 98–100% [32, 33] (**Figure 2**). Lipid chromatography-tandem mass spectrometry (LC-MS/MS) is another, more recent technology which determines the presence of mutant peptides with rather high accuracy [33–35]. However, LC-MS/MS had a sensitivity of 84% in picking up mutations that were detected in the genetic testing in a recent US study on 56 patients with fATTR cardiomyopathy [36]. Eight of the nine patients with mismatch between genetic testing and LC-MS/MS in the aforementioned study

(a) (b)

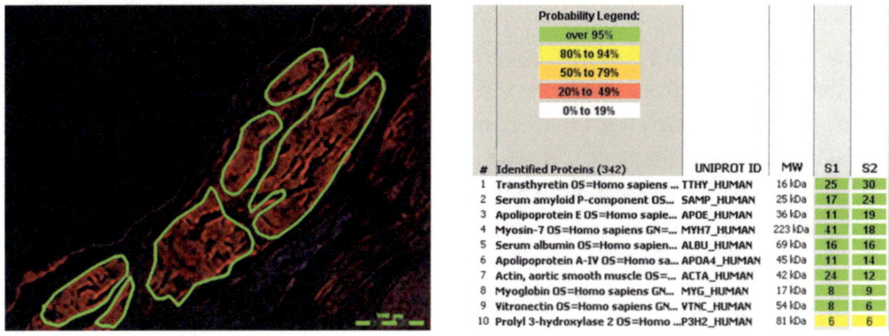

#	Identified Proteins (342)	UNIPROT ID	MW	S1	S2
1	Transthyretin OS=Homo sapiens ...	TTHY_HUMAN	16 kDa	25	30
2	Serum amyloid P-component OS...	SAMP_HUMAN	25 kDa	17	24
3	Apolipoprotein E OS=Homo sapie...	APOE_HUMAN	36 kDa	11	19
4	Myosin-7 OS=Homo sapiens GN=...	MYH7_HUMAN	223 kDa	41	18
5	Serum albumin OS=Homo sapien...	ALBU_HUMAN	69 kDa	16	16
6	Apolipoprotein A-IV OS=Homo sa...	APOA4_HUMAN	45 kDa	11	14
7	Actin, aortic smooth muscle OS=...	ACTA_HUMAN	42 kDa	24	12
8	Myoglobin OS=Homo sapiens GN...	MYG_HUMAN	17 kDa	8	9
9	Vitronectin OS=Homo sapiens GN...	VTNC_HUMAN	54 kDa	8	6
10	Prolyl 3-hydroxylase 2 OS=Homo ...	P3H2_HUMAN	81 kDa	6	6

Figure 2.
Laser microdissection of amyloid deposits and mass spectroscopy. (a) Congo red-stained section of the postmortem heart specimen viewed under fluorescent light source. Bright red areas represent amyloid deposits. Areas microdissected for mass spectrometry-based proteomic analysis are indicated by purple-colored lines. (b) The results of mass spectrometry-based proteomics analysis of amyloid plaques obtained by microdissection. The identified proteins are listed according to the relative abundance they were represented in two independent microdissections. The top 10 proteins are shown. The columns show the protein name, the UnitProt identifier (protein accession number in the UniProt database, http://www.uniprot.org/), the molecular weight of the protein (MW) and two microdissections (S1-S2). The numbers indicate number of total peptide spectra identified for each protein. The most abundant protein is TTR. Apolipoprotein E, serum amyloid P-component and apolipoprotein A-IV are constituents of many amyloid types. In contrast, the peptides representing TTR (The top hit) are only seen in ATTR amyloidosis [from [91] with permission].

were African Americans, two of whom were homozygote to Val122Ile mutation. Sensitivity of LC-MS/MS to pick up mutations is diminished in instances that mutation does not result in significant mass shift, or is located in regions of the gene with short tryptic peptides [34, 37]. Nuclear imaging studies, using bone avid tracers 99mTc-DPD (technetium-3,3-diphosphono-1,2-propanodicarboxylic acid), 99mTc-PYP (technetium-pyrophosphate) and 99mTc-HMDP (technetium-hydroxymethylene diphosphonate) have been increasingly used to diagnose ATTR related cardiomyopathy as they are widely available, have good sensitivity and are not costly [38, 39]. Demonstration of cardiac uptake using the aforementioned methods in a patient with neuropathy and heart disease strongly suggests ATTR if AL amyloidosis is excluded using serum and urine immunoelectrophoresis/immunofixation and assessment of serum free light chains [29].

3.2.2 Familial leptomeningeal and oculomeningeal amyloidosis

Leptomeningeal and meningovascular amyloidosis, often with concomitant vitreous opacity, are rare neurological manifestations of fATTR. Leptomeningeal amyloidosis has been reported with different TTR mutations (Val30Met, Val30Gly, Leu12Pro, Phe64Ser, Ala36Pro, Gly53Glu, Tyr69His, Ala25Thr, Tyr114Cys, Asp18Gly), sometimes in combination with FAP [40–47]. CNS symptoms include stroke, subarachnoid hemorrhage, dementia, hydrocephalus, ataxia, seizures, and sensorineural hearing loss. MRI studies may demonstrate leptomeningeal enhancement and superficial siderosis (sequela of intracranial bleedings) and there may be markedly elevated CSF protein [46, 48]. Ocular and meningovascular manifestations are specially common after liver transplantation, as the patient lives longer and mutant TTR is still being ecreted from the retinal cells and choroid plexus [49]. A previous study demonstrated that 27/87 (31%) of patients with Val30Met related FAP had focal neurological episodes, which occurred on average >14 years after the onset of FAP; more common after liver transplantation but also in patients with milder phenotypes which have a longer survival [47].

3.3 Treatment of familial ATTR

Disease modifying treatments have become available for FAP since 1990s, starting with liver transplantation (**Figure 3**). Treatment strategies include: (1), depleting the source of mutant TTR (liver transplantation); (2), inhibition of formation of TTR (wild type and mutant), by preventing translation of mRNA with antisense oligonucleotide (ASO) or with small interfering RNA (siRNA) technologies; (3), stabilization of TTR tetramere by small molecules (diflunisal and tafamidis); and (4), therapy directed to remove the amyloid deposits [19]. Currently approved disease modifying treatments by US food and drug administration (FDA) include inotersen and patisiran; with tafamidis approval under FDA review.

3.3.1 Liver transplantation

Removing the source of mutant TTR (liver) was the first disease modifying treatment for FAP. Liver transplantation, however, involves a major surgery, which is not tolerated with patients with significant underlying cardiovascular disease, and necessitates lifelong immunosuppression. Overall 5 year survival after liver transplantation is ~80% [50]. The 5 and 10 years survival rates post- transplantation were significantly better after Val30Met cases (82 and 74%) than the other mutations [50, 51]. Cardiomyopathy is a major determinant of prognosis with 10-year survival rates of 92 and 64% post-transplantation for patients without and with cardiomyopathy in a previous study [52]. Furthermore, liver transplant is more effective in changing the natural course of the disease in early onset Val30Met than the late onset cases, which could be due to more severe cardiomyopathy in the latter subtype [53]. Liver transplant is not an effective treatment for ATTRwt, leptomeningeal and ocular amyloidosis. Although ~90% of patients with early sensory neuropathy demonstrate disease stability after a liver transplant, organ involvement is not usually reversed, furthermore, FAP, and specially cardiomyopathy often deteriorate gradually post-transplant due to the deposition of ATTRwt [54, 55]. Advanced age and malnutrition are also risk factors for poor outcome/survival after liver transplantation [53, 56], partly because there is more predisposition to deposition of wild-type TTR in older age.

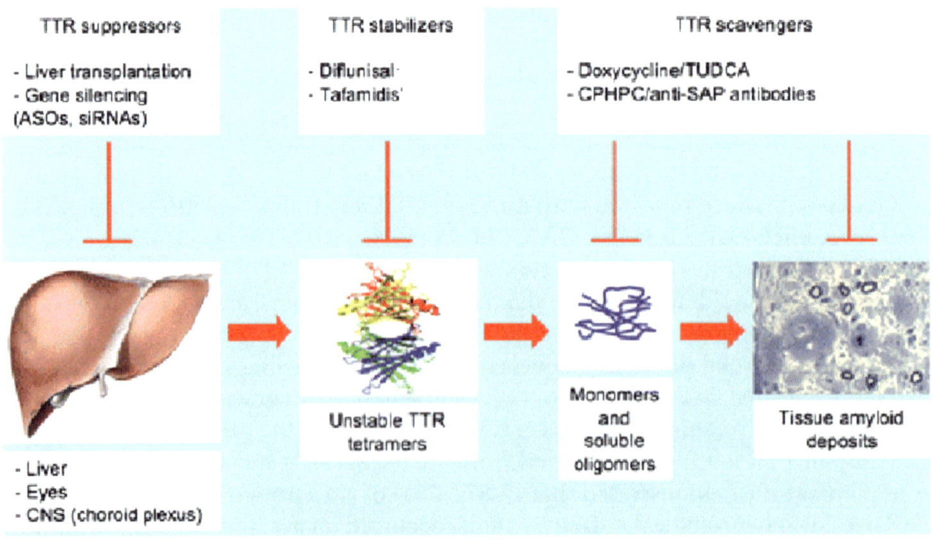

Figure 3.
Treatment strategies for fATTR (modified, from [92], with permission).

Combined liver-kidney or liver-heart, and rarely liver-heart-kidney transplantation has been used for FAP patients with advanced renal or heart disease [55].

3.3.2 Stabilizers of TTR tetramere

Nonsteroidal anti-inflammatory drugs (NSAIDs) and tafamidis meglumine inhibit TTR tetramere degradation and therefore formation of amyloidogenic monomers. NSAIDs have structural resemblance to thyroxine, a natural tetramere stabilizer. Diflunisal and tafamidis are disease modifying treatments for fATTR.

3.3.2.1 Diflunisal

In a randomized, double blinded, placebo controlled trial on 130 patients with FAP, diflunisal 250 mg twice a day was well tolerated and slowed the progression of neuropathy over a period of 2 years [57]. In that study, the Neuropathy Impairment +7 (NIS + 7) score increased by an average of 25.0 points in the placebo group versus 8.7 points in the diflunisal group (increase indicates deterioration of neuropathy). On the other hand, diflunisal also had a favorable effect on the quality of life; average of 36-Item Short-Form Health Survey (SF-36) physical scores decreased by 4.9 points in the placebo group and increased by 1.5 points in the diflunisal group. Modified body mass index (BMI), the product of serum albumin concentration (measured in grams per liter) and BMI (calculated as weight in kilograms divided by height in meters squared), which is an indicator of malnutrition and correlates with survival in FAP [58, 59], was the only endpoint which did not show improvement with diflunisal. In another study on 40 Japanese patients with fATTR, diflunisal was effective on neurological and cardiological manifestations after a period of 24 months, 3 patients could not tolerate diflunisal because of declining renal function or thrombocytopenia [60]. Diflunisal is inexpensive and widely available, but some of the potential problems associated with NSAIDs in general, such as gastrointestinal adverse effects including bleeding, limit its use, and caution is to be exercised in its use in the setting of underlying heart or kidney disease [61].

3.3.2.2 Tafamidis (Vyndaqel)

Tafamidis was the approved in European Union in 2011, for adult patients with early FAP regardless of the type of mutation [12]. It has since also been approved in Argentina, Japan and Mexico, for delaying the neurological disabilities of FAP [62]. Tafamidis binds selectively to the two normally unoccupied thyroxine-binding sites of the tetramer, and kinetically stabilizes TTR, including the less stable mutant TTR tetramers, preventing the tetramer dissociation, which is the rate-limiting step in the generation of amyloidogenic monomers [63] (**Figure 1**). In a previous study, 98% of the patients had TTR stabilization after 18 months of tafamidis [64]. Tafamidis is more effective in early onset Val30Met cases than late onset Val30Met and non-Val3 Met mutations, there was progression of disability score in 55% and deterioration of neuropathy score of most of patients with late-onset ATTR V30 M involved in a nonrandomized controlled trial [13]. In a double blinded multicenter study, tafamidis 20 mg per day, was compared to placebo in an 18-month study in adult patients with early-stage Val30Met TTR-FAP [64]. There were no statistically significant differences between tafamidis and placebo for the coprimary endpoints (changes of the Neuropathy Impairment Score-Lower Limb (NIS-LL) and Norfolk Quality-of- Life (QOL) Diabetic-Neuropathy Questionnaire) in the intent to treat population, which included patients who dropped out for liver transplantation. On the other hand, in the efficacy evaluable population, tafamidis patients had significantly better outcomes with the primary endpoints. Furthermore, tafamidis group had more favorable outcomes in the secondary endpoints which included changes in neurologic function, nutritional status, and TTR stabilization. Tafamidis is generally well tolerated including in long term, post-marketing, extension studies, with the majority of adverse effects of mild to moderate severity [64, 65].

3.3.3 Gene therapies

Inhibiting the transcription of TTR mRNA by gene silencing technologies such as antisense oligonucleotides (ASO) and small interfering RNAs (siRNA) constitute most promising approaches in the treatment of FAP. Inotersen and patisiran were approved by FDA in 2018.

3.3.3.1 Inotersen

Inotersen is a 2′-O-methoxyethyl-modified ASO, which selectively binds to the TTR complementary RNA and inhibits the liver synthesis of both wild-type and mutant TTR. In a double blinded 15 months study, NEURO-TTR, FAP patients in earlier neuropathy stages (ambulatory with or without assistance) received weekly subcutaneous injections of inotersen 300 mg after loading dose of 3 doses in the first week, versus placebo [66]. All of the patients also received daily Vitamin A supplementation 3000 IU. The serum TTR level in the inotersen group significantly dropped from its baseline with a median nadir of 79.0% from week 13 to 65. Inotersen recipients did significantly better in the primary endpoints: there was a difference in the least-square mean of 19.7 points in modified Neuropathy Impairment Score+7 (mNIS+7) and 11.7 points in Norfolk Quality of Life-Diabetic Neuropathy (QOL-DN), favoring inotersen group, after 66 weeks of treatment. Inotersen also slowed the weight loss with a statistical trend towards efficacy on decline of BMI. Improvement of the course of FAP and quality of life in the patients who received inotersen occurred regardless of the mutation type or the presence of cardiomyopathy. This study did not have sufficient power to assess efficacy of inotersen on cardiomyopathy. Significant side effects of inotersen included glomerulonephritis and thrombocytopenia. 23% of inotersen recipients developed a platelet count below 100×10^9/L, and three patients had platelet counts to $<25 \times 10^9$/L, one of whom died of brain hemorrhage. Antiplatelet antibodies were positive in all of the 3 patients with severe thrombocytopenia pointing to the immune mediated nature of this complication. As thrombocytopenia associated with ASO treatment can be severe and fatal, platelet counts should be closely monitored in patients who receive inotersen. Patients who developed nephropathy had a crescentic glomerulonephritis on the background of amyloidosis, kidney function in one patients improved after treatment with prednisone and cyclophosphamide; therefore, monitoring of kidney function and urine protein are also necessary during treatment with inotersen. As a matter of fact, there was no additional cases of severe thrombocytopenia, and only a single patient developed a mild glomerulonephritis after the implementation of enhanced monitoring in the NEURO-TTR study. Local skin reactions were generally mild and did not result in discontinuation of the treatment in any patient.

3.3.3.2 Patisiran

Patisiran is a siRNA oligonucleotide wrapped in nanoparticles for specialized delivery to the liver, where it targets the 3′ untranslated region of TTR's messenger RNA, resulting its cleavage, and therefore lack of transcription of TTR mRNA to a protein product. Treatment with patisiran therefore results in reduction in the production of both wild-type and mutant TTR. After preliminary studies showed dose dependent reduction of serum TTR in normal subjects and patients with FAP who received patisiran, and possible favorable effect on the course of neuropathy in a phase 2 study [67, 68], a recent phase 3 double blinded (APOLLO) study compared patisiran 0.3 mg/kg every 3 weeks intravenously to placebo in patients with FAP [69]. Patients who had undergone liver transplantation or those with advanced heart failure were excluded. Treatment with patisiran resulted in sustained reduction of serum TTR over a period of 18 months (median 81%, range – 38–95). Patisiran recipients did significantly did better in all primary endpoints: the least-squares mean mNIS+7 change from baseline was −6.0 in the patisiran versus + 28.0 in the placebo group (difference of 34.0 points favoring the patisiran group; $P < 0.001$) and the effect could be seen as early as 9 months; The least-squares mean change from baseline in Norfolk QOL-DN was −6.7 in patisiran versus 14.4 in the placebo group (difference, −21.1 points, $P < 0.001$); patisiran recipients also did better with the modified BMI and gait speed. Fifty one percent of patients who received patisiran versus 10% of those on placebo had improvement in the Norfolk QOL-DN score after 18 months. Treatment efficacy included patients with Val30Met as well as other mutations, and included sensory, motor and autonomic aspects of neuropathy. Patients in the patisiran group also had better cardiac outcomes, i.e. changes in NT-proBNP, left ventricular wall thickness and longitudinal stress, than those on placebo. The side effects that were more common in the patisiran than the placebo included infusion-related reactions (19%) and peripheral edema (30%). Infusion reactions (back pain, flushing, abdominal pain, and nausea) were mild to moderate and only one patient dropped from the study as their result. Thrombocytopenia and nephropathy were not among the patisiran related side effects in that study.

3.3.4 Other potential treatments

A combination of doxycycline, which is proposed to disrupt deposited fibrillar TTR amyloid fibrils [19, 55, 70] and tauroursodeoxycholic acid (a biliary acid, and also a disrupter of nonfibrillar TTR) has been effective in removal of amyloid deposits in a mouse model [71]. Another promising approach to resolve existing amyloid deposits is targeting serum amyloid P (SAP) component, which has an avid binding to all amyloid fibril types, resulting in stabilization of the amyloid fibrils and preventing their proteolysis [72]; antibodies to SAP have been promising in animal models of amyloidosis [73], and are being investigated in different forms of human amyloidosis.

4. Wild-type ATTR (ATTRwt), aka. senile systemic amyloidosis

Systemic Deposition of ATTRwt is a rather common process associated with aging. Previous studies have reported a prevalence of 12–25% for tissue deposition of ATTRwt in people older than 80 year old [74, 75]. Despite very common prevalence in postmortem and tissue studies, ATTRwt is not a very recognized entity among the community physicians and therefore it is rather underdiagnosed. Patients with ATTRwt typically present with cardiac manifestations, including congestive heart failure, atrial fibrillation and other arrhythmias. ATTRwt is increasingly diagnosed as a cause of heart failure with preserved ejection fraction (HFpEF) [76]. Embolic evens are frequently encountered, mean survival period from the onset of congestive heart failure symptoms is ~75 months [19]. There are differences between fATTR and ATTRwt in the pattern and shape of tissue amyloid deposition [74]. In fATTR deposits are predominantly localized in the pericardium and surrounding muscle fascicles, on the other hand, they have patchy plaque-like shapes and mostly appear inside the ventricular wall in ATTRwt cases. Differences also exist between the shape of deposited amyloid fibrils between fATTR and ATTRwt in electron microscopy: in fATTR, long, straight fibrils are arranged in parallel, whereas short, rigid fibrils with haphazard arrangement are noted in ATTRwt, with endocardial region more involved than epicardium [74]. ATTRwt also involves other organs, often subclinically. In the pathological study by Ueda, et al., amyloid deposits were noted in bladder in 5/6 cases; deposits in the thyroid, pancreas, liver, gallbladder, adrenal gland, and gastrointestinal tract were mainly located in the walls of small arteries [74].

4.1 Diagnosis of ATTRwt

It should be noted that significant amount of ATTRwt deposition, not a mere presence, is needed to establish a pathogenic role [77]. ATTRwt is most commonly diagnosed in the setting of a late onset cardiomyopathy. Tissue deposition of amyloid with Congo Red staining and subsequent immunohistochemical or proteomic analysis of the amyloid deposits along with a TTR gene sequencing (which does not show a pathogenic Mutation) are usually needed to diagnose ATTRwt. On the other hand, Technetium-labeled bone scintigraphy tracers are long to be known to be able to detect myocardial amyloid deposits, and use of this imaging modality for the diagnosis of cardiac ATTR amyloidosis has been increasingly. In a recent study on 857 patients with histologically proven cardiac amyloid (374 with endomyocardial biopsies) and 360 patients with nonamyloid cardiomyopathies, myocardial radiotracer uptake on bone scintigraphy was >99% sensitive and 86% specific for cardiac ATTR amyloid, with false positives exclusively due to cases with AL amyloidosis [29]. Therefore cardiac ATTR can be diagnosed without a tissue biopsy and exclusion of AL amyloidosis based on serum and urine immunofixation and free lambda and kappa levels. Similar to the situation with fATTR, high prevalence of MGUS in ATTRwt poses a diagnostic challenge. About one fourth to 50% of patients with ATTRwt have a monoclonal gammopathy in the serum or urine and ~10% have a high serum kappa/lambda ratio [30, 78, 79]. It should be noted that abdominal fat pad aspiration and biopsy have a low sensitivity for ATTRwt, 12–14% on some of the previous studies [80, 81], although using abdominal fat pad biopsy, sensitivity of 73% has also been reported in another study [82].

4.2 Neurological manifestations of ATTRwt

ATTRwt is generally not associated with a polyneuropathy. A previous report suggested ATTRwt as a cause of a rapidly progressive neuropathy in an elderly woman; amyloid deposits were present in the gastrocnemius, but not the sural nerve of that patient [83]. On the other hand, ATTRwt is rather commonly associated with late onset musculoskeletal problems, particularly carpal tunnel syndrome and lumbar spinal stenosis, but overall it is underdiagnosed. ATTRwt deposits have been demonstrated in about one third of tenosynovial tissues obtained during carpal tunnel release operation in elderly patients [84, 85], as well as in 30–45% of the resected tissues harvested during decompression surgeries for lumbar spinal stenosis [77, 86].

The ATTRwt deposits are frequently minimal and may not be important from the pathogenesis standpoint [77]. On the other hand, more prominent amyloid deposition may play a role in spinal stenosis as they cause increased thickness of ligamentum flavum or abnormal spinal stability [86]. Examination of tenosynovial tissue on 100 patients with idiopathic CTS showed positive Congo Red staining on 34 patients, all also positively staining with anti TTR antibody with negative gene sequencing, consistent with ATTRwt [84]. On the other hand, in a single center study involving 31 ATTRwt patients, CTS was the most common presenting symptom in more than 50% of the patients [87]. In another recent prospective study on 98 patients with idiopathic CTS in men >60 year and women >50, who underwent decompressive surgery, amyloid deposits were found in 10 patients, 5 of which turned out to be due to ATTRwt [88]. Spinal cord compression secondary to ATTRwt has also been rarely reported [89, 90]. Myopathy is rarely reported as a feature of ATTRwt, but in the author's opinion it is underdiagnosed. We previously reported a patient who presented with bent spine syndrome due to ATTRwt related myopathy affecting the thoracic paraspinal muscles [91]. That patient succumbed as the result of consequences of cardiomyopathy and a cardioembolic stroke.

4.3 Treatment of ATTRwt

Although TTR stabilizers and suppressors of gene expression will likely suppress ATTRwt deposition, there are no current FDA approved disease modifying therapies for ATTRwt and the management remains to be symptomatic, such as medical treatment of heart failure and arrhythmias, including insertion of defibrillator/pacemaker, and heart transplantation if necessary. Treatment of neuromuscular complications remains to be symptomatic as well, i.e. decompression surgeries of myelopathy and lumbar spinal stenosis and carpal tunnel syndrome release. The reasons for lack of disease modifying treatments include the fact that ATTRwt is underdiagnosed and the natural history of its neuromuscular complications is unknown. Furthermore, ATTRwt is a disease of older population and neuromuscular complications are likely overshadowed by other medical comorbidities specially heart disease [78], and therefore the effect of disease modifying treatments would be difficult to assess.

5. Conclusions

Familial amyloid polyneuropathy is a rare, but treatable cause of neuropathy, diagnosis in an early stage is essential to establish disease modifying treatment at a stage which the disability can be prevented from progression or potentially reversed. Diagnosis should be suspected when red-flag symptomatology is present in a patient with neuropathy; and can possibly be established by sequencing of transthyretin gene. Musculoskeletal disease such as carpal tunnel syndrome and spinal stenosis are early manifestations and underdiagnosed causes of wild-type transthyretin amyloidosis. Increased cardiac uptake on nuclear imaging studies is a sensitive, widely available diagnostic modality for early diagnosis of familial and wild-type transthyretin amyloidosis.

Conflict of interest

Dr. Rezania has received funding from Amyotrophic Lateral Sclerosis Association (ALSA) and National Institute of Neurological Disorders and Stroke; has served on the advisory boards of Alnylam, Alexion and MT Pharma; has received honoraria for giving speeches from Alexion, MT Pharma Tanabe, Kabafusion, Option Care, Sanofi-Genzyme, and American Association of Neuromuscular and Electrodiagnostic Medicine; has received loyalties from Medlink.

Acronyms and abbreviations

TTR	transthyretin
ATTR	transthyretin related amyloidosis
fATTR	familial transthyretin related amyloidosis
ATTRwt	wild-type transthyretin related amyloidosis
CIDP	chronic inflammatory demyelinating polyneuropathy
FAP	familial amyloid polyneuropathy

Author details

Kourosh Rezania[1*] and Laleh Saadat[2]

1 Department of Neurology, University of Chicago Medical Center, Chicago, IL, USA

2 Department of Surgery, University of Chicago Medical Center, Chicago, IL, USA

*Address all correspondence to: krezania@neurology.bsd.uchicago.edu

References

[1] Lachmann HJ, Hawkins PN. Systemic amyloidosis. Current Opinion in Pharmacology. 2006;**6**(2):214-220

[2] Sipe JD, Benson MD, Buxbaum JN, Ikeda SI, Merlini G, Saraiva MJ, et al. Amyloid fibril proteins and amyloidosis: Chemical identification and clinical classification International Society of Amyloidosis 2016 Nomenclature Guidelines. Amyloid. 2016;**23**(4):209-213

[3] Wechalekar AD, Gillmore JD, Hawkins PN. Systemic amyloidosis. Lancet. 2016;**387**(10038):2641-2654

[4] Wallace MR, Naylor SL, Kluve-Beckerman B, Long GL, McDonald L, Shows TB, et al. Localization of the human prealbumin gene to chromosome 18. Biochemical and Biophysical Research Communications. 1985;**129**(3):753-758

[5] Episkopou V, Maeda S, Nishiguchi S, Shimada K, Gaitanaris GA, Gottesman ME, et al. Disruption of the transthyretin gene results in mice with depressed levels of plasma retinol and thyroid hormone. Proceedings of the National Academy of Sciences of the United States of America. 1993;**90**(6):2375-2379

[6] Palha JA. Transthyretin as a thyroid hormone carrier: Function revisited. Clinical Chemistry and Laboratory Medicine. 2002;**40**(12):1292-1300

[7] Suhr OB, Lundgren E, Westermark P. One mutation, two distinct disease variants: Unravelling the impact of transthyretin amyloid fibril composition. Journal of Internal Medicine. 2017;**281**(4):337-347

[8] Fandrich M, Nystrom S, Nilsson KPR, Bockmann A, LeVine H, 3rd, Hammarstrom P. Amyloid fibril polymorphism: A challenge for molecular imaging and therapy. Journal of Internal Medicine. 2018;**283**(3):218-237

[9] Plante-Bordeneuve V, Ferreira A, Lalu T, Zaros C, Lacroix C, Adams D, et al. Diagnostic pitfalls in sporadic transthyretin familial amyloid polyneuropathy (TTR-FAP). Neurology. 2007;**69**(7):693-698

[10] Sekijima Y, Ueda M, Koike H, Misawa S, Ishii T, Ando Y. Diagnosis and management of transthyretin familial amyloid polyneuropathy in Japan: Red-flag symptom clusters and treatment algorithm. Orphanet Journal of Rare Diseases. 2018;**13**(1):6

[11] Schmidt HH, Waddington-Cruz M, Botteman MF, Carter JA, Chopra AS, Hopps M, et al. Estimating the global prevalence of transthyretin familial amyloid polyneuropathy. Muscle & Nerve. 2018;**57**(5):829-837

[12] Ando Y, Coelho T, Berk JL, Cruz MW, Ericzon BG, Ikeda S, et al. Guideline of transthyretin-related hereditary amyloidosis for clinicians. Orphanet Journal of Rare Diseases. 2013;**8**:31

[13] Adams D, Theaudin M, Cauquil C, Algalarrondo V, Slama M. FAP neuropathy and emerging treatments. Current Neurology and Neuroscience Reports. 2014;**14**(3):435

[14] Holmgren G, Costa PM, Andersson C, Asplund K, Steen L, Beckman L, et al. Geographical distribution of TTR met30 carriers in northern Sweden: Discrepancy between carrier frequency and prevalence rate. Journal of Medical Genetics. 1994;**31**(5):351-354

[15] Sousa A, Coelho T, Barros J, Sequeiros J. Genetic epidemiology of familial amyloidotic polyneuropathy (FAP)-type I in Povoa do Varzim and

Vila do Conde (north of Portugal). American Journal of Medical Genetics. 1995;**60**(6):512-521

[16] Jacobson DR, Alexander AA, Tagoe C, Buxbaum JN. Prevalence of the amyloidogenic transthyretin (TTR) V122I allele in 14 333 African-Americans. Amyloid. 2015;**22**(3):171-174

[17] Carr AS, Pelayo-Negro AL, Evans MR, Laura M, Blake J, Stancanelli C, et al. A study of the neuropathy associated with transthyretin amyloidosis (ATTR) in the UK. Journal of Neurology, Neurosurgery, and Psychiatry. 2016;**87**(6):620-627

[18] Plante-Bordeneuve V, Lalu T, Misrahi M, Reilly MM, Adams D, Lacroix C, et al. Genotypic-phenotypic variations in a series of 65 patients with familial amyloid polyneuropathy. Neurology. 1998;**51**(3):708-714

[19] Sekijima Y. Transthyretin (ATTR) amyloidosis: Clinical spectrum, molecular pathogenesis and disease-modifying treatments. Journal of Neurology, Neurosurgery, and Psychiatry. 2015;**86**(9):1036-1043

[20] Koike H, Misu K, Ikeda S, Ando Y, Nakazato M, Ando E, et al. Type I (transthyretin Met30) familial amyloid polyneuropathy in Japan: Early- vs late-onset form. Archives of Neurology. 2002;**59**(11):1771-1776

[21] Koike H, Tanaka F, Hashimoto R, Tomita M, Kawagashira Y, Iijima M, et al. Natural history of transthyretin Val30Met familial amyloid polyneuropathy: Analysis of late-onset cases from non-endemic areas. Journal of Neurology, Neurosurgery, and Psychiatry. 2012;**83**(2):152-158

[22] Cappellari M, Cavallaro T, Ferrarini M, Cabrini I, Taioli F, Ferrari S, et al. Variable presentations of TTR-related familial amyloid polyneuropathy in seventeen patients. Journal of the Peripheral Nervous System. 2011;**16**(2):119-129

[23] Mathis S, Magy L, Diallo L, Boukhris S, Vallat JM. Amyloid neuropathy mimicking chronic inflammatory demyelinating polyneuropathy. Muscle & Nerve. 2012;**45**(1):26-31

[24] Buxbaum JN, Ruberg FL. Transthyretin V122I (pV142I)* cardiac amyloidosis: An age-dependent autosomal dominant cardiomyopathy too common to be overlooked as a cause of significant heart disease in elderly African Americans. Genetics in Medicine. 2017;**19**(7):733-742

[25] Quarta CC, Buxbaum JN, Shah AM, Falk RH, Claggett B, Kitzman DW, et al. The amyloidogenic V122I transthyretin variant in elderly black Americans. The New England Journal of Medicine. 2015;**372**(1):21-29

[26] Carr AS, Pelayo-Negro AL, Jaunmuktane Z, Scalco RS, Hutt D, Evans MR, et al. Transthyretin V122I amyloidosis with clinical and histological evidence of amyloid neuropathy and myopathy. Neuromuscular Disorders. 2015;**25**(6):511-515

[27] Wang AK, Fealey RD, Gehrking TL, Low PA. Patterns of neuropathy and autonomic failure in patients with amyloidosis. Mayo Clinic Proceedings. 2008;**83**(11):1226-1230

[28] Conceicao I, Gonzalez-Duarte A, Obici L, Schmidt HH, Simoneau D, Ong ML, et al. "Red-flag" symptom clusters in transthyretin familial amyloid polyneuropathy. Journal of the Peripheral Nervous System. 2016;**21**(1):5-9

[29] Gillmore JD, Maurer MS, Falk RH, Merlini G, Damy T, Dispenzieri A, et al. Nonbiopsy diagnosis of cardiac

transthyretin amyloidosis. Circulation. 2016;**133**(24):2404-2412

[30] Phull P, Sanchorawala V, Connors LH, Doros G, Ruberg FL, Berk JL, et al. Monoclonal gammopathy of undetermined significance in systemic transthyretin amyloidosis (ATTR). Amyloid. 2018;**25**(1):62-67

[31] Halushka MK, Eng G, Collins AB, Judge DP, Semigran MJ, Stone JR. Optimization of serum immunoglobulin free light Chain analysis for subclassification of cardiac amyloidosis. Journal of Cardiovascular Translational Research. 2015;**8**(4):264-268

[32] Gilbertson JA, Theis JD, Vrana JA, Lachmann H, Wechalekar A, Whelan C, et al. A comparison of immunohistochemistry and mass spectrometry for determining the amyloid fibril protein from formalin-fixed biopsy tissue. Journal of Clinical Pathology. 2015;**68**(4):314-317

[33] Vrana JA, Gamez JD, Madden BJ, Theis JD, Bergen HR, 3rd, Dogan A. Classification of amyloidosis by laser microdissection and mass spectrometry-based proteomic analysis in clinical biopsy specimens. Blood. 2009;**114**(24):4957-4959

[34] Dasari S, Theis JD, Vrana JA, Zenka RM, Zimmermann MT, Kocher JP, et al. Clinical proteome informatics workbench detects pathogenic mutations in hereditary amyloidoses. Journal of Proteome Research. 2014;**13**(5):2352-2358

[35] Klein CJ, Vrana JA, Theis JD, Dyck PJ, Dyck PJ, Spinner RJ, et al. Mass spectrometric-based proteomic analysis of amyloid neuropathy type in nerve tissue. Archives of Neurology. 2011;**68**(2):195-199

[36] Brown EE, Lee YZJ, Halushka MK, Steenbergen C, Johnson NM, Almansa J, et al. Genetic testing improves identification of transthyretin amyloid (ATTR) subtype in cardiac amyloidosis. Amyloid. 2017;**24**(2):92-95

[37] Vrana JA, Theis JD, Dasari S, Mereuta OM, Dispenzieri A, Zeldenrust SR, et al. Clinical diagnosis and typing of systemic amyloidosis in subcutaneous fat aspirates by mass spectrometry-based proteomics. Haematologica. 2014;**99**(7):1239-1247

[38] Rapezzi C, Quarta CC, Guidalotti PL, Pettinato C, Fanti S, Leone O, et al. Role of (99m)Tc-DPD scintigraphy in diagnosis and prognosis of hereditary transthyretin-related cardiac amyloidosis. JACC: Cardiovascular Imaging. 2011;**4**(6):659-670

[39] Bokhari S, Castano A, Pozniakoff T, Deslisle S, Latif F, Maurer MS. (99m) Tc-pyrophosphate scintigraphy for differentiating light-chain cardiac amyloidosis from the transthyretin-related familial and senile cardiac amyloidoses. Circulation. Cardiovascular Imaging. 2013;**6**(2):195-201

[40] Herrick MK, DeBruyne K, Horoupian DS, Skare J, Vanefsky MA, Ong T. Massive leptomeningeal amyloidosis associated with a Val30Met transthyretin gene. Neurology. 1996;**47**(4):988-992

[41] Garzuly F, Vidal R, Wisniewski T, Brittig F, Budka H. Familial meningocerebrovascular amyloidosis, Hungarian type, with mutant transthyretin (TTR Asp18Gly). Neurology. 1996;**47**(6):1562-1567

[42] Petersen RB, Goren H, Cohen M, Richardson SL, Tresser N, Lynn A, et al. Transthyretin amyloidosis: A new mutation associated with dementia. Annals of Neurology. 1997;**41**(3):307-313

[43] Uemichi T, Uitti RJ, Koeppen AH, Donat JR, Benson

MD. Oculoleptomeningeal amyloidosis associated with a new transthyretin variant Ser64. Archives of Neurology. 1999;**56**(9):1152-1155

[44] Mascalchi M, Salvi F, Pirini MG, D'Errico A, Ferlini A, Lolli F, et al. Transthyretin amyloidosis and superficial siderosis of the CNS. Neurology. 1999;**53**(7):1498-1503

[45] Ellie E, Camou F, Vital A, Rummens C, Grateau G, Delpech M, et al. Recurrent subarachnoid hemorrhage associated with a new transthyretin variant (Gly53Glu). Neurology. 2001;**57**(1):135-137

[46] Jin K, Sato S, Takahashi T, Nakazaki H, Date Y, Nakazato M, et al. Familial leptomeningeal amyloidosis with a transthyretin variant Asp18Gly representing repeated subarachnoid haemorrhages with superficial siderosis. Journal of Neurology, Neurosurgery, and Psychiatry. 2004;**75**(10):1463-1466

[47] Maia LF, Magalhaes R, Freitas J, Taipa R, Pires MM, Osorio H, et al. CNS involvement in V30M transthyretin amyloidosis: Clinical, neuropathological and biochemical findings. Journal of Neurology, Neurosurgery, and Psychiatry. 2015;**86**(2):159-167

[48] Horowitz S, Thomas C, Gruener G, Nand S, Shea JF. MR of leptomeningeal spinal and posterior fossa amyloid. AJNR. American Journal of Neuroradiology. 1998;**19**(5):900-902

[49] Sekijima Y. Transthyretin-type cerebral amyloid angiopathy: A serious complication in post-transplant patients with familial amyloid polyneuropathy. Journal of Neurology, Neurosurgery, and Psychiatry. 2015;**86**(2):124

[50] Wilczek HE, Larsson M, Ericzon BG, FAPWTR. Long-term data from the Familial Amyloidotic Polyneuropathy World Transplant Registry (FAPWTR). Amyloid. 2011;**18**(Suppl 1):193-195

[51] Herlenius G, Wilczek HE, Larsson M, Ericzon BG. Familial Amyloidotic Polyneuropathy World Transplant R. Ten years of international experience with liver transplantation for familial amyloidotic polyneuropathy: Results from the Familial Amyloidotic Polyneuropathy World Transplant Registry. Transplantation. 2004;**77**(1):64-71

[52] Okamoto S, Wixner J, Ericzon BG, Friman S, Lindqvist P, Henein M, et al. Prognostic value of pre-transplant cardiomyopathy in Swedish liver transplanted patients for familial amyloidotic polyneuropathy. Amyloid. 2011;**18**(Suppl 1):171-173

[53] Okamoto S, Wixner J, Obayashi K, Ando Y, Ericzon BG, Friman S, et al. Liver transplantation for familial amyloidotic polyneuropathy: Impact on Swedish patients' survival. Liver Transplantation. 2009;**15**(10):1229-1235

[54] Yazaki M, Tokuda T, Nakamura A, Higashikata T, Koyama J, Higuchi K, et al. Cardiac amyloid in patients with familial amyloid polyneuropathy consists of abundant wild-type transthyretin. Biochemical and Biophysical Research Communications. 2000;**274**(3):702-706

[55] Carvalho A, Rocha A, Lobato L. Liver transplantation in transthyretin amyloidosis: Issues and challenges. Liver Transplantation. 2015;**21**(3):282-292

[56] Suhr OB, Ericzon BG, Friman S. Long-term follow-up of survival of liver transplant recipients with familial amyloid polyneuropathy (Portuguese type). Liver Transplantation. 2002;**8**(9):787-794

[57] Berk JL, Suhr OB, Obici L, Sekijima Y, Zeldenrust SR, Yamashita T, et al. Repurposing diflunisal for familial amyloid polyneuropathy: A randomized clinical trial. Journal of the American Medical Association. 2013;**310**(24):2658-2667

[58] Suhr O, Danielsson A, Holmgren G, Steen L. Malnutrition and gastrointestinal dysfunction as prognostic factors for survival in familial amyloidotic polyneuropathy. Journal of Internal Medicine. 1994;**235**(5):479-485

[59] Suhr OB, Holmgren G, Steen L, Wikstrom L, Norden G, Friman S, et al. Liver transplantation in familial amyloidotic polyneuropathy. Follow-up of the first 20 Swedish patients. Transplantation. 1995;**60**(9):933-938

[60] Sekijima Y, Tojo K, Morita H, Koyama J, Ikeda S. Safety and efficacy of long-term diflunisal administration in hereditary transthyretin (ATTR) amyloidosis. Amyloid. 2015;**22**(2):79-83

[61] Harirforoosh S, Asghar W, Jamali F. Adverse effects of nonsteroidal antiinflammatory drugs: An update of gastrointestinal, cardiovascular and renal complications. Journal of Pharmacy & Pharmaceutical Sciences. 2013;**16**(5):821-847

[62] Scott LJ. Tafamidis: A review of its use in familial amyloid polyneuropathy. Drugs. 2014;**74**(12):1371-1378

[63] Bulawa CE, Connelly S, Devit M, Wang L, Weigel C, Fleming JA, et al. Tafamidis, a potent and selective transthyretin kinetic stabilizer that inhibits the amyloid cascade. Proceedings of the National Academy of Sciences of the United States of America. 2012;**109**(24):9629-9634

[64] Coelho T, Maia LF, Martins da Silva A, Waddington Cruz M, Plante-Bordeneuve V, Lozeron P, et al. Tafamidis for transthyretin familial amyloid polyneuropathy: A randomized, controlled trial. Neurology. 2012;**79**(8):785-792

[65] Coelho T, Maia LF, da Silva AM, Cruz MW, Plante-Bordeneuve V, Suhr OB, et al. Long-term effects of tafamidis for the treatment of transthyretin familial amyloid polyneuropathy. Journal of Neurology. 2013;**260**(11):2802-2814

[66] Benson MD, Waddington-Cruz M, Berk JL, Polydefkis M, Dyck PJ, Wang AK, et al. Inotersen Treatment for Patients with Hereditary Transthyretin Amyloidosis. The New England Journal of Medicine. 2018;**379**(1):22-31

[67] Coelho T, Adams D, Silva A, Lozeron P, Hawkins PN, Mant T, et al. Safety and efficacy of RNAi therapy for transthyretin amyloidosis. The New England Journal of Medicine. 2013;**369**(9):819-829

[68] Suhr OB, Coelho T, Buades J, Pouget J, Conceicao I, Berk J, et al. Efficacy and safety of patisiran for familial amyloidotic polyneuropathy: A phase II multi-dose study. Orphanet Journal of Rare Diseases. 2015;**10**:109

[69] Adams D, Gonzalez-Duarte A, O'Riordan WD, Yang CC, Ueda M, Kristen AV, et al. Patisiran, an RNAi Therapeutic, for Hereditary Transthyretin Amyloidosis. The New England Journal of Medicine. 2018;**379**(1):11-21

[70] Cardoso I, Saraiva MJ. Doxycycline disrupts transthyretin amyloid: Evidence from studies in a FAP transgenic mice model. The FASEB Journal. 2006;**20**(2):234-239

[71] Cardoso I, Martins D, Ribeiro T, Merlini G, Saraiva MJ. Synergy of combined doxycycline/TUDCA treatment in lowering Transthyretin deposition and associated biomarkers: Studies in FAP mouse models. Journal of Translational Medicine. 2010;**8**:74

[72] Pepys MB, Dyck RF, de Beer FC, Skinner M, Cohen AS. Binding of serum amyloid P-component (SAP) by amyloid fibrils. Clinical and Experimental Immunology. 1979;**38**(2):284-293

[73] Bodin K, Ellmerich S, Kahan MC, Tennent GA, Loesch A, Gilbertson JA, et al. Antibodies to human serum amyloid P component eliminate visceral amyloid deposits. Nature. 2010;**468**(7320):93-97

[74] Ueda M, Horibata Y, Shono M, Misumi Y, Oshima T, Su Y, et al. Clinicopathological features of senile systemic amyloidosis: An ante- and post-mortem study. Modern Pathology. 2011;**24**(12):1533-1544

[75] Tanskanen M, Peuralinna T, Polvikoski T, Notkola IL, Sulkava R, Hardy J, et al. Senile systemic amyloidosis affects 25% of the very aged and associates with genetic variation in alpha2-macroglobulin and tau: A population-based autopsy study. Annals of Medicine. 2008;**40**(3):232-239

[76] Ton VK, Bhonsale A, Gilotra NA, Halushka MK, Steenbergen C, Almansa J, et al. Baseline characteristics predict the presence of amyloid on endomyocardial biopsy. Journal of Cardiac Failure. 2017;**23**(4):340-344

[77] Westermark P, Westermark GT, Suhr OB, Berg S. Transthyretin-derived amyloidosis: Probably a common cause of lumbar spinal stenosis. Upsala Journal of Medical Sciences. 2014;**119**(3):223-228

[78] Pinney JH, Whelan CJ, Petrie A, Dungu J, Banypersad SM, Sattianayagam P, et al. Senile systemic amyloidosis: Clinical features at presentation and outcome. Journal of the American Heart Association. 2013;**2**(2):e000098

[79] Geller HI, Singh A, Mirto TM, Padera R, Mitchell R, Laubach JP, et al. Prevalence of monoclonal gammopathy in wild-type transthyretin amyloidosis. Mayo Clinic Proceedings. 2017;**92**(12):1800-1805

[80] Fine NM, Arruda-Olson AM, Dispenzieri A, Zeldenrust SR, Gertz MA, Kyle RA, et al. Yield of noncardiac biopsy for the diagnosis of transthyretin cardiac amyloidosis. The American Journal of Cardiology. 2014;**113**(10):1723-1727

[81] Garcia Y, Collins AB, Stone JR. Abdominal fat pad excisional biopsy for the diagnosis and typing of systemic amyloidosis. Human Pathology. 2018;**72**:71-79

[82] Ikeda S, Sekijima Y, Tojo K, Koyama J. Diagnostic value of abdominal wall fat pad biopsy in senile systemic amyloidosis. Amyloid. 2011;**18**(4):211-215

[83] Lam L, Margeta M, Layzer R. Amyloid polyneuropathy caused by wild-type transthyretin. Muscle & Nerve. 2015;**52**(1):146-149

[84] Sekijima Y, Uchiyama S, Tojo K, Sano K, Shimizu Y, Imaeda T, et al. High prevalence of wild-type transthyretin deposition in patients with idiopathic carpal tunnel syndrome: A common cause of carpal tunnel syndrome in the elderly. Human Pathology. 2011;**42**(11):1785-1791

[85] Gioeva Z, Urban P, Meliss RR, Haag J, Axmann HD, Siebert F, et al. ATTR amyloid in the carpal tunnel ligament is frequently of wildtype transthyretin origin. Amyloid. 2013;**20**(1):1-6

[86] Yanagisawa A, Ueda M, Sueyoshi T, Okada T, Fujimoto T, Ogi Y, et al. Amyloid deposits derived from transthyretin in the ligamentum flavum as related to lumbar spinal canal stenosis. Modern Pathology. 2015;**28**(2):201-207

[87] Nakagawa M, Sekijima Y, Yazaki M, Tojo K, Yoshinaga T, Doden T, et al. Carpal tunnel syndrome: A common initial symptom of systemic wild-type ATTR (ATTRwt) amyloidosis. Amyloid. 2016;**23**(1):58-63

[88] Sperry BW, Reyes BA, Ikram A, Donnelly JP, Phelan D, Jaber WA, et al. Tenosynovial and cardiac amyloidosis in patients undergoing carpal tunnel release. Journal of the American College of Cardiology. 2018;**72**(17):2040-2050

[89] Sueyoshi T, Ueda M, Sei A, Misumi Y, Oshima T, Yamashita T, et al. Spinal multifocal amyloidosis derived from wild-type transthyretin. Amyloid. 2011;**18**(3):165-168

[90] Rezania K, Pytel P, Highsmith WE, Gabikian P. Cervicomedullary compression as the main manifestation of wild-type transthyretin amyloidosis. Amyloid. 2017;**24**(2):133-134

[91] Rezania K, Pytel P, Smit LJ, Mastrianni J, Dina MA, Highsmith WE, et al. Systemic transthyretin amyloidosis in a patient with bent spine syndrome. Amyloid. 2013;**20**(2):131-134

[92] Kerschen P, Plante-Bordeneuve V. Current and future treatment approaches in transthyretin familial amyloid polyneuropathy. Current Treatment Options in Neurology. 2016;**18**(12):53

Chapter 7

Serum Amyloid A and Immunomodulation

Yu Fan, Chi Teng Vong and Richard D. Ye

Abstract

Serum amyloid A1 (SAA1), a major isoform of acute-phase SAA, is a well-known precursor of amyloid A (AA) that contributes to secondary amyloidosis with its tissue deposition. Acute-phase SAA is also a biomarker of inflammation. Recent studies have focused on the roles for acute-phase SAA in the regulation of immunity and inflammation. *In vitro* characterization of recombinant human SAA identified its chemotactic and cytokine-like properties, whereas the use of SAA isoform-specific transgenic and knockout mice has led to the discovery of new functions of SAA proteins in host defense and tissue homeostasis. Characterization of SAA-derived peptides has shown that fragments of SAA, generated through proteolysis, are bioactive and may contribute to a growing list of functions related to inflammation. This chapter summarizes recent progress in the studies of acute-phase SAA and its fragments in inflammation and immunomodulation.

Keywords: SAA, inflammation, immunity

1. Introduction

Serum amyloid A (SAA) was identified in early studies as the precursor of amyloid A (AA), the tissue deposit of which causes secondary amyloidosis [1–4]. SAA was also found as one of the major acute-phase proteins that are produced in large quantities by hepatocytes and released to blood circulation in response to trauma, infection, late-stage malignancy and severe stress [5, 6]. Extending from these early findings, increased levels of SAA were found both in plasma and in injured and inflammatory tissues. A large body of literature reports SAA as a biomarker in a variety of diseases ranging from acute inflammation, chronic inflammation, type-2 diabetes, malignancy and postsurgical complications [7–9]. However, the biological functions of SAA remained largely unknown for many years [10] despite efforts in it biochemical characterization, gene cloning of its isoforms, studies of the interactions between SAA and high-density lipoprotein (HDL), and delineation of its regulatory activities in inflammation and immunity. The widespread use of recombinant human SAA proteins has accelerated the characterization of the biological functions of SAA *in vitro*, but at the same time produced data that are not fully compatible with those obtained from *in vivo* studies. In the past decade, mice with genetically altered genes were prepared and their use in a number of diseases models has begun to delineate the pathophysiological functions of SAA *in vivo*. This chapter provides an overview of the studies of SAA that have been published and summarizes recent findings of the immunomodulatory functions of different SAA proteins. For other functions of SAA, the interested reader is referred to several excellent reviews that have been published recently [9, 11–15].

2. SAA and its role in amyloidosis

SAA is the general name of a family of proteins with high sequence homology but encoded by distinct genes [16]. Both humans and mice have 4 SAA genes, but in human the *SAA3* is a pseudogene that does not express [17]. SAA4 is constitutively expressed in both humans and mice. In contrast, the expression of SAA1, SAA2 and in mice, SAA3, is highly inducible [18]. These SAA proteins are therefore termed acute-phase SAAs based on their induced expression during the acute-phase response [18, 19]. The human SAA genes are located on chromosome 11 while the mouse SAA genes are found in a cluster on chromosome 7 [20, 21].

At the primary sequence level, the human and mouse SAA proteins share high sequence homology (**Figure 1**), suggesting that these proteins may have similar functions although their modes of expression vary. Of note, although mouse SAA3 has an expression profile different from that of SAA1 and SAA2, its sequence is as homologous to human SAA1 as mouse SAA1 and SAA2 (**Figure 1**). The sequence homology suggests that the functions of SAA3, expressed upon induction by inflammatory cues in various mouse tissues, may be similar to those of human SAA1 and SAA2.

Human SAA1 has been widely studied for its functions. SAA1 was first identified as a serum component recognized by antibodies raised against the amyloid fibril protein known as amyloid A (AA). In one of the studies, antisera were prepared against the major nonimmunoglobulin component of secondary amyloidosis. The antisera were able to detect a serum component that was present at much higher levels in more than half of the pathological samples collected from

```
                10         20         30         40         50
hSAA1   RSFFSFLGEA FDGARDMWRA YSDMREANYI GSDKYFHARG NYDAAKRGPG
hSAA2   RSFFSFLGEA FDGARDMWRA YSDMREANYI GSDKYFHARG NYDAAKRGPG
mSAA1   -GFFSFIGEA FQGAGDMWRA YTDMKEAGWK DGDKYFHARG NYDAAQRGPG
mSAA2   -GFFSFVHEA FQGAGDMWRA YTDMKEANWK NSDKYFHARG NYDAAQRGPG
mSAA3   -RWVQFMKEA GQGSRDMWRA YSDMKKANWK NSDKYFHARG NYDAARRGPG
             *  **   *  ***** * **  *      ******** ***** ****

                60         70         80
hSAA1   GAWAAEVISD ARENIQRFFG HGAEDSLADQ
hSAA2   GAWAAEVISN ARENIQRLTG RGAEDSLADQ
mSAA1   GVWAAEKISD ARESFQEFFG RGHEDTMADQ
mSAA2   GVWAAEKISD GREAFQEFFG RGHEDTIADQ
mSAA3   GAWAAKVISD AREAVQKFTG HGAEDSRADQ
        * ***  **   **  *   *  * **  ***

                90        100
hSAA1   AANEWGRSGK DPNHFRPAGL PEKY
hSAA2   AANKWGRSGR DPNHFRPAGL PEKY
mSAA1   EANRHGRSGK DPNYYRPPGL PAKY
mSAA2   EANRHGRSGK DPNYYRPPGL PDKY
mSAA3   FANEWGRSGK DPNHFRPAGL PARY
         **  ****  ***  ** ** *  *
```

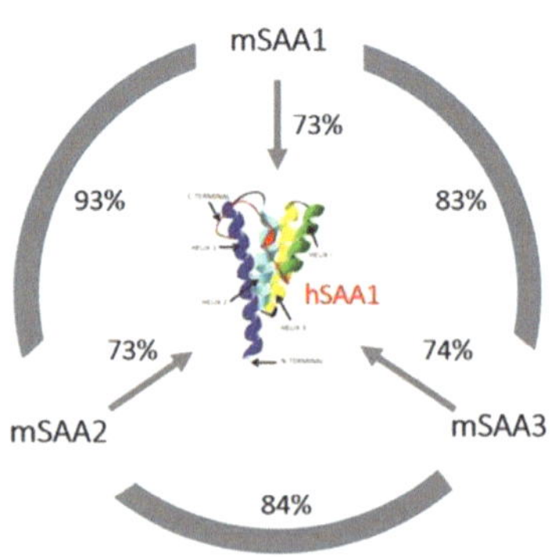

Figure 1.
Comparison of the amino acid sequence of human and mouse inducible SAA proteins. The amino acid sequences of mature SAA protein (without signal peptides) are shown, and identical amino acids are marked with asterisks (*). Inset shows the percent of sequence homology between the 3 inducible mouse SAA proteins and human SAA1.

patients compared to only 7% of normal controls [1]. Husby and Natvig found that the serum component detected by the antisera against AA was larger and its circulation level was increased with age and during pregnancy [2]. The protein immuoprecipitated by the antisera was of low molecular weight with similar but not identical amino acid composition of the AA fibrils [22]. It was thought that AA could be a subunit of the SAA protein [22], which was identified as a cleavage product of SAA.

Amyloidosis develops when insoluble amyloid fibrils accumulate in the extracellular space of the tissues and organs in the body. Patients with chronic inflammatory diseases may develop AA amyloidosis, also termed secondary amyloidosis [23, 24]. SAA as an amyloid protein has the propensity of fibril formation. However, how SAA forms fibril is not fully understood. A number of observations suggest that SAA produced in inflammatory tissues is endocytosed into macrophages [25], where the acidic environment of lysosome promotes fibril formation [26]. The small amount of fibril formed is then exocytosed to the cell surface, prompting a nucleation-dependent incorporation of additional SAA into fibrils [27]. More recent studies have shown that SAA forms stable oligomers at pH of 3.5–4.5, that are resistant to proteolysis and undergo α-helix to β-sheet conversion. The SAA accumulated in lysosomes eventually escape from the cells [28]. Based on these studies, AA fibril formation is a biphasic process [27, 29] that involves an intracellular phase and an extracellular phase. Proteolysis is involved probably in both phases [27, 30]. In the second phase, additional SAA proteins may be recruited with nucleation of AA fibrils, and cleavage of SAA may be a post-fibrillogenic event [31].

Recent delineation of the crystal structure of human SAA1 provides a structural basis for AA amyloidosis [32]. Despite high levels of sequence homology, different SAA isoforms have different propensity in forming AA fibrils. Human SAA1.1 has a high tendency of amyloidogenicity, whereas SAA2.2 found in the CE/J mice did not form amyloid fibrils [33, 34] despite sequence homology as high as 94% with SAA1.1. It was found that the structural determinants for amyloidogenicity reside in the first 10–15 residues of mature SAA protein [35]. In a more recent study, SAA2.2 was found to form small fibrils within a few hours, in contrast to the long lag time of SAA1.1 that was characteristically oligomer-rich [36]. These fibrils exhibited different morphology and the fibrils of SAA1.1 were found to be pathogenic. The results of this study suggest that fibrillation kinetics and prefibrillar oligomers of different SAA isoforms may determine their pathogenicity even though they all possess intrinsic amyloidogenicity.

3. Production and characterization of SAA fragments

In AA amyloidosis, the insoluble AA amyloid protein is derived from the proteolytic cleavage of SAA, generating an N-terminal fragment of SAA. In some cases, this AA amyloid protein lacks amino acids at both N- and C-terminus compared to the full-length SAA. One reported study found that the AA fibril protein purified from rheumatoid arthritis patients with secondary amyloidosis contained 2 fragments with residues 1–50 and 1–45 [37]. However, a SAA fragment with residues 1–76 (or 2–76) was most commonly found in amyloid fibrils, such as those from the livers and spleens of patients with familial Mediterranean fever (FMF), tuberculosis, Hodgkin's diseases and bronchiectasis [24, 38].

In patients with rheumatoid arthritis, higher serum levels of metalloproteinases (MMPs)-1, -2, -3 and -9 were detected compared to healthy controls [39, 40], and the production of these enzymes could be stimulated by SAA [41, 42]. Besides, these MMPs were shown to cleave SAA and AA amyloid protein *in vitro* to produce various sizes of SAA fragments (see **Table 1**). In addition to generating the AA fragments commonly identified in secondary amyloidosis, MMP-1, -2 and -3 cleaved SAA into fragments with residues 1–57, 1–51 and 8–55, respectively [43]. The spanning region (residues 51–57) contains sites that may be cleaved by all three MMPs. In addition, MMP-2 and MMP-3 can also cleave at other residues including residues 7–8 (MMP-2 and -3), 16–17 (MMP-3) and 23–24 (MMP-3). In other species studied, MMP-1 and -3 are able to cleave rabbit SAA3 at residues 50–57, showing conservation between the rabbit SAA3 and human SAA1 [44]. Therefore it was suggested that these MMPs might contribute to the pathogenesis of AA amyloidosis by generating SAA fragments.

In addition to their roles in AA amyloidosis, SAA-derived fragments may have other biological functions. A recent study demonstrated that MMP-9 could rapidly cleave human SAA1 within 30 minutes *in vitro* to produce COOH-terminal fragments, SAA1 (58–104), SAA1 (52–104) and SAA1 (57–104) [46]. These fragments account for 50, 30 and 20% of the total cleaved fragments by MMP-9, respectively. The synthetic peptides of these fragments failed to induce CXCL8 production in human monocytes and diploid fibroblasts, as well as neutrophil chemotaxis; however they potentiated CXCL8-induced neutrophil chemotaxis in a dose-dependent manner via FPR2 [46]. The authors of this report suggested that intact SAA first initiates the inflammatory response and induces the release of MMP-9, which cleaves SAA and modulates the response of SAA by potentiating activities of selected chemokines to prolong the inflammation process. In addition to MMPs,

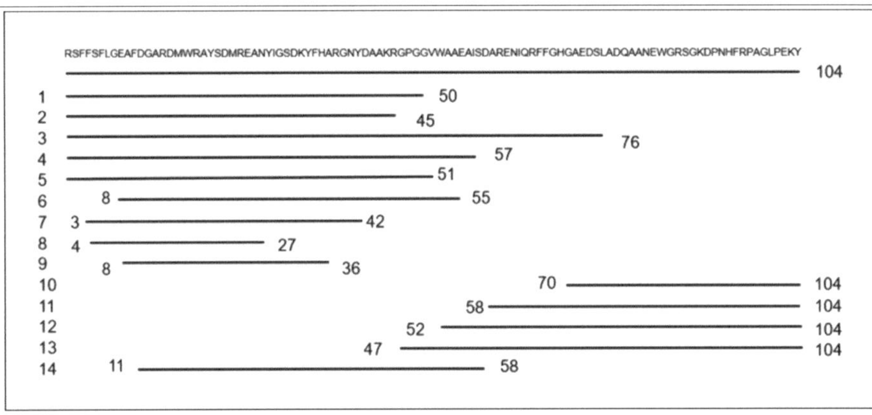

Numbers	Sources of SAA fragments	References
1–2	An AA amyloidosis patient with rheumatoid arthritis	[37]
3	Patients with FMF, tuberculosis, Hodgkin's disease and bronchiectasis	[38]
4–6	Degradation products of human SAA with MMP1, MMP2, MMP3	[43]
7–10	Recombinant SAA cleaved with cathepsin B and cathepsin L	[45]
11–12	MMP-9 cleaved recombinant SAA1	[46]
13	Chemically synthesized fragment based on bovine serum SAA1 fragment	[47]
14	Recombinant protein based on human SAA1 sequence	[48]

The table lists known SAA fragments and synthetic peptides that have been identified. References are provided on the column to the right.

Table 1.
Generation of SAA fragments.

cathepsins, endosomal and lysosomal proteases, were also shown to cleave SAA and might also be involved in AA amyloidosis. Cathepsin B was shown to cleave SAA at residues 76–77 to produce the most common form of AA found in amyloidosis [49]. Another study also reported that both cathepsin B and L completely cleaved SAA, and cathepsin B could produce 9 AA amyloid-like proteins; however, cathepsin L produced no fragments resembling AA amyloid proteins by cleaving within the N-terminus [45]. All amyloid-like SAA fragments described to date have either an intact N-terminus or one that only lacks 1–2 amino acids. Elastase and cathepsin D that cleave SAA further along the N-terminus can prevent the formation of AA amyloid protein [35, 49, 50].

Accumulating evidence suggests that some of the observed biological functions of SAA, other than those related to amyloidosis, may be attributed to SAA-derived fragments rather than the intact protein. In some of these studies, synthetic peptides based on SAA protein sequence were prepared to verify or identify the potential functions. SAA-derived peptides with IFNγ-inducing capability were found in human rheumatic synovial fluid [51]. An SAA2-derived peptide with chemotactic activity for B lymphocytes was found in cow milk [52]. In a recent study, a fragment of SAA1 (46–112) was found in bovine serum and is equivalent to human SAA1 (47–104). The synthetic peptides of this fragment failed to directly induce chemotaxis and chemokine production (CXCL8 and CCL3) in human neutrophils and monocytes, but it synergized with CXCL8 or CCL3 to induce chemotaxis via FPR2 [47]. Studies were also conducted to examine potential functions of SAA and its peptides in LPS-induced inflammatory response. SAA-derived fragments lacking both N- and C-terminal residues were expressed as recombinant proteins and texted for their activities *in vitro*. Fragments such as one with amino acids 11–58 of human SAA1 exhibited minimal proinflammatory activity but enhanced ability to induce IL-10 expression and to counteract LPS-induced inflammation and lung injury [48]. In a recent study, a peptide consisting amino acids 32–47 of human SAA1 was found to disrupt the binding of SAA1 to LPS, suggesting the involvement of this region of SAA1 in LPS binding [53].

4. The cytokine-like activities of recombinant SAA

Recombinant SAA was used in an early study that identified the SAA protein as a chemoattractant for phagocytes [54]. Xu et al. reported that SAA also induced the migration and adhesion of lymphocytes [55]. These studies were among the first to identify leukocyte-activating activities of the recombinant SAA protein. SAA differs from chemokines as it lacks the characteristic cysteine residues that form disulfide bonds for structural stabilization. It was not until 2014 when the crystal structures of two SAA proteins were solved [32, 56]. The 4-helix bundle structure of the SAA monomers and the propensity of forming multimers [32, 56] are strikingly different from the known structural properties of chemokines [57].

Studies conducted by Patel et al. [58] and Fulaneto et al. [59] revealed cytokine-like activities of SAA for its induction of IL-1β, TNFα, IL-1RA and IL-8. Of note, the study conducted by Patel and coworkers used both the recombinant human SAA (rhSAA) and purified SAA-HDL complex, although they found that the cytokine-inducing activity of the SAA-HDL complex was much lower than that of rhSAA. These studies were followed by reports that SAA in neutrophils could induce IL-8 expression through one of the chemoattractant receptors [60] that also mediates anti-inflammatory activities when stimulated by the eicosanoid lipoxin A4 [61, 62]. In addition to proinflammatory cytokines, rhSAA was found to stimulate monocyte expression of tissue factor [63]. Injection of rhSAA to mice increased G-CSF production and neutrophil expansion [64]. SAA also induced the expression of immunomodulatory cytokines including selective induction of IL-23 over IL-12 [65] and the induction of IL-33 expression [66]. The transcription factors NF-κB, IRF4 and IRF7 have been implicated in SAA-induced gene expression [66, 67]. In addition, SAA appears to be involved in epigenetic regulation of gene expression [68].

One of the cellular targets of SAA is macrophages, a major source of cytokines and most if not all SAA receptors. Macrophages may be differentiated into M1 or M2 phenotypes. Studies have shown that SAA may influence macrophage differentiation. Anthony et al. examined the effects of SAA *in vitro*, using human blood monocytes from chronic obstructive pulmonary disease patients and healthy controls, and *in vivo* using a mouse model with airway SAA challenge [69]. Their work showed that SAA-rendered human monocytes secrete IL-6 and IL-1β concurrently with the M2 markers CD163 and IL-10. Moreover, these cells responded to subsequent LPS stimulation with markedly higher levels of IL-6 and IL-1β. In the mouse model, SAA induced a $CD11c^{high}$ $CD11b^{high}$ macrophage population in a CSF-1R signaling-dependent manner, with concurrent inhibition of neutrophilic inflammation. Sun et al. investigated the potential effect of SAA on macrophage plasticity, and found that SAA treatment led to increased expression of macrophage M2 markers including IL-10, Ym1, Fizz-1, MRC1, IL-1Rn, and CCL17 [67]. Moreover, SAA enhanced efferocytosis of mouse macrophages. Silencing IRF4 by small interfering RNA abrogated the SAA-induced expression of M2 markers, suggesting a potential role for SAA to alter macrophage phenotype and modulate macrophage functions.

SAA has been identified as an endogenous activator of the NLRP3 inflammasome, which is critical to the process of pro-IL-1β. Niemi et al. reported that SAA provided a signal for pro-IL-1β expression and for inflammasome activation [70]. At least 3 SAA receptors, including TLR2, TLR4 and the ATP receptor P2X7, were involved. Interestingly, inflammasome activation was dependent on the activity of cathepsin B, the expression of which was induced by SAA. Therefore, SAA-induced secretion of cathepsin B could facilitate extracellular processing of SAA and development of AA amyloidosis. Ather et al. showed SAA3 expression in the lungs of mice exposed to mixed Th2/Th17-polarizing allergic sensitization regimens [71]. SAA instillation into the lungs elicited pulmonary neutrophilic inflammation and activation of the NLRP3 inflammasome, thereby promoting IL-1β secretion by dendritic cells and macrophages. SAA administered into the lungs also served as an adjuvant that sensitized mice to inhaled OVA, promoting IL-17 production from restimulated splenocytes and leukocyte influx. Collectively, these findings illustrate a stimulatory function of SAA in the induced expression of IL-1β.

5. SAA receptors

It has long been suspected that the diverse functions of SAA are mediated by cell surface receptors. Studies conducted in the past 20 years have led to the identification of several cell surface receptors for SAA in addition to a number of binding proteins (**Figure 2**). In 1999, Su et al. reported the involvement of formyl peptide receptor 2 (FPR2, also termed FPRL1 [72, 73]), in the chemotactic activity of SAA [74]. FPR2 is a G protein-coupled chemoattractant receptor initially identified as a homolog of human FPR1 with low-affinity binding of formylated peptide [75–77]. The identification of FPR2 as a receptor for SAA is consistent with reports that SAA induces migration of phagocytes and to a lesser extent, lymphocytes [54, 55]. Subsequent studies have shown that a number of biological functions of SAA, ranging from chemotaxis and superoxide generation to induced expression of proinflammatory cytokines and matrix metalloproteases, are mediated through FPR2 [47, 60, 78–85].

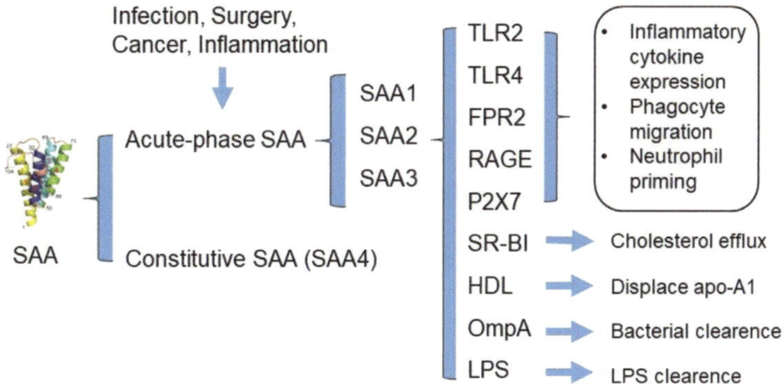

Figure 2.
SAA receptors. The major receptors of human and mouse SAA proteins and their projected functions are listed. Also shown in the figure are selected binding partners of SAA. OmpA, bacterial outer membrane protein a; HDL, high-density lipoprotein. Permission from the publisher was obtained for the use of the crystal structure of SAA1 [32].

The identification of cytokine-like activities of recombinant SAA protein suggests the involvement of receptors that typically mediate phagocyte cytokine production. The finding that SAA selectively induces IL-23 but not IL-12 expression suggests a pattern similar to that of Toll-like receptor (TLR)-mediated cytokine induction [65]. In 2008, two of the TLRs were identified as SAA receptors. TLR2, and more specifically the TLR2-TLR1 heterodimer, was found to mediate SAA-induced NF-κB activation leading to the expression of several proinflammatory cytokines and chemokines [86]. TLR2 is also responsible for SAA-induced neutrophil expansion through upregulation of G-CSF [64]. TLR4 was found to mediate SAA-induced expression of iNOS and activation of the related signaling pathways [87]. Despite differences in primary and high-level structures between SAA and the microbial ligands for these receptors, the two TLRs mediate SAA functions both in transfected cells expressing the receptors and *in vivo* [48, 71, 79, 88–92]. The identification of the two TLRs as SAA receptors illustrates the possible roles for TLRs in detecting host-derived molecules as a mechanism for alerting immune cells upon exposure to environmental stress.

RAGE (receptor for advanced glycation end product) is a multiligand immunoglobulin superfamily cell surface molecule. In a study of AA amyloidosis, RAGE was identified as a receptor of SAA [93]. The expression of RAGE and its interaction with SAA coincide with cell stress, and RAGE has been shown to mediate the NF-κB activating effect of SAA [93, 94]. SAA also binds to soluble RAGE [63]. NF-κB activation induced by SAA interaction with RAGE apparently contributed to the expression of tissue factor in monocytes through MAP kinase activation. Inhibition of RAGE by a RAGE competitor, by soluble RAGE, and by anti-RAGE IgG reduced the SAA-stimulated tissue factor expression [63]. RAGE is also reported to mediate the proinflammatory activity of SAA in uremia-related atherosclerosis, based on a study using the *Apoe*$^{-/-}$ and *Ager*$^{-/-}$ mice [95]. These studies identify RAGE as an endothelial and monocyte-expressed molecule that mediates selected activities of SAA.

Scavenger receptors on macrophages play important roles in the removal of debris during tissue injury and in macrophage transport of lipids. The scavenge-receptor SR-BI has been known for mediating cholesterol efflux, in which SAA plays a role [96]. Two independent studies published in the same year reported the identification of SR-BI as an SAA receptor [97, 98]. Direct binding assays using radiolabeled SAA found its interaction with SR-B1 in cells that express this receptor [97]. SR-BI and its human homolog CLA-I mediate SAA uptake and its downstream signaling, including the activation of ERK and p38 MAPK that leads to IL-8 expression [98]. A more recent study reported that SR-BII, a splice variant of SR-BI, also serves as a SAA receptor for uptake and proinflammatory signaling through MAP kinase signaling [99].

The human P2X7 purinergic receptor is an ionotropic receptor found at high expression levels in immune cells such as macrophages and microglia. Activation of P2X7 receptor by extracellular ATP opens a cation channel, allowing K^+ efflux that is associated with processing of pro-interleukin IL-1β and IL-18. Christenson et al. found that SAA, either recombinant or purified from the plasma of rheumatoid arthritis patients, could suppress apoptosis of human neutrophils, an effect abrogated by antagonizing the nucleotide receptor P2X7 [100]. Niemi et al. reported that the P2X7 receptor plays a role in SAA-mediated activation of NLRP3, thereby explaining the involvement of SAA in the processing of pro-IL-1β [70]. However, a recently published work indicates that in murine J774 and bone marrow-derived macrophages, SAA stimulates IL-1β secretion through a mechanism that depends on NLRP3 expression and caspase-1 activity but not the P2X7 receptor [101].

Collectively, published reports have identified several functional receptors that mediate SAA signaling. It is likely that these receptors and their downstream signaling pathways have substantial cross-talk that together contributes to the diverse immunomodulatory and homeostatic functions of SAA.

Recent studies have shown that recombinant human SAA, which has been widely used in in *vitro* studies throughout the last two decades, has properties that differ from those of native SAA purified from human samples [102–104]. The rhSAA differs from human SAA1 in two sites, with amino acid substitutions at positions 60 and 71 in addition to gaining a methionine at the N-terminus. Since the rhSAA is made by *Escherichia coli* expression, the bacterial contaminants in the preparation may contribute to the observed cytokine-like activity. This is especially a concern because the contaminating bacterial products can activate the two TLRs that are known as the SAA receptors. A careful analysis of published literature found evidence that both support the use of the two TLRs by SAA and detract from the claim. Many of the published studies have included controls for LPS contamination, showing that the SAA protein is necessary for the reported biological functions. A recent study has shown that the bacterial contaminants may not be LPS that acts through TLR4 but lipoproteins that activate TLR2 [105]. The study also showed that adding bacterial lipopeptides into mammalian cell-expressed SAA1 protein could restore the cytokine-like activity that otherwise was missing from the SAA1 protein [105]. It is however unclear how much lipoproteins are carried by the *E. coli*-derived recombinant SAA. The *E. coli* expression system has been widely used in the production of reagents including proinflammatory cytokines such as TNFα and IL-1β, and there were not previous concerns over bacterial product contamination with these cytokines. Whereas the authors attributed the previously reported NLRP3 inflammasome-activating property of SAA to bacterial lipoprotein contaminants in the *E. coli*-derived SAA [105], another recent study demonstrated that SAA purified from human samples was able to stimulate NLRP3 inflammasome activation [101]. Taken together, these findings raise the possibility that bacterial contaminants may modify the biological properties of human SAA1 for a potent cytokine-inducing effect. Exactly how much bacterial contaminant is associated with a recombinant human SAA1 is still unknown, but published studies have shown that *E. coli*-produced SAA proteins can be processed to sufficient purity so they can form crystals [32, 56]. Moreover, CHO cell-derived SAA in the form of secreted Fc fusion protein has been shown to bind to the ectodomain of TLR2 [86]. While the contaminating lipoproteins may contribute to the cytokine-inducing activity through TLR2, these contaminants have not been known to stimulate the G protein-coupled FPR2 that mediates some of the biological activities of SAA [47, 60, 74, 78–85]. Based on available data, it is postulated that some of the observed functions of rhSAA are attributable to bacterial contaminants. *In vivo* studies conducted in various models of diseases are therefore important for confirming the biological functions of SAA under physiologically relevant conditions.

6. Immunomodulatory functions of SAA in disease models

Since most of the early studies were conducted using cell lines and isolated primary cells such as monocytes and neutrophils, these experimental findings are now examined in an *in vivo* setting. An early model created for the *in vivo* studies of SAA employed adenoviral expression of human SAA1, raising the circulatory levels of human SAA1 in the infected mice [106]. This approach was used in studies of the involvement of SAA1 in lipid metabolism [106] and fibril formation [107]. In a more recent study, the same group that created the adenoviral approach found a role for SAA3 in atherosclerosis [108].

Transgenic expression of human SAA1 in mice is another approach used in studies of the *in vivo* functions of SAA. Ji et al. reported transgenic expression of human SAA1 in mouse liver [89]. These mice exhibited more severe liver injury, increased hepatocyte apoptosis, and higher levels of hepatic enzymes than in their wildtype controls. After induction of hepatitis, liver infiltration of $CD4^+$ T cells and macrophages was also increased more in the transgenic mice than in wildtype mice, along with elevated expression of several chemokines. The aggravated liver injury, increased hepatocyte apoptosis and elevated levels of hepatic enzymes in the transgenic mice were eased with the use of a TLR2 antagonist, suggesting that TLR2 mediates the effects of the transgenic SAA1. In a more recent study, Cheng et al. placed the human SAA1 under an inducible promoter of SR-A receptor, generating transgenic mice with elevated local production of SAA1 upon inflammatory stimulation [53]. The transgenic SAA1 was most abundant in mouse lungs and protected mice against acute lung injury caused by LPS administration and cecal ligation and puncture (CLP). Transgenic expression of SAA1 did not protect mice against acute lung injury induced by intratracheal instillation of TNFα. Binding studies showed that human SAA1, purified from either *E. coli* or transfected HEK293 cells, bound to LPS and formed a complex that promoted LPS clearance by macrophages. As a result, serum endotoxin concentration was significantly reduced in the transgenic mice than in their wildtype controls that went through the CLP procedure. Of note, injection of a SAA1-derived peptide that disrupted LPS-SAA1 interaction diminished the endotoxin-lowering effect in the SAA1 transgenic mice and increased serum endotoxin level in wildtype mice after CLP [53]. These findings suggest a mechanism by which acute-phase SAA protects host against bacterial infection-induced injury.

SAA gene knockout mice were generate to examine the physiological functions of the individual SAA proteins. After observing SAA1 and SAA2 expression in intestinal epithelial cells and conforming their cell-protecting effect in epithelial cell line co-cultured with *E. coli*, Eckhardt et al. examined the effect of Saa1/2 double knockout (DKO) in dextran sodium sulfate (DSS) induced colitis model [109]. They found that that epithelial expression of SAA1 and SAA2 protected colonic epithelium against bacterial infection. A more recent study using Saa3 gene knockout mice found that SAA3 is the predominant isoform of inducible SAA proteins in colonic epithelium following chemical injury [92]. Compared to wildtype mice, $Saa3^{-/-}$ mice exposed to DSS showed more severe damage to the colonic epithelial structure, significantly reduced expression of the anti-microbial peptides Reg3β and Reg3γ, and reduced lifespan of afflicted mice if not treated. Administration of exogenous SAA3 protein or adoptive transfer of SAA3-treated neutrophils partially ameliorated symptoms of DSS-induced colitis in part due to SAA3-induced neutrophil expression of IL-22, a cytokine with epithelia-protection function [110]. Together, these results suggest that epithelial expression of SAA1 and SAA2 in healthy mice may be important for homeostasis of gut functions including host defense, whereas inducible expression of SAA3 serves to combat acute injury to the colonic epithelium.

A role for SAA as a mediator of local immune response has been reported recently. In a study of segmented filamentous bacteria (SFB) for its involvement in mucosal defenses and autoimmune diseases through RORγ^{+} Th17 cells, Sano et al. found that direct contact of SFB with epithelium in the ileum could induce SAA1 and SAA2 expression and promote local IL-17A expression in RORγ$^{(+)}$ T cells. The mechanisms involved an IL-23R/IL-22 circuit and the participation of type 3 innate lymphoid cells (ILC3) that secretes IL-22 [111]. Likewise, Atarashi et al. investigated a group of intestinal microbes for their ability to induce Th17 response, and found that SFB could stimulate intestinal epithelial cells to generate SAA and ROS, creating an amplification loop for sustained production of SAA by both epithelial cells and myeloid cells that led to local Th17 response [112]. These findings provide direct evidence for the contribution of epithelial SAA to intestinal homeostasis in an environment where host interaction with gut microbiota influences the health states of individuals.

In addition to studies of the *in vivo* functions of SAA in innate immunity and inflammation, mice with genetically altered SAA genes were used in the investigation of these acute-phase proteins in animal models of atherosclerosis, osteoclast activation, adipogenesis, and neurodegenerative disorders such as Alzheimer's disease. Ahlin et al. generated transgenic mouse model expressing human SAA1 in the adipose tissue, and used the hSAA1$^{+/-}$ mice in studies of the effect of SAA1 on glucose metabolism and insulin resistance [114]. They found no evidence that adipose tissue-derived hSAA1 could influence the development of insulin resistance or obesity-related inflammation. The potential involvement of SAA in atherogenesis was investigated using the Saa1/2 DKO mice in the *Apoe*$^{-/-}$ background [115]. Surprisingly, the absence of *Saa1.1* and *Saa2.1* did not affect atherosclerotic lesion in the ApoE-deficient mice that were fed with Western diets. It was later reported that SAA3, instead of SAA1/2, is pro-atherogenic based on experiments using adeno-associated virus for overexpression of SAA3 and antisense oligonucleotide-mediated suppression of Saa3 expression [108]. Using SAA3 KO mice, Liu et al. reported elevated Tau phosphorylation (hyperphosphorylation) compared to wildtype mice upon systemic LPS administration. Overexpression of SAA by intracerebral injection attenuated tau hyperphosphorylation in the brain, suggesting that SAA3 may be neuroprotective in the mouse AD model [116].

Several studies of the *in vivo* functions of SAA were conducted in wildtype mice. De Santo et al. reported that systemic SAA1 plays a role in the regulation of neutrophil plasticity through induction of the anti-inflammatory IL-10 and promotion of the interaction of invariant natural killer T cells (iNKT cells) with neutrophils. As a result, SAA1 indirectly limits the suppressive activity by diminishing IL-10 production and enhancing IL-12 production [113].

Collectively, results from the studies of SAA proteins in mice identified important functions of SAA that were previous unknown from *in vitro* studies. There are other functions revealed from the *in vivo* studies using genetically altered mice that are consistent with the *in vitro* findings. For example, the ability of SAA to interact with Gram-negative bacterial wall components [117] is consistent with the *in vivo* findings that SAA1 protects mice against LPS- and CLP-induced acute lung injury [53]. The *in vivo* findings strongly suggest that acute-phase SAA protects host against environmental insults such as chemical-induced intestinal epithelial injury and bacterial infection. Four of the animal models used in studies of SAA are

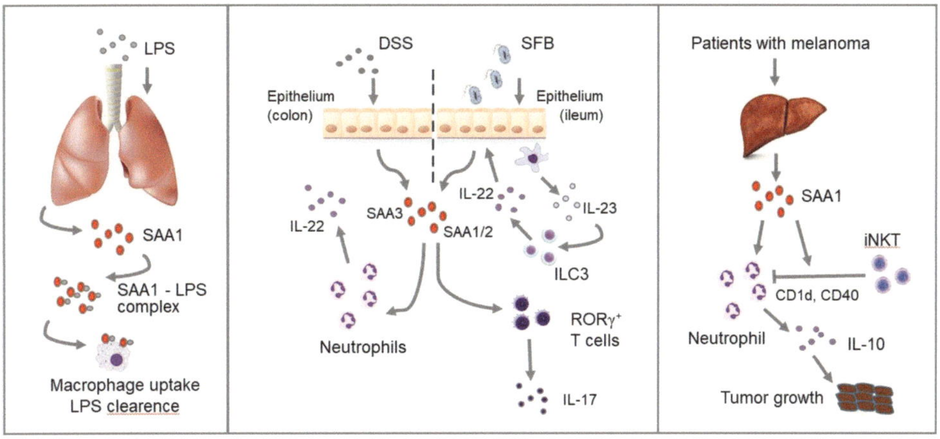

Figure 3.
Immunomodulatory functions of SAA in selected mouse models. Left: transgenic expression of human SAA1 in the lung tissue protects mice against LPS-induced acute lung injury [53]. The protection is conferred in part through SAA binding to LPS, forming a complex that promotes LPS clearance by macrophages. Middle: SAA1 and SAA2 expressed in epithelium of the ileum serves as a mediator of segmented filamentous bacteria-induced local Th17 response [111, 112], contributing to homeostasis of the microenvironment in the intestine [109]. In response to acute injury such as dextran sodium sulfate (DSS) treatment, SAA3 is induced in mouse colonic epithelium and serves as an inducer for neutrophil IL-22 expression [92]. Right: SAA1-producing melanomas induce neutrophil secretion of IL-10 for its suppressive effect. SAA1 also promotes neutrophil interaction with invariant natural killer T (iNKT) cells, thereby limiting IL-10 production but enhancing IL-12 production [113]. This mechanism may be explored to reduce the immunosuppressive neutrophils and restore tumor-specific immunity.

summarized in **Figure 3**. Due to page limitation, *in vivo* studies on SAA functions other than those related to immunomodulation are not discussed in this chapter.

7. Conclusion remarks

SAA has emerged from a precursor of AA to a modulator of immunity and inflammation. Several developments, including the ability to express recombinant SAA proteins, the generation of genetically altered mice expressing SAA transgenes or deletion of a specific SAA gene, and the availability of crystal structures of SAA proteins, have helped to advance our understanding of SAA for its functions in host defense, lipid metabolism, adipogenesis, and neuroprotection. In coming years, studies will likely focus on the comparison of SAA functions *in vitro* to those identified *in vivo,* and on the possible modifications and proteolytic processing of newly synthesized SAA in order to address several questions that remain unanswered today. A better understanding of SAA for its biological functions is expected to benefit human health through development of new diagnostic approaches and therapies.

Acknowledgements

This work was supported in part by grants from the Science and Technology Development Fund of Macau (026/2016/A1) and the University of Macau (MYRG2016-00152-ICMS-QRCM and CPG2015-00018-ICMS).

Conflict of interest

The authors declare that they have no conflict of interest.

Author details

Yu Fan, Chi Teng Vong and Richard D. Ye*
State Key Laboratory of Quality Research in Chinese Medicine and Institute of Chinese Medical Sciences, University of Macau, Macau Special Administrative Region, China

*Address all correspondence to: richardye@umac.mo

References

[1] Levin M, Pras M, Franklin EC. Immunologic studies of the major nonimmunoglobulin protein of amyloid. I. Identification and partial characterization of a related serum component. The Journal of Experimental Medicine. 1973;**138**(2):373-380

[2] Husby G, Natvig JB. A serum component related to nonimmunoglobulin amyloid protein AS, a possible precursor of the fibrils. The Journal of Clinical Investigation. 1974;**53**(4):1054-1061

[3] Rosenthal CJ, Franklin EC. Variation with age and disease of an amyloid A protein-related serum component. The Journal of Clinical Investigation. 1975;**55**(4):746-753

[4] Rosenthal CJ, Franklin EC, Frangione B, Greenspan J. Isolation and partial characterization of SAA-an amyloid-related protein from human serum. Journal of Immunology. 1976;**116**(5):1415-1418

[5] Kushner I. The phenomenon of the acute phase response. Annals of the New York Academy of Sciences. 1982;**389**:39-48

[6] Gabay C, Kushner I. Acute-phase proteins and other systemic responses to inflammation. The New England Journal of Medicine. 1999;**340**(6):448-454

[7] Urieli-Shoval S, Linke RP, Matzner Y. Expression and function of serum amyloid A, a major acute-phase protein, in normal and disease states. Current Opinion in Hematology. 2000;**7**(1):64-69

[8] Dalla Vestra M, Mussap M, Gallina P, Bruseghin M, Cernigoi AM, Saller A, et al. Acute-phase markers of inflammation and glomerular structure in patients with type 2 diabetes. Journal of the American Society of Nephrology. 2005;**16**(Suppl 1):S78-S82

[9] Malle E, Sodin-Semrl S, Kovacevic A. Serum amyloid A: An acute-phase protein involved in tumour pathogenesis. Cellular and Molecular Life Sciences. 2009;**66**(1):9-26

[10] Kisilevsky R. Serum amyloid A (SAA), a protein without a function: Some suggestions with reference to cholesterol metabolism. Medical Hypotheses. 1991;**35**(4):337-341

[11] Getz GS, Reardon CA. SAA, HDL biogenesis, and inflammation. Journal of Lipid Research. 2008;**49**(2):269-270

[12] Kisilevsky R, Manley PN. Acute-phase serum amyloid A: Perspectives on its physiological and pathological roles. Amyloid. 2012;**19**(1):5-14

[13] De Buck M, Gouwy M, Wang JM, Van Snick J, Proost P, Struyf S, et al. The cytokine-serum amyloid A-chemokine network. Cytokine & Growth Factor Reviews. 2016;**30**:55-69. DOI: 10.1016/j.cytogfr.2015.12.010

[14] Sun L, Ye RD. Serum amyloid A1: Structure, function and gene polymorphism. Gene. 2016;**583**(1):48-57. DOI: 10.1016/j.gene.2016.02.044

[15] Sack GH Jr. Serum amyloid A—A review. Molecular Medicine. 2018;**24**(1):46. DOI: 10.1186/s10020-018-0047-0

[16] Uhlar CM, Burgess CJ, Sharp PM, Whitehead AS. Evolution of the serum amyloid A (SAA) protein superfamily. Genomics. 1994;**19**(2):228-235

[17] Kluve-Beckerman B, Drumm ML, Benson MD. Nonexpression of the human serum amyloid A three (SAA3) gene. DNA and Cell Biology. 1991;**10**(9):651-661

[18] Uhlar CM, Whitehead AS. Serum amyloid A, the major vertebrate acute-phase reactant. European Journal of Biochemistry. 1999;**265**(2):501-523

[19] Kushner I, Rzewnicki D. Acute phase response. In: Gallin JI, Snyderman R, editors. Inflammation: Basic Principles and Clinical Correlates. 3rd ed. Philadelphia: Lippincott Williams & Wilkins; 1999. pp. 317-329

[20] Butler A, Whitehead AS. Mapping of the mouse serum amyloid A gene cluster by long-range polymerase chain reaction. Immunogenetics. 1996;**44**(6):468-474

[21] Mori M, Tian G, Ishikawa A, Higuchi K. Diversity and complexity of the mouse Saa1 and Saa2 genes. Experimental Animals. 2014;**63**(1):99-106

[22] Anders RF, Natvig JB, Michaelsen TE, Husby G. Isolation and characterization of amyloid-related serum protein SAA as a low molecular weight protein. Scandinavian Journal of Immunology. 1975;**4**(4):397-401

[23] Pinney JH, Hawkins PN. Amyloidosis. Annals of Clinical Biochemistry. 2012;**49**(Pt 3):229-241. DOI: 10.1258/acb.2011.011225

[24] Westermark GT, Fändrich M, Westermark M. AA amyloidosis: Pathogenesis and targeted therapy. Annual Review of Pathology: Mechanisms of Disease. 2015;**10**(1):321-344. DOI: 10.1146/annurev-pathol-020712-163913

[25] Chan SL, Chronopoulos S, Murray J, Laird DW, AliKhan Z. Selective localization of murine ApoSAA(1)/SAA(2) in endosomes-lysosomes in activated macrophages and their degradation products. Amyloid-International Journal of Experimental and Clinical Investigation. 1997;**4**(1):40-48. DOI: 10.3109/13506129708995267

[26] Kluve-Beckerman B, Manaloor J, Liepnieks JJ. Binding, trafficking and accumulation of serum amyloid A in peritoneal macrophages. Scandinavian Journal of Immunology. 2001;**53**(4):393-400

[27] Magy N, Benson MD, Liepnieks JJ, Kluve-Beckerman B. Cellular events associated with the initial phase of AA amyloidogenesis: Insights from a human monocyte model. Amyloid. 2007;**14**(1):51-63. DOI: 10.1080/13506120601116575

[28] Jayaraman S, Gantz DL, Haupt C, Gursky O. Serum amyloid A forms stable oligomers that disrupt vesicles at lysosomal pH and contribute to the pathogenesis of reactive amyloidosis. Proceedings of the National Academy of Sciences of the United States of America. 2017;**114**(32):E6507-E6515. DOI: 10.1073/pnas.1707120114

[29] Sipe JD, McAdam KP, Uchino F. Biochemical evidence for the biphasic development of experimental amyloidosis. Laboratory Investigation. 1978;**38**(1):110-114

[30] Phipps-Yonas H, Pinard G, Ali-Khan Z. Humoral proinflammatory cytokine and SAA generation profiles and spatio-temporal relationship between SAA and lysosomal cathepsin B and D in murine splenic monocytoid cells during AA amyloidosis. Scandinavian Journal of Immunology. 2004;**59**(2):168-176

[31] Kisilevsky R, Narindrasorasak S, Tape C, Tan R, Boudreau L. During Aa-Amyloidogenesis is proteolytic attack on serum amyloid-a a pre-fibrillogenic or post-fibrillogenic event. Amyloid-International Journal of Experimental and Clinical Investigation. 1994;**1**(3):174-183. DOI: 10.3109/13506129409148449

[32] Lu J, Yu Y, Zhu I, Cheng Y, Sun PD. Structural mechanism of serum amyloid A-mediated inflammatory amyloidosis. Proceedings of the National Academy of Sciences of the United States of America. 2014;**111**(14):5189-5194

[33] de Beer MC, de Beer FC, McCubbin WD, Kay CM, Kindy MS. Structural prerequisites for serum amyloid A fibril formation. The Journal of Biological Chemistry. 1993;**268**(27):20606-20612

[34] Sipe JD, Carreras I, Gonnerman WA, Cathcart ES, Debeer MC, Debeer FC. Characterization of the inbred Ce/J mouse strain as amyloid resistant. American Journal of Pathology. 1993;**143**(5):1480-1485

[35] Westermark GT, Engstrom U, Westermark P. The N-terminal segment of protein AA determines its fibrillogenic property. Biochemical and Biophysical Research Communications. 1992;**182**(1):27-33

[36] Srinivasan S, Patke S, Wang Y, Ye Z, Litt J, Srivastava SK, et al. Pathogenic serum amyloid A 1.1 shows a long oligomer-rich fibrillation lag phase contrary to the highly amyloidogenic non-pathogenic SAA2.2. The Journal of Biological Chemistry. 2013;**288**(4):2744-2755. DOI: 10.1074/jbc.M112.394155

[37] Westermark GT, Westermark P, Sletten K. Amyloid fibril protein AA. Characterization of uncommon subspecies from a patient with rheumatoid arthritis. Laboratory Investigation. 1987;**57**(1):57-64

[38] Levin M, Franklin EC, Frangione B, Pras M. The amino acid sequence of a major nonimmunoglobulin component of some amyloid fibrils. The Journal of Clinical Investigation. 1972;**51**(10):2773-2776. DOI: 10.1172/JCI107098

[39] Keyszer G, Lambiri I, Keysser M, Keysser C, Nagel R, Burmester GR, et al. Matrix metalloproteinases, but not cathepsins B, H, and L or their inhibitors in peripheral blood of patients with rheumatoid arthritis are potentially useful markers of disease activity. Zeitschrift für Rheumatologie. 1998;**57**(6):392-398

[40] Keyszer G, Lambiri I, Nagel R, Keysser C, Keysser M, Gromnica-Ihle E, et al. Circulating levels of matrix metalloproteinases MMP-3 and MMP-1, tissue inhibitor of metalloproteinases 1 (TIMP-1), and MMP-1/TIMP-1 complex in rheumatic disease. Correlation with clinical activity of rheumatoid arthritis versus other surrogate markers. The Journal of Rheumatology. 1999;**26**(2):251-258

[41] Migita K, Kawabe Y, Tominaga M, Origuchi T, Aoyagi T, Eguchi K. Serum amyloid A protein induces production of matrix metalloproteinases by human synovial fibroblasts. Laboratory Investigation. 1998;**78**(5):535-539

[42] Mullan RH, Bresnihan B, Golden-Mason L, Markham T, O'Hara R, Fitz Gerald O, et al. Acute-phase serum amyloid A stimulation of angiogenesis, leukocyte recruitment, and matrix degradation in rheumatoid arthritis through an NF-kappa B-dependent signal transduction pathway. Arthritis and Rheumatism. 2006;**54**(1):105-114

[43] Stix B, Kahne T, Sletten K, Raynes J, Roessner A, Rocken C. Proteolysis of AA amyloid fibril proteins by matrix metalloproteinases-1, -2, and -3. The American Journal of Pathology. 2001;**159**(2):561-570. DOI: 10.1016/S0002-9440(10)61727-0

[44] Mitchell TI, Jeffrey JJ, Palmiter RD, Brinckerhoff CE. The acute phase reactant serum amyloid A (SAA3) is a novel substrate for degradation by the metalloproteinases collagenase and

stromelysin. Biochimica et Biophysica Acta. 1993;**1156**(3):245-254

[45] Röcken C, Menard R, Bühling F, Vöckler S, Raynes J, Stix B, et al. Proteolysis of serum amyloid A and AA amyloid proteins by cysteine proteases: Cathepsin B generates AA amyloid proteins and cathepsin L may prevent their formation. Annals of the Rheumatic Diseases. 2005;**64**(6):808

[46] Gouwy M, De Buck M, Abouelasrar Salama S, Vandooren J, Knoops S, Pörtner N, et al. Matrix metalloproteinase-9-generated COOH-, but not NH(2)-terminal fragments of serum amyloid A1 retain potentiating activity in neutrophil migration to CXCL8, with loss of direct chemotactic and cytokine-inducing capacity. Frontiers in Immunology. 2018;**9**:1081. DOI: 10.3389/fimmu.2018.01081

[47] De Buck M, Gouwy M, Berghmans N, Opdenakker G, Proost P, Struyf S, et al. COOH-terminal SAA1 peptides fail to induce chemokines but synergize with CXCL8 and CCL3 to recruit leukocytes via FPR2. Blood. 2018;**131**(4):439-449. DOI: 10.1182/blood-2017-06-788554

[48] Zhou H, Chen M, Zhang G, Ye RD. Suppression of lipopolysaccharide-induced inflammatory response by fragments from serum amyloid A. Journal of Immunology. 2017;**199**(3):1105-1112. DOI: 10.4049/jimmunol.1700470

[49] Yamada T, Liepnieks JJ, Kluve-Beckerman B, Benson MD. Cathepsin B generates the most common form of amyloid A (76 residues) as a degradation product from serum amyloid A. Scandinavian Journal of Immunology. 1995;**41**(1):94-97

[50] Yamada T, Kluve-Beckerman B, Liepnieks JJ, Benson MD. In vitro degradation of serum amyloid A by cathepsin D and other acid proteases: Possible protection against amyloid fibril formation. Scandinavian Journal of Immunology. 1995;**41**(6):570-574

[51] Yavin EJ, Preciado-Patt L, Rosen O, Yaron M, Suessmuth RD, Levartowsky D, et al. Serum amyloid A-derived peptides, present in human rheumatic synovial fluids, induce the secretion of interferon-gamma by human CD(4)(+) T-lymphocytes. FEBS Letters. 2000;**472**(2-3):259-262

[52] de Jesus Rodriguez B, Chevaleyre C, Henry G, Molle D, Virlogeux-Payant I, Berri M, et al. Identification in milk of a serum amyloid A peptide chemoattractant for B lymphoblasts. BMC Immunology. 2009;**10**:4. DOI: 10.1186/1471-2172-10-4

[53] Cheng N, Liang Y, Du X, Ye RD. Serum amyloid A promotes LPS clearance and suppresses LPS-induced inflammation and tissue injury. EMBO Reports. 2018;**19**(10). pii:e45517. DOI: 10.15252/embr.201745517

[54] Badolato R, Wang JM, Murphy WJ, Lloyd AR, Michiel DF, Bausserman LL, et al. Serum amyloid A is a chemoattractant: Induction of migration, adhesion, and tissue infiltration of monocytes and polymorphonuclear leukocytes. The Journal of Experimental Medicine. 1994;**180**(1):203-209

[55] Xu L, Badolato R, Murphy WJ, Longo DL, Anver M, Hale S, et al. A novel biologic function of serum amyloid A. Induction of T lymphocyte migration and adhesion. Journal of Immunology. 1995;**155**(3):1184-1190

[56] Derebe MG, Zlatkov CM, Gattu S, Ruhn KA, Vaishnava S, Diehl GE, et al. Serum amyloid A is a retinol binding protein that transports retinol during bacterial infection. eLife. 2014;**3**:e03206

[57] Clore GM, Gronenborn AM. Three-dimensional structures of alpha and beta chemokines. The FASEB Journal. 1995;**9**(1):57-62

[58] Patel H, Fellowes R, Coade S, Woo P. Human serum amyloid A has cytokine-like properties. Scandinavian Journal of Immunology. 1998;**48**(4):410-418

[59] Furlaneto CJ, Campa A. A novel function of serum amyloid A: A potent stimulus for the release of tumor necrosis factor-alpha, interleukin-1beta, and interleukin-8 by human blood neutrophil. Biochemical and Biophysical Research Communications. 2000;**268**(2):405-408

[60] He R, Sang H, Ye RD. Serum amyloid A induces IL-8 secretion through a G protein-coupled receptor, FPRL1/LXA4R. Blood. 2003;**101**(4):1572-1581

[61] Sodin-Semrl S, Spagnolo A, Mikus R, Barbaro B, Varga J, Fiore S. Opposing regulation of interleukin-8 and NF-kappaB responses by lipoxin A4 and serum amyloid A via the common lipoxin A receptor. International Journal of Immunopharmacology. 2004;**17**(2):145-156

[62] Bozinovski S, Uddin M, Vlahos R, Thompson M, McQualter JL, Merritt AS, et al. Serum amyloid A opposes lipoxin A(4) to mediate glucocorticoid refractory lung inflammation in chronic obstructive pulmonary disease. Proceedings of the National Academy of Sciences of the United States of America. 2012;**109**(3):935-940. DOI: 10.1073/pnas.1109382109

[63] Cai H, Song C, Endoh I, Goyette J, Jessup W, Freedman SB, et al. Serum amyloid A induces monocyte tissue factor. Journal of Immunology. 2007;**178**(3):1852-1860

[64] He RL, Zhou J, Hanson CZ, Chen J, Cheng N, Ye RD. Serum amyloid A induces G-CSF expression and neutrophilia via Toll-like receptor 2. Blood. 2009;**113**(2):429-437. DOI: 10.1182/blood-2008-03-139923

[65] He R, Shepard LW, Chen J, Pan ZK, Ye RD. Serum amyloid A is an endogenous ligand that differentially induces IL-12 and IL-23. Journal of Immunology. 2006;**177**(6):4072-4079

[66] Sun L, Zhu Z, Cheng N, Yan Q, Ye RD. Serum amyloid A induces interleukin-33 expression through an IRF7-dependent pathway. European Journal of Immunology. 2014;**44**(7):2153-2164

[67] Sun L, Zhou H, Zhu Z, Yan Q, Wang L, Liang Q, et al. Ex vivo and in vitro effect of serum amyloid A in the induction of macrophage m2 markers and efferocytosis of apoptotic neutrophils. Journal of Immunology. 2015;**194**(10):4891-4900. DOI: 10.4049/jimmunol.1402164

[68] Yan Q, Sun L, Zhu Z, Wang L, Li S, Ye RD. Jmjd3-mediated epigenetic regulation of inflammatory cytokine gene expression in serum amyloid A-stimulated macrophages. Cellular Signalling. 2014;**26**(9):1783-1791

[69] Anthony D, McQualter JL, Bishara M, Lim EX, Yatmaz S, Seow HJ, et al. SAA drives proinflammatory heterotypic macrophage differentiation in the lung via CSF-1R-dependent signaling. The FASEB Journal. 2014;**28**(9):3867-3877. DOI: 10.1096/fj.14-250332

[70] Niemi K, Teirila L, Lappalainen J, Rajamaki K, Baumann MH, Oorni K, et al. Serum amyloid A activates the NLRP3 inflammasome via P2X7 receptor and a cathepsin B-sensitive pathway. Journal of Immunology. 2011;**186**(11):6119-6128

[71] Ather JL, Ckless K, Martin R, Foley KL, Suratt BT, Boyson JE, et al. Serum amyloid A activates the NLRP3 inflammasome and promotes Th17 allergic asthma in mice. Journal of Immunology. 2011;**187**(1):64-73. DOI: 10.4049/jimmunol.1100500

[72] Migeotte I, Communi D, Parmentier M. Formyl peptide receptors: A promiscuous subfamily of G protein-coupled receptors controlling immune responses. Cytokine & Growth Factor Reviews. 2006;**17**(6):501-519

[73] Ye RD, Boulay F, Wang JM, Dahlgren C, Gerard C, Parmentier M, et al. International union of basic and clinical pharmacology. LXXIII. Nomenclature for the formyl peptide receptor (FPR) family. Pharmacological Reviews. 2009;**61**(2):119-161. DOI: 10.1124/pr.109.001578

[74] Su SB, Gong W, Gao JL, Shen W, Murphy PM, Oppenheim JJ, et al. A seven-transmembrane, G protein-coupled receptor, FPRL1, mediates the chemotactic activity of serum amyloid A for human phagocytic cells. The Journal of Experimental Medicine. 1999;**189**(2):395-402

[75] Ye RD, Cavanagh SL, Quehenberger O, Prossnitz ER, Cochrane CG. Isolation of a cDNA that encodes a novel granulocyte N-formyl peptide receptor. Biochemical and Biophysical Research Communications. 1992;**184**(2):582-589

[76] Murphy PM, Ozcelik T, Kenney RT, Tiffany HL, Mcdermott D, Francke U. A structural homolog of the N-formyl peptide receptor-characterization and chromosome mapping of a peptide chemoattractant receptor family. Journal of Biological Chemistry. 1992;**267**(11):7637-7643

[77] Lu B, Gerard NP, Eddy RL, Shows TB, Gerard C. Mapping of genes for the human-C5a receptor (C5ar), human Fmlp receptor (Fpr), and 2 Fmlp receptor homolog orphan receptors (Fprh1, Fprh2) to Chromosome-19. Genomics. 1992;**13**(2):437-440

[78] Bjorkman L, Karlsson J, Karlsson A, Rabiet MJ, Boulay F, Fu H, et al. Serum amyloid A mediates human neutrophil production of reactive oxygen species through a receptor independent of formyl peptide receptor like-1. Journal of Leukocyte Biology. 2008;**83**(2):245-253. DOI: 10.1189/jlb.0607-408

[79] Chen M, Zhou H, Cheng N, Qian F, Ye RD. Serum amyloid A1 isoforms display different efficacy at Toll-like receptor 2 and formyl peptide receptor 2. Immunobiology. 2014;**219**(12):916-923

[80] Lee HY, Kim MK, Park KS, Bae YH, Yun J, Park JI, et al. Serum amyloid A stimulates matrix-metalloproteinase-9 upregulation via formyl peptide receptor like-1-mediated signaling in human monocytic cells. Biochemical and Biophysical Research Communications. 2005;**330**(3):989-998

[81] Lee HY, Kim SD, Baek SH, Choi JH, Bae YS. Role of formyl peptide receptor 2 on the serum amyloid A-induced macrophage foam cell formation. Biochemical and Biophysical Research Communications. 2013;**433**(2):255-259

[82] Lee HY, Kim SD, Shim JW, Lee SY, Lee H, Cho KH, et al. Serum amyloid A induces CCL2 production via formyl peptide receptor-like 1-mediated signaling in human monocytes. Journal of Immunology. 2008;**181**(6):4332-4339

[83] Lee MS, Yoo SA, Cho CS, Suh PG, Kim WU, Ryu SH. Serum amyloid A binding to formyl peptide receptor-like 1 induces synovial hyperplasia and angiogenesis. Journal of Immunology. 2006;**177**(8):5585-5594

[84] O'Hara R, Murphy EP, Whitehead AS, Fitz Gerald O, Bresnihan B. Local

expression of the serum amyloid A and formyl peptide receptor-like 1 genes in synovial tissue is associated with matrix metalloproteinase production in patients with inflammatory arthritis. Arthritis and Rheumatism. 2004;**50**(6):1788-1799

[85] Ren SW, Qi X, Jia CK, Wang YQ. Serum amyloid A and pairing formyl peptide receptor 2 are expressed in corneas and involved in inflammation-mediated neovascularization. International Journal of Ophthalmology. 2014;**7**(2):187-193

[86] Cheng N, He R, Tian J, Ye PP, Ye RD. Cutting edge: TLR2 is a functional receptor for acute-phase serum amyloid A. Journal of Immunology. 2008;**181**(1):22-26

[87] Sandri S, Rodriguez D, Gomes E, Monteiro HP, Russo M, Campa A. Is serum amyloid A an endogenous TLR4 agonist? Journal of Leukocyte Biology. 2008;**83**:1174-1180

[88] Hansen MT, Forst B, Cremers N, Quagliata L, Ambartsumian N, Grum-Schwensen B, et al. Oncogene. 2015;**34**(4):424-435. DOI: 10.1038/onc.2013.568

[89] Ji YR, Kim HJ, Bae KB, Lee S, Kim MO, Ryoo ZY. Hepatic serum amyloid A1 aggravates T cell-mediated hepatitis by inducing chemokines via Toll-like receptor 2 in mice. The Journal of Biological Chemistry. 2015;**290**(20):12804-12811. DOI: 10.1074/jbc.M114.635763

[90] Lee JM, Kim EK, Seo H, Jeon I, Chae MJ, Park YJ, et al. Serum amyloid A3 exacerbates cancer by enhancing the suppressive capacity of myeloid-derived suppressor cells via TLR2-dependent STAT3 activation. European Journal of Immunology. 2014;**44**(6):1672-1684

[91] O'Reilly S, Cant R, Ciechomska M, Finnigan J, Oakley F, Hambleton S, et al. Serum amyloid A induces interleukin-6 in dermal fibroblasts via Toll-like receptor 2, interleukin-1 receptor-associated kinase 4 and nuclear factor-kappaB. Immunology. 2014;**143**(3):331-340. DOI: 10.1111/imm.12260

[92] Zhang G, Liu J, Wu L, Fan Y, Sun L, Qian F, et al. Elevated expression of serum amyloid A 3 protects colon epithelium against acute injury through TLR2-dependent induction of neutrophil IL-22 expression in a mouse model of colitis. Frontiers in Immunology. 2018;**9**(1503):1-11. DOI: 10.3389/fimmu.2018.01503

[93] Yan SD, Zhu H, Zhu A, Golabek A, Du H, Roher A, et al. Receptor-dependent cell stress and amyloid accumulation in systemic amyloidosis. Nature Medicine. 2000;**6**(6):643-651

[94] Okamoto H, Katagiri Y, Kiire A, Momohara S, Kamatani N. Serum amyloid A activates nuclear factor-kappaB in rheumatoid synovial fibroblasts through binding to receptor of advanced glycation end-products. The Journal of Rheumatology. 2008;**35**(5):752-756

[95] Belmokhtar K, Robert T, Ortillon J, Braconnier A, Vuiblet V, Boulagnon-Rombi C, et al. Signaling of serum amyloid A through receptor for advanced glycation end products as a possible mechanism for uremia-related atherosclerosis. Arteriosclerosis, Thrombosis, and Vascular Biology. 2016;**36**(5):800-809. DOI: 10.1161/ATVBAHA.115.306349

[96] van der Westhuyzen DR, Cai L, de Beer MC, de Beer FC. Serum amyloid A promotes cholesterol efflux mediated by scavenger receptor B-I. The Journal of Biological Chemistry. 2005;**280**(43):35890-35895

[97] Cai L, de Beer MC, de Beer FC, van der Westhuyzen DR. Serum amyloid

A is a ligand for scavenger receptor class B type I and inhibits high density lipoprotein binding and selective lipid uptake. The Journal of Biological Chemistry. 2005;**280**(4):2954-2961

[98] Baranova IN, Vishnyakova TG, Bocharov AV, Kurlander R, Chen Z, Kimelman ML, et al. Serum amyloid A binding to CLA-1 (CD36 and LIMPII analogous-1) mediates serum amyloid A protein-induced activation of ERK1/2 and p38 mitogen-activated protein kinases. The Journal of Biological Chemistry. 2005;**280**(9):8031-8040

[99] Baranova IN, Souza ACP, Bocharov AV, Vishnyakova TG, Hu X, Vaisman BL, et al. Human SR-BII mediates SAA uptake and contributes to SAA pro-inflammatory signaling in vitro and in vivo. PLoS One. 2017;**12**(4):e0175824. DOI: 10.1371/journal.pone.0175824

[100] Christenson K, Bjorkman L, Tangemo C, Bylund J. Serum amyloid A inhibits apoptosis of human neutrophils via a P2X7-sensitive pathway independent of formyl peptide receptor-like 1. Journal of Leukocyte Biology. 2008;**83**(1):139-148

[101] Shridas P, De Beer MC, Webb NR. High-density lipoprotein inhibits serum amyloid A-mediated reactive oxygen species generation and NLRP3 inflammasome activation. The Journal of Biological Chemistry. 2018;**293**(34):13257-13269. DOI: 10.1074/jbc.RA118.002428

[102] Bjorkman L, Raynes JG, Shah C, Karlsson A, Dahlgren C, Bylund J. The proinflammatory activity of recombinant serum amyloid A is not shared by the endogenous protein in the circulation. Arthritis and Rheumatism. 2010;**62**(6):1660-1665

[103] Kim MH, de Beer MC, Wroblewski JM, Webb NR, de Beer FC. SAA does not induce cytokine production in physiological conditions. Cytokine. 2013;**61**(2):506-512

[104] Christenson K, Bjorkman L, Ahlin S, Olsson M, Sjoholm K, Karlsson A, et al. Endogenous acute phase serum amyloid A lacks pro-inflammatory activity, contrasting the two recombinant variants that activate human neutrophils through different receptors. Frontiers in Immunology. 2013;**4**:92

[105] Burgess EJ, Hoyt LR, Randall MJ, Mank MM, Bivona JJ 3rd, Eisenhauer PL, et al. Bacterial lipoproteins constitute the TLR2-stimulating activity of serum amyloid A. Journal of Immunology. 2018. DOI: 10.4049/jimmunol.1800503. [Epub ahead of print]

[106] Webb NR, de Beer MC, van der Westhuyzen DR, Kindy MS, Banka CL, Tsukamoto K, et al. Adenoviral vector-mediated overexpression of serum amyloid A in apoA-I-deficient mice. Journal of Lipid Research. 1997;**38**(8):1583-1590

[107] Kindy MS, King AR, Yu J, Gerardot C, Whitley J, de Beer FC. Adenoviral expression of murine serum amyloid A proteins to study amyloid fibrillogenesis. The Biochemical Journal. 1998;**332**(Pt 3):721-728

[108] Thompson JC, Wilson PG, Shridas P, Ji A, de Beer M, de Beer FC, et al. Serum amyloid A3 is pro-atherogenic. Atherosclerosis. 2018;**268**:32-35. DOI: 10.1016/j.atherosclerosis.2017.11.011

[109] Eckhardt ER, Witta J, Zhong J, Arsenescu R, Arsenescu V, Wang Y, et al. Intestinal epithelial serum amyloid A modulates bacterial growth in vitro and pro-inflammatory responses in mouse experimental colitis. BMC Gastroenterology. 2010;**10**:133. DOI: 10.1186/1471-230X-10-133

[110] Sugimoto K, Ogawa A, Mizoguchi E, Shimomura Y, Andoh A, Bhan AK,

et al. IL-22 ameliorates intestinal inflammation in a mouse model of ulcerative colitis. The Journal of Clinical Investigation. 2008;**118**(2):534-544. DOI: 10.1172/JCI33194

[111] Sano T, Huang W, Hall JA, Yang Y, Chen A, Gavzy SJ, et al. An IL-23R/IL-22 circuit regulates epithelial serum amyloid A to promote local effector Th17 responses. Cell. 2015;**163**(2): 381-393. DOI: 10.1016/j.cell.2015.08.061

[112] Atarashi K, Tanoue T, Ando M, Kamada N, Nagano Y, Narushima S, et al. Th17 cell induction by adhesion of microbes to intestinal epithelial cells. Cell. 2015;**163**(2):367-380. DOI: 10.1016/j.cell.2015.08.058

[113] De Santo C, Arscott R, Booth S, Karydis I, Jones M, Asher R, et al. Invariant NKT cells modulate the suppressive activity of IL-10-secreting neutrophils differentiated with serum amyloid A. Nature Immunology. 2010;**11**(11):1039-1046. DOI: 10.1038/ni.1942

[114] Ahlin S, Olsson M, Olsson B, Svensson PA, Sjoholm K. No evidence for a role of adipose tissue-derived serum amyloid A in the development of insulin resistance or obesity-related inflammation in hSAA1(+/−) transgenic mice. PLoS One. 2013;**8**(8):e72204

[115] De Beer MC, Wroblewski JM, Noffsinger VP, Rateri DL, Howatt DA, Balakrishnan A, et al. Deficiency of endogenous acute phase serum amyloid A does not affect atherosclerotic lesions in apolipoprotein E-deficient mice. Arteriosclerosis, Thrombosis, and Vascular Biology. 2014;**34**(2):255-261. DOI: 10.1161/ATVBAHA.113.302247

[116] Liu J, Wang D, Li SQ, Yu Y, Ye RD. Suppression of LPS-induced tau hyperphosphorylation by serum amyloid A. Journal of Neuroinflammation. 2016;**13**:28. DOI: 10.1186/s12974-016-0493-y

[117] Shah C, Hari-Dass R, Raynes JG. Serum amyloid A is an innate immune opsonin for Gram-negative bacteria. Blood. 2006;**108**(5):1751-1757

Section 3

Onset and Development of Amyloidosis

Chapter 8

Neuropathology of Traumatic Brain Injury and Its Role in the Development of Alzheimer's Disease

Sonia Villapol

Abstract

The devastating deficiencies that result from brain injury stem from multiple overlapping mechanisms, exacerbated by the fact that there are no effective treatments. Traumatic brain injury (TBI) is recognized as the most influential environmental risk factor for neurodegenerative disease later in life, including dementia of Alzheimer's disease (AD)-type. However, exactly how TBI triggers and strengthens the neurodegenerative cascade of events in AD remains controversial. Amyloid deposits and fibril precursor protein are extracellular in systemic amyloid A (AA) amyloidosis. In this chapter, I will discuss the neuropathology following TBI connected to AD. Additionally, I critically review recent animal and human studies regarding how brain trauma affects the potential risks factors for AD progression. Furthermore, it will be shown investigate the principal pathological features of dementia or AD, specifically focusing on axonal damage and consequent cleavage of the amyloid precursor protein (APP), amyloid β plaque formation, or phosphorylation and aggregation of tau, neurofibrillary tangles formation, and TDP-43 accumulation. In summary, despite recent progress more studies are required to (1) further understanding of the basic mechanisms and pathophysiology of TBI, (2) elucidate the precise association between TBI and neurodegenerative disease, and (3) to identify treatments and therapies that can mitigate long-term consequences.

Keywords: tau, TDP-43, neurodegenerative, dementia, amyloid beta, plaques, amyloid beta deposition

1. Introduction

Traumatic brain injury (TBI) affects millions of individuals worldwide, with 1.7 million new cases in the US each year [1]. Although many patients survive the initial lesion, TBI initiates a wide variety of pathologies such as neurological deficits, short and long-term brain damage, neuroinflammation, cognitive and emotional impairments, all of which depend on the severity of the injury and other various factors [2, 3]. Brain injuries are most frequently caused by motor vehicle crashes, sports injuries, or simple falls; males are about twice as likely as females to experience a brain trauma [4]. At least 5.3 million Americans, or approximately 2% of the total US population, currently are burdened with disabilities resulting from TBI [5].

Functional deficits caused by TBI result from an initial impact and secondary damage that continue to develop over time and provide a therapeutic window for treatment to prevent or ameliorate many of the damaging consequences of injury [6]. While single compounds have been reported to be effective for short periods in standardized rodent models of TBI, therapeutic tools currently available to clinicians to treat patients with TBI are minimal.

The neuroinflammatory cascade following TBI contributes to neurodegeneration and death through the cumulative action of multiple damaging processes [7]. TBI is one of the most consistent candidates for initiating the molecular cascades that result in neurodegenerative diseases, such as Parkinson's disease (PD) or amyotrophic lateral sclerosis (ALS) [8–11]. Notably, there exists a strong epidemiological relationship between the occurrence of TBI and the development of Alzheimer's disease (AD) later in life [12–15]. The link between TBI and AD is strengthened through the identification of acute and chronic AD-like pathologies in the brain in both TBI survivors and animal models of brain injury.

AD is a progressive neurodegenerative disease, which can only be fully diagnosed at autopsy. It is characterized, histologically, by the presence of amyloid plaques and intracellular neurofibrillary tangles (NFT) in the brain [16]. The amyloid plaques consist of aggregated proteinaceous material, a significant component of amyloid β (Aβ). The tangles are composed of paired helical filaments (PHF) of the microtubule-associated phosphoprotein tau [16, 17]. In this chapter, I will describe the main pathological similarities, and differences, between TBI and AD. Although the evidence suggests that TBI is a risk factor for dementia, very little is known about what type, frequency, or severity of trauma is necessary to induce dementia [18].

A chronic disease process is initiated after TBI, known as the secondary injury cascade, and as part of this process, neuroinflammation, neuronal loss, or the production, aggregation and clearance of Aβ peptides occurs [19]. Several of these pathophysiological features have been characterized in patients with AD with similar neuropathology. Furthermore, epidemiological studies have shown how repetitive injury, or a single mild, moderate, or severe TBI, can cause a wide range of proteinopathies [20], and likely contribute to the later onset of debilitating neurodegenerative diseases. Indeed, the human pathology of survival from TBI is best described as a "polypathology", featuring Aβ, tau, and TDP-43 pathologies, together with white matter degradation, neuronal loss, and neuroinflammation [21]. There exist many pathological features common to both acute brain injury and AD, including Aβ deposition, tau phosphorylation, neurite degeneration, synapse loss and microgliosis [22]. Besides, the susceptibility of the patient may be predetermined by multiple factors such as age, sex and the interplay of several genetic factors [23–25].

The purpose of this chapter is to discuss the neuropathology and genetic risk factors associated with TBI that may collectively shed some light on the risk of developing dementia or AD following head trauma, as well as possible treatments in animal models and human studies.

2. Traumatic brain injury, neuroinflammation, and its link with Alzheimer's disease

Postmortem studies in human populations have shown microglia activation many years after TBI. Innate activation of microglia generally leads to amyloidogenic APP processing and the generation of Aβ plaques. Aβ plaques formed during the initial weeks after injury may regress with time. In this case, a continuously renewed store of Aβ in degenerating axons can be kept in check through degeneration by endogenous mediators or anti-inflammatory phagocytic microglia, or macrophages. A deficiency in microglia clearance of Aβ could possibly account for this balance shift, especially since aging microglia are known to have a reduction in phagocytic capacity and this is also observed in AD, the most common age-related dementia [13].

Compelling epidemiological evidence indicates that moderate and severe TBI is associated with increased risk of development of progressive disorders of cognitive impairment leading to dementia or AD [15, 26–28]. Therefore, TBI is considered as a strong epigenetic risk factor for AD [29, 30]. Aβ plaques, a hallmark of AD, are found in 30% of patients who do not survive TBI [13]. A history of TBI is a strong risk factor for AD, although there remains a lack of clear consensus around this topic since a few epidemiological studies have not uncovered such an association [31]. However, there exists strong evidence linking TBI to AD-related pathologies [32, 33]. Moderate and severe head injury increased the risk of AD for 2.3 and 4.5 times, respectively [30]. Although there is clinical evidence linking TBI and AD pathologies, there is an important lack of knowledge specific to the mechanisms driving this link.

In follow up studies, an increased incidence of head trauma in those with AD has been found only in males, not in females, and the risk of developing AD after TBI focused on injury severity [4, 25]. In studies where these criteria are more broadly defined, we can analyze the relative risk from head trauma of differing severity; it has been suggested [8] that a prior history of TBI accelerates the onset of AD and that the higher the incidence of severe the injury, the higher the risk of developing AD. Roberts et al. provided one of the first studies to closely examine Aβ deposition after TBI [34] (**Table 1**). Data from subsequent studies have suggested that even a single moderate to severe TBI event is a significant risk factor for the later onset of dementia or AD [35, 36].

However, it remains unknown whether patients with prior brain damage instead develop a distinct clinical phenotype of dementia, different from that of the typical AD. Examination of human brain samples confirmed that TBI

Patients (N)	Category of TBI	Pathology associated, postmortem tissue	Time after injury	References
16	Severe TBI	38% Aβ deposits, diffuse plaques	18 days of TBI	[34]
152	Severe TBI	30% Aβ diffuse deposits 20% (under 40) Aβ plaques 70% (60–80 age) Aβ plaques (50% controls)	Several times	[96]
7	TBI	Aβ42 peptide 30% Aβ diffuse deposits	Several times	[97]
18	Severe TBI	33% Aβ deposits, Aβ42 peptide, diffuse plaques 80% neuronal/glial intracellular Aβ peptides tau (PHF-1) axons	2–19 h	[36]
18	TBI	Aβ42 peptide, axonal damage, APP deposits, neurofilament, β-secretase, g-secretase Tau-positive astrocytes	4 h–5 days	[22]
11	TBI	Tau-positive oligodendrocytes	2 h	[107]

Table 1.
Patients with TBI and associated AD pathology.

Animals	Animal injury model	Pathology associated to AD	Time post-injury	Brain regions	References
Mouse (Tg2576)	Controlled cortical impact	Increase Aβ40 and Aβ42 levels	9–16 weeks	Cortex	[92]
Mouse (wild-type)	Controlled cortical impact	Increase Aβ40 oligomers and Aβ42 levels Increase pTau	3 days	Hippocampus	[37]
Mouse (3xTg-AD)	Repetitive mild TBI	Increase pTau	1 day	Fimbria	[93]
Mouse (3xTg-AD)	Controlled cortical impact	Increase Aβ40 levels Increase total Tau and pTau	1–24 h and 7 days	Cortex	[76, 108]
Mouse (h-Tau)	Repetitive mTBI	Increase pTau	21 d	Cortex	[77]
Mouse (APP-YAC)	Controlled cortical impact	Decrease Aβ40 levels, but not Aβ42	1 week	Cortex	[109]
Mouse (APPNLh/NLh)	Controlled cortical impact	Decrease of caspase-3 by administration of a pan-caspase inhibitor Reduction of caspase-cleaved APP, Aβ40 and Aβ40 Improved histological outcome	24 h 14 days	Cortex	[43]
	Controlled cortical impact	Administration of simvastatin resulted in decreased Aβ levels Decreased hippocampal tissue loss Behavioural outcome improved	3 h	Hippocampus	[110]
Mouse (BACE knock-out)	Controlled cortical impact	Increase Aβ40 Improved histological, behavioural outcomes following injury Administration of a γ-secretase inhibitor (DAPT) in non-transgenic mice improved outcomes	1–7 days	Cortex and hippocampus	[19]
	Controlled cortical impact	Increase Aβ40	23 days	Hippocampus	[111]
Mouse (PDAPP)	Controlled cortical impact	Increase Aβ40 and Aβ42 levels Increase neuronal death and memory impairment No Aβ plaques	2 h–2 months	Cortex and hippocampus	[90]
	Controlled cortical impact	Decrease in Aβ plaques	2, 5 and 8 months	Cortex and Hippocampus	[91]
	Controlled cortical impact	Decrease in Aβ plaques	16 weeks	Hippocampus	[103]

Animals	Animal injury model	Pathology associated to AD	Time post-injury	Brain regions	References
Mouse (PDAPP) and Tg2576	Controlled cortical impact	Increase Aβ baseline in transgenic and decrease Aβ after injury	2–24 h	Interstitial fluid	[112]
Mouse (PDAPP) crossed with apoE3 and apoE4	Controlled cortical impact	56% apoE4:PDAPP: increase Aβ deposition and amyloid plaques 20% apoE3:PDAPP: increase Aβ deposition and amyloid plaques	3 months	Hippocampus	[100]
Mouse (ApoE3/ApoE4), or ApoE null mice	Closed head injury	ApoE4 Die or poorer outcomes than apoE3	11 days	Cortex	[113]
Rat (Sprague Dawley)	Weight drop (open skull)	APP accumulation in damaged axons No accumulating Aβ observed intracellularly or in plaques	1, 3 and 21 days	Cortex and thalamus	[94]
	Lateral fluid percussion	APP accumulation in damaged axons No accumulating Aβ observed intracellularly or in plaques	1 h, 2 h, 48 h, 1 week, or 2 weeks	Cortex, striatum, cingulum, and hippocampus	[95]
	Lateral fluid percussion	Reduction of Aβ accumulated in damage axons according with severity of injury	2 days–1 year	White matter, cortex and thalamus	[114]
	Lateral fluid percussion	Increase pTau	6 months	White matter, cortex	[115]
	Weight drop (open skull)	APP and Aβ identified in damaged axons No Aβ plaques observed	6 h–10 days	White matter	[44]
	Controlled cortical impact	Increase cleaved Tau	6–168 h	Cortex	[116]
Swine	Rotational acceleration (model of DAI)	APP and Aβ accumulation Diffuse Aβ plaques Increase total Tau	3–10 days	White matter and cortex	[117]
	Rotational acceleration (model of DAI)	Aβ, APP, BACE and presenilin-1 accumulation in damaged axons Diffuse Aβ plaques	3h, 3 days, 6 months	Subcortical white matter	[65]

Table 2.
Animal studies on TBI and associated AD pathology.

processes were the principal driver of accumulation of Aβ peptides in swollen axons shortly after TBI, which persisted for years following the initial trauma [13]. In addition to such clinical studies, there exist multiple types of brain injuries in different animal models of AD. These animal models have been used to examine the formation, aggregation, and accumulation of Aβ after injury; almost all of these are demonstrated an elevation in Aβ levels after TBI (**Table 2**).

3. Neuropathology of TBI: related proteins

TBI regulates the expression patterns of several proteins commonly associated with neurodegenerative diseases, such as α-synuclein, amyloid precursor protein, Aβ, TDP-43, and tau [37–40] (**Figure 1**). Besides, the ApoE4 gene and their cleaved products are implicated in neurodegenerative disorders, axonal pathology, and apoptosis following TBI [41, 42]. TBI also induces caspase-3, which is involved in APP processing, contributing to AD [43, 44]. This increase in APP expression and neuroinflammatory response following injury may contribute to a cycle of Aβ deposition and microglial activation that ultimately result in chronic neuropathology [45, 46]. In this section, I will summarize the principal proteins involved in TBI and AD and their associated factors in the neurodegenerative process.

3.1 Amyloid precursor protein (APP)

APP and its proteolytic derivatives are important mediators of neuronal synaptogenesis and synapse maintenance [47]. APP functions in the axonal transport of vesicles and presenilin (PS) regulate intracellular protein trafficking, highlighting the role of APP as a synaptic vesicle protein [47]. TBI leads to overexpression

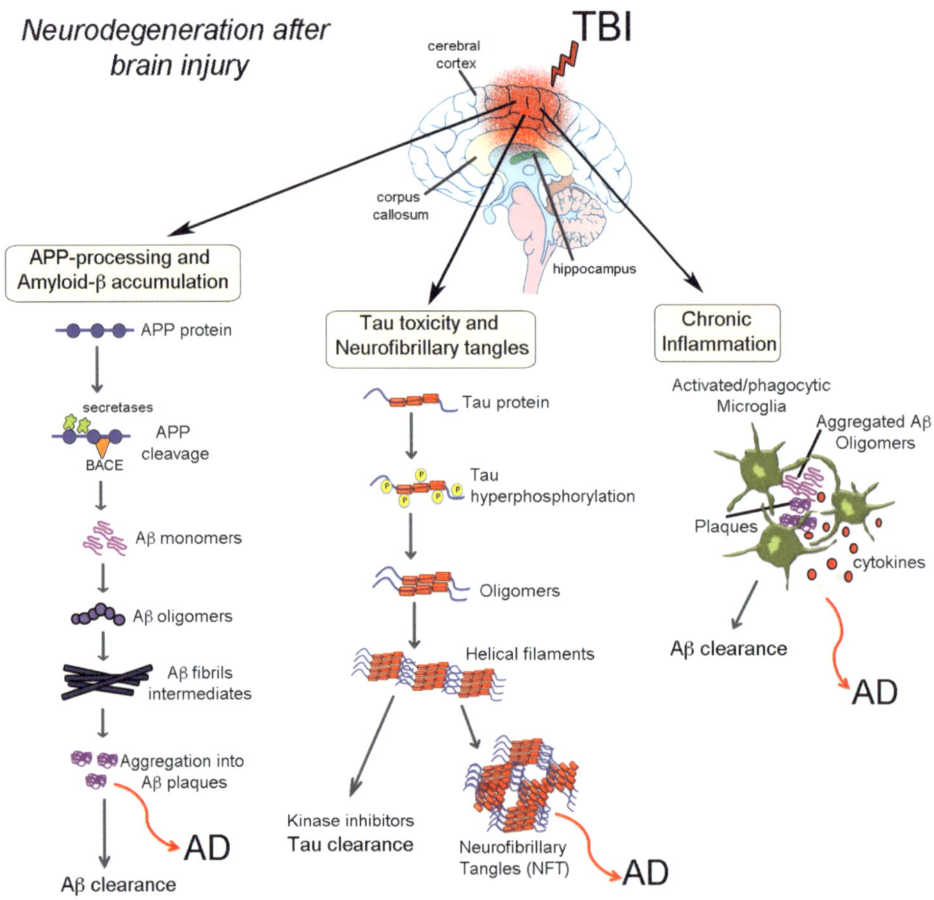

Figure 1.
Relationship between neuropathological proteins induced after brain injury and the onset of Alzheimer's disease. Schematic diagram showing that traumatic brain injury (TBI) and Alzheimer's disease (AD) share similar pathological pathways (such Aβ pathologies and TDP-43 proteinopathy) and neuroinflammatory responses that potentially could explain the vulnerability of TBI patients to the onset of dementia/AD.

of APP within neuronal cell bodies and APP accumulation within injured axons [48] (**Figure 2C**). Postmortem studies on human brain tissue samples from patients who have sustained mild TBI, but died due to other causes, have shown that APP accumulation occurs very rapidly (within a few hours) after brain [49]. Once mature, APP can be processed by two mutually exclusive complex pathways, either the non-amyloidogenic or the amyloidogenic pathway [50]. The non-amyloidogenic pathway accounts for the majority of APP processing and results in the secreted APP (sAPPα) via α-secretase cleavage [51]. The β- and γ-secretase pathway is responsible for producing secreted APPβ (sAPPβ) and the toxic Aβ, which is found within amyloid plaques in AD [52]. Both axonal APP accumulation and long-term accumulation of Aβ has been reported in injured axons following TBI [53]. This large reservoir of APP in axons might be aberrantly cleaved to form Aβ [49]. Evidence for the role of caspase-3 in APP cleavage and Aβ production has come from recent studies examining the effects of caspase inhibition following trauma [43]. APP undergoes sequential proteolysis to produce plaque-forming Aβ peptides.

3.2 Amyloid β formation and amyloid plaques

3.2.1 Protein amyloid-β

Amyloid is a highly-ordered filamentous protein aggregate generally regarded as a misfolding event in which proteins that are soluble accumulate into fibrous structures [54]. However, determinants of amyloid formation and toxicity are largely unknown.

Edema, inflammatory response, vasculature changes, and deposition of Aβ have all been found to be localized pathological changes after TBI [55]. As such, an understanding of the mechanism promoting AD risk is important. Although TBI is typically believed to be a static pathological insult from a single event, new clinical unrecognized clinical symptoms can arise many years after the initial injury. In human studies, TBI has been shown to result in amyloid deposits reminiscent of AD pathology.

Aβ immunoreactivity and protein expression increase for as long as a year after injury, indicating that Aβ aggregation and plaques formation may continue long after APP gene expression returns to normal. Plaques found in TBI patients are strikingly similar to those observed in the early stages of AD [13, 14]. However, TBI-associated plaques can appear rapidly (within hours) after injury, whereas plaques in AD develop slowly and are found predominantly in the elderly [13].

Monomeric forms of Aβ can aggregate to form oligomers, protofibrils; these fibrils deposit as amyloid plaque (**Figure 1**), unaggregated oligomeric forms of Aβ may contribute to toxicity after TBI [56]. Aβ causes apoptotic cell death of neuronal cells in culture by the induction of caspases, known instigators of apoptotic cell death [57]. Accumulation of Aβ deposits, hippocampal damage, and chronic inflammation were found mainly in subcortical regions [18]. Early microglial accumulation in AD delays disease progression by promoting clearance of neurotoxic Aβ peptides before the formation of senile plaques. However, as AD mice age, microglia become dysfunctional, producing proinflammatory cytokines in response to Aβ aggregation downregulate genes involved in Aβ clearance [58].

3.2.2 Mechanisms of post-traumatic amyloid-β formation

The intracellular accumulation of Aβ, extracellular deposition of soluble Aβ plaques, and aggregation of tau protein have all been observed in patients, sometimes within hours after severe brain injury [59, 60]. Aβ accumulation and amyloid

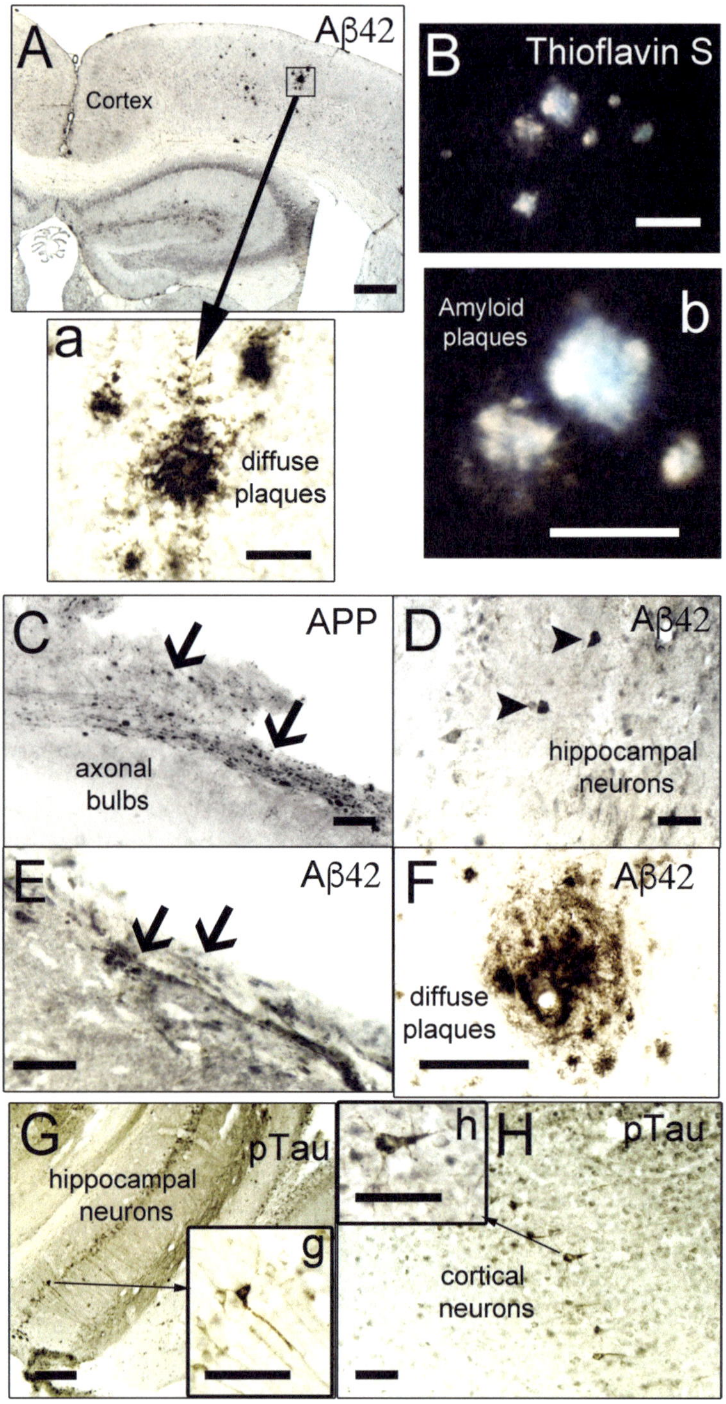

Figure 2.
Representative immunohistochemical images showing neurodegenerative markers in a mouse model of Alzheimer's disease after brain injury. (A) Aβ plaques detected using Aβ42 antibody in the cortex of AD model mice (3xTg-AD, 9 months old mice) (inset in A, high magnification in a). (B) Aβ plaques detected using Thioflavin-S staining in the cortex of old 3xTg-AD (B, high magnification in b). (C) Representative broken axons stained with APP showing axonal bulbs found acutely following TBI in wild-type mice. (D–F) Aβ42 diffuse plaques were identifying using an antibody specific for Aβ42 and were not detected by Thioflavin-S staining, in the CA1 hippocampal region (D), in the corpus callosum (E), and in the cortex (F) of wild-type mice. (G–H) Hippocampal neurons were stained using an antibody for phosphorylated tau in the CA1 hippocampus (G, high magnification in g) and cortical pyramidal layer (H, high magnification in h) after TBI in old 3xTg-AD mice. Scale bars: 200 μm (A), 50 μm (B–H), and 20 μm (a, b, f, g, and h).

deposition precede the cognitive decline in Alzheimer's disease, with the pathology arriving later, and is associated with non-Alzheimer's disease dementia. Deposition of amyloid plaques from Aβ peptide in Alzheimer's disease or acute phase of TBI have previously been reported to involve either mononuclear phagocytes, endocytic uptake, or proteolytic processing of the APP during fibril formation [61, 62]. Levels of Aβ were found to be high days after TBI and then declined towards control levels in the subsequent 2 weeks. It has been suggested that a long-term process of Aβ metabolism is initiated by TBI, which can be cleaved to form Aβ. Both species of Aβ, Aβ40, and Aβ42, are increased in the first week after injury in the CSF of TBI patients; other studies have shown comparatively lower Aβ40 levels compared to high levels of Aβ42 [63]. Intracellular Aβ accumulation of non-plaque species of Aβ is more common than plaque deposition after TBI. Aβ is produced by sequential cleavage of the amyloid precursor protein APP via two enzymes, β- and γ-secretase. Depending on the cleavage point of γ-secretase, Aβ peptides of different amino acid length are produced. The two most closely linked to AD are Aβ40 and Aβ42 [64]. The accumulation of Aβ peptides is thought to be a major initiator event in AD pathogenesis (**Figure 1**). TBI leading to impaired axonal transport induces a long-term pathological co-accumulation of APP with β-site APP-cleavage enzyme 1 (BACE1), presenilin 1 and activated caspases, thus providing a possible mechanism for APP cleavage and production of Aβ within axons following TBI [65]. The release of Aβ (especially Aβ42) into tissue and plaque formation around damaged axons occurs after APP accumulation and Aβ production in damaged axons. Both presenilin-1 (PS1) and BACE were found in swollen axons in the swine model and in humans (**Table 2**). Targeting the APP secretase enzymes can prevent the increase in Aβ after TBI [19], specifically, Aβ42 was found to accumulate in the axonal bulbs of injured brains [22]. BACE1 and PS1 were increased in the damaged axons of TBI patients, and our previous studies have also shown that BACE1 and PS1 are considered the promising targets for the treatment of TBI [19].

Plaques have also been observed in pericontusional tissue surgically excised from survivors of TBI. Nevertheless, the key pathological similarity between TBI with AD is the observation that Aβ plaques are found in up to 30% of patients who die of acute TBI [14]. While TBI-associated plaques largely appear in the gray matter, they have also been identified in white matter. Amyloid plaques consist primarily of aggregated Aβ peptides, which are surrounded by dystrophic neurites, microglia, and reactive astrocytes [66, 67].

3.3 Tau protein and neurofibrillary tangles

The tau protein is associated with microtubules and plays a role in the outgrowth of neuronal processes and the development of neuronal polarity [68]. Misfolded and aggregated tau causes a gain of toxic function by hindering normal and axonal processes; axonal neurodegeneration due to the loss of tau is caused by a decrease in tau microtubule binding capabilities [69, 70]. Tau oligomerization is known as a critical mechanism in the development of NFTs, consisting of hyperphosphorylated tau proteins with pathological function [71]. AD is also characterized by intracellular hyperphosphorylated tau that constitutes the NFTs and senile plaques and is one of the most common tauopathies [72]. Furthermore, toxic tau proteins increase within hours after clinical brain injury [22], and their release and spreading effect may also contribute to the development of tauopathy following TBI [73]. It was described that the spatial pattern of the tau-immunoreactive pathology observed in chronic traumatic encephalopathy (CTE) is typical of the tauopathies [74]. The tau from both TBI and AD brains is phosphorylated at the same amino acids, resulting in the proteolytic cleavage of six isoforms known as cleaved tau (c-tau), including the AT8 epitope [75]. Hyperphosphorylated Tau has been shown to increase between 1 and 7 days after moderate TBI in triple transgenic AD mice [76] and at 3 weeks after repetitive mild TBI in the human Tau (hTau) tauopathy mouse model [77] (**Table 2**). Experimental studies in animal models suggest that intra-axonal tau accumulation and tau phosphorylation may be in fact the consequences of repeated brain trauma or dementia pugilistica/CTE [78]. Today, CTE is used to define the neurological sequelae and neuropathological changes that occur as a result of repeat concussive or subconcussive blows to the head. Besides, the pathology of CTE is also characterized as a tauopathy, a class of neurodegenerative disease caused by the pathological aggregation of tau protein [78]. In CTE, NFTs also consist of hyperphosphorylated and ubiquitinated tau [79, 80]. Tau degradation in boxers with CTE are structurally and chemically similar to those seen in AD and frontotemporal lobar degeneration (FTLD) [80]. Treatment with γ-secretase inhibitors diminishes amyloid pathology but does not affect TBI-induced tangle formation, suggesting that TBI-induced tau pathology is not a downstream event of Aβ and plaque formation [81].

3.4 TDP-43 pathology

TAR DNA-binding protein (TDP-43) protein has been identified as a regulator of gene expression and exon splicing with DNA and RNA binding capabilities. Hence, though TDP-43 is synthesized in the cytoplasm and resides in the nucleus of neurons and glia, under pathological conditions TDP-43 is accumulated in the cytoplasm in the form of ubiquitinated and hyperphosphorylated inclusions [82] (**Figure 1**). Pathological TDP-43 has been identified as the main disease-associated protein in ALS and FTLD. It has also been recognized as a secondary feature in many other neurodegenerative diseases, including Huntington disease, AD and PD [83]. Axonal damage results in an upregulation of TDP-43 expression, together with a redistribution of TDP-43 from the nuclear compartment to the cytoplasm [33, 84]. TBI induces TDP-43 abnormalities that can contribute to the neurological consequences of TBI, such as worse cell death, and cognitive deficits [85]. TDP-43 proteinopathy is also part of the acute or delayed pathological sequelae of repetitive mild, concussive TBI or CTE pathogenesis [86, 87]. The TDP-43 proteinopathy associated with CTE is similar to that found in FTLD with TDP-43 inclusions [87]. Intraneuronal accumulation of non-phosphorylated TDP-43 after a single TBI has also been reported [88]. Contrarily, related studies failed to demonstrate an association between single TBI and TDP-43 proteinopathy, only with repetitive TBI, indicating that just many insults reinforcing acute upregulation are sufficient to cause TDP-43 aggregation. Importantly, aggregates of phospho-TDP-43 were not increased long-term following TBI [88]. To the best of our knowledge, a clear functional role of altered TDP-43 expression levels after TBI has not been demonstrated, though this might disrupt signaling pathways involved in neuronal dysfunction, as some authors have suggested [89].

4. AD pathology in animal models of brain trauma

Several experimental animal models of TBI have been utilized in the attempt to replicate amyloid and tau pathologies, as well as other proteinopathies associated to AD. Some of these have been summarized in **Table 2**. Animal models of TBI show elevated Aβ levels, Aβ production, and Aβ deposition, specific to the brain region and anatomy and varying with the type of injury. Observed in mice that overexpress normal human APP, there is an increase in tissue concentrations of Aβ after injury, associated with an increase in hippocampal neuronal death and memory impairment [43]. However, TBI alone does not seem to induce acute plaque formation systematically. Controlled cerebral impact (CCI) injury in an APP transgenic mouse model (PDAPP) has been shown to result in a spike in Aβ40 and Aβ42, peaking at 2 h post-injury and returning to baseline by 6 h [90]. Studies in PDAPP mice over greater intervals have shown that CCI can decrease the deposition of Aβ in the ipsilateral cortex and hippocampus, up to 4–8 months after injury, compared to the uninjured side of the brain [91]. Additionally, CCI injuries, using in a different APP transgenic mouse model (Tg2576), have been shown cause elevated soluble and insoluble cortical Aβ40 and Aβ42 levels as well as amyloid plaque deposition [92]. Finally, studies in $APP^{NLh/NLh}$ mice, a gene-targeted mouse model that expresses normal levels of human APP, yielded elevated Aβ40 levels via inhibition of caspase-3 activity, only for the first 24 h after CCI, while Aβ42 levels remain elevated through 14 days [43]. Repetitive TBI is known to cause cumulative damage. After mild TBI in mice, during two consecutive days, studies have reported delayed recovery from fine motor coordination deficits as well as evidence of enhanced blood-brain barrier breakdown accompanied by axonal injury [21]. A recent study in an animal model using a triple-transgenic mouse model of Alzheimer's disease (3xTg-AD), the effect of repetitive mild TBI caused an increase of tau hyperphosphorylation and activation of asparaginyl endopeptidase (AEP), a cysteine proteinase which is known to be involved in tau phosphorylation [93].

In contrast, repetitive TBI in a Tg2576 APP-transgenic mice model did result in greater Aβ deposition as well as an increase in the production of both soluble and insoluble cortical Aβ40 and Aβ42, which may be a result of the higher levels of oxidative stress after repetitive TBI [92]. However, TBI does not lead to early amyloid plaque formation in transgenic mice, and at later times there is a reduction in amyloid plaques in ipsilateral injury regions [90, 91]. Also, Aβ accumulation was identified in damaged axons shortly after brain injury, albeit still in the absence of Aβ plaques [94, 95]. However, the lack of evidence of Aβ deposition in non-transgenic animals was attributed, in part, to differences in the Aβ peptides found in different species. Experimental results of moderate and severe TBI studies in transgenic models of AD are also contrasted with that seen in human TBI (**Table 1**). First, rapid Aβ deposition has not been demonstrated in any of the described transgenic models, unlike human studies [34, 36, 96, 97]. Second, increased severity of the injury does not result in increased Aβ deposition; instead, it seems to correlate with reduced Aβ deposition or possibly resolution of previously established plaques, as reported by [98]. In summary, all the animal models mentioned above provide important information regarding the potentially detrimental consequences of elevated Aβ levels following TBI. However, post-traumatic Aβ deposition has not been observed in the majority of non-transgenic animal studies; most failed to identify plaque pathology that is commonly observed following human TBI. To better understand the effects of repeat trauma on the brain, an animal model that can model the disease after repetitive trauma is required. Unfortunately, such an experimental model does not yet exist and will be challenging to generate.

5. Apolipoprotein E4 allele and TBI increase the risk of developing AD

The epidemiology of both AD and TBI are dominated by a single genetic risk factor, the APOE genotype. In humans, there are three distinct isoforms of the protein: apoE2, apoE3, and apoE4, distinguished by three alleles [99]. The apoE ε4 allele confers strong susceptibility for AD and is also the factor for the development of amyloid plaques after TBI. Furthermore, the apoE ε4 allele has been associated with increased Aβ in the cerebral cortex and unfavorable outcome after TBI [100]. ApoE4 individuals were over 10 times more likely to develop AD after severe TBI than those who did not posse the allele [101], and the presence of an apoE4 allele is linked to poor recovery from extended coma. Professional boxers containing the apoE ε4 allele were at increased risk of CTE compared to boxers without the apoE ε4 allele [102]. This finding suggests that genetic factors may strongly influence the risk of CTE after brain injury. However, the possibility remains that certain boxers may be innately 'resistant' to developing AD or dementia following CTE; definitely, not all boxers go on to develop AD, despite repetitive injury and having the higher risk genotype. Consistent with a role of ApoE protein in amyloid deposition in humans, apoE4 also increases amyloid plaque formation in mice. Aβ deposition is also significantly increased following head trauma in PDAPP (platelet-derived growth factor promoter expressing amyloid precursor protein) mice carrying the human apoE ε4 allele versus those carrying apoE ε3 or no apoE (**Table 2**) [103]. Finally, transgenic APOE ε4 mice, which also overexpress APP, show accelerated deposition of Aβ following injury, suggesting apoE ε4 may reduce the clearance of Aβ, thereby favoring its deposition [100] (**Table 2**). Some recent reports are controversial clinical and preclinical studies about the link between poor outcome after severe and mild TBI and the APOE4 gene [11, 16, 30, 104, 105].

6. Similarities and differences in the neuropathology of TBI and AD

The similarities and differences in the neuropathology associated to TBI and AD are complex. Aβ formation and aggregation, tau phosphorylation, including other proteins found in the brain and CSF following TBI, share a lot of similarities with AD, but also several evident differences. Principally, the localization and distribution of proteins in TBI patients are fundamentally distinct from the characteristic pattern commonly observed in AD [13]. However, one strong similarity between TBI and AD is in the Aβ plaque formation; both are primarily composed of Aβ 41–42, furthermore, CSF levels of Aβ are increased similarly for both [106]. However, in AD there are numerous, compact, core Aβ aggregates in addition to neurofibrillary tangles and neuropil threads, this in contrast to TBI where there appears to be a higher prevalence of diffuse Aβ plaques [34, 36]. Notably, Aβ plaques in TBI are typically described as diffuse and do not display the histochemical or morphological features of the senile plaques that are characteristic of AD [35]. Aβ toxicity only emerges when levels exceed a certain threshold, and unaggregated oligomeric forms of Aβ may contribute to toxicity. As such, rapid aggregation of Aβ into plaques may be a protective event following TBI [73]. In CTE, the tau inclusions are morphologically most similar to those found in AD, with pyramidal neurons maintaining their shape, and tangles consisting of hyperphosphorylated and ubiquitinated tau [84]. This phospho-tau staining was also observed in axons and clusters of neuronal cell bodies in the cerebral cortex and hippocampus (**Figure 2G** and **H**). Such studies have also noted the existence of tau-positive reactive astrocytes in AD, a pathology that is not usually associated with AD. Finally, the tau immunoreactive profile of CTE is characteristically very patchy and irregular, with preferential deposition in the superficial neocortical layers, while tangles in AD are found in deep and in superficial layers [33]. In summary, while there are certain important differences between mild, moderate, and severe TBI and dementia or AD, given the significant overlap in neuropathology, there is still much that can be gleaned by closely comparing the molecular and cellular mechanisms involved in both of these neuropathological processes.

7. Conclusions

The association between trauma and the onset of neurodegenerative diseases, such as AD, is extremely convoluted, further complicated by the absence of appropriate animal models able to reproduce human pathologies. Elucidation of this nature of this link remains in its infancy, requiring extensive further research to chip away at the underlying relationship. Moreover, quantification of the relative contributions of various risk factors for developing these pathologies, such as cellular and molecular mechanisms, frequency and severity of the injury, age, sex, and potential genetic predisposition, remain mostly imprecise. Although we do not know how TBI fundamentally impacts the long-term outcome and affects the risk of dementia, it remains clear that amyloid pathways play an important role in secondary injury and acute cell death after trauma. Continued efforts to investigate why TBI, and repeat concussions, may lead to AD and other associated dementias are required. Further understanding of the molecular mechanism underlying these events is required, achievable via better designed animal models able to more closely and accurately mimic the observed behavioral and pathological changes. Only then will we be well equipped to precisely evaluate novel therapeutic agents that may intervene in the disease process. Future research will be required to uncover the mechanisms through which TBI increases the risk of AD, opening the door to designer treatment strategies for the full scope of post-traumatic injuries.

Acknowledgements

This work was supported by R21NS106640 (SV) and R03NS09503 (SV) from the National Institute for Neurological Disorders and Stroke (NINDS).

Conflict of interest

There are no conflicts of interest to disclose.

Author details

Sonia Villapol[1,2]

1 Center for Neuroregeneration and Department of Neurosurgery, Institute for Academic Medicine, Houston Methodist Research Institute, Houston, TX, USA

2 Department of Neuroscience in Neurological Surgery, Weill Cornell Medical College, NY, USA

*Address all correspondence to: svillapol@houstonmethodist.org

References

[1] Zitnay GA. Lessons from national and international TBI societies and funds like NBIRTT. Acta Neurochirurgica. Supplement. 2005;**93**:131-133

[2] Chua KS, Ng YS, Yap SG, Bok CW. A brief review of traumatic brain injury rehabilitation. Annals of the Academy of Medicine, Singapore. 2007;**36**(1):31-42

[3] Kibby MY, Long CJ. Minor head injury: Attempts at clarifying the confusion. Brain Injury. 1996;**10**(3):159-186

[4] Taylor CA, Bell JM, Breiding MJ, Xu L. Traumatic brain injury-related emergency department visits, hospitalizations, and deaths—United States, 2007 and 2013. MMWR Surveillance Summaries. 2017;**66**(9):1-16

[5] Langlois JA, Rutland-Brown W, Wald MM. The epidemiology and impact of traumatic brain injury: A brief overview. The Journal of Head Trauma Rehabilitation. 2006;**21**(5):375-378

[6] Clausen T, Bullock R. Medical treatment and neuroprotection in traumatic brain injury. Current Pharmaceutical Design. 2001;**7**(15):1517-1532

[7] Mendez MF. What is the relationship of traumatic brain injury to dementia? Journal of Alzheimer's Disease. 2017;**57**(3):667-681

[8] Little DM, Geary EK, Moynihan M, Alexander A, Pennington M, Glang P, et al. Imaging chronic traumatic brain injury as a risk factor for neurodegeneration. Alzheimer's & Dementia. 2014;**10**(3 Suppl):S188-S195

[9] Mouzon BC, Bachmeier C, Ferro A, Ojo JO, Crynen G, Acker CM, et al. Chronic neuropathological and neurobehavioral changes in a repetitive mild traumatic brain injury model. Annals of Neurology. 2014;**75**(2):241-254

[10] Gavett BE, Stern RA, Cantu RC, Nowinski CJ, McKee AC. Mild traumatic brain injury: A risk factor for neurodegeneration. Alzheimer's Research & Therapy. 2010;**2**(3):18

[11] Jellinger KA. Head injury and dementia. Current Opinion in Neurology. 2004;**17**(6):719-723

[12] Breunig JJ, Guillot-Sestier MV, Town T. Brain injury, neuroinflammation and Alzheimer's disease. Frontiers in Aging Neuroscience. 2013;**5**:26

[13] Johnson VE, Stewart W, Smith DH. Traumatic brain injury and amyloid-beta pathology: A link to Alzheimer's disease? Nature Reviews. Neuroscience. 2010;**11**(5):361-370

[14] Sivanandam TM, Thakur MK. Traumatic brain injury: A risk factor for Alzheimer's disease. Neuroscience and Biobehavioral Reviews. 2012;**36**(5):1376-1381

[15] Van Den Heuvel C, Thornton E, Vink R. Traumatic brain injury and Alzheimer's disease: A review. Progress in Brain Research. 2007;**161**:303-316

[16] Jellinger KA, Bancher C. Neuropathology of Alzheimer's disease: A critical update. Journal of Neural Transmission. Supplementum. 1998;**54**:77-95

[17] Dickson DW. Neuropathological diagnosis of Alzheimer's disease: A perspective from longitudinal clinicopathological studies. Neurobiology of Aging. 1997;**18**(4 Suppl):S21-S26

[18] Wang HK, Lin SH, Sung PS, Wu MH, Hung KW, Wang LC, et al. Population based study on patients with traumatic brain injury suggests increased risk of dementia. Journal of Neurology, Neurosurgery, and Psychiatry. 2012;**83**(11):1080-1085

[19] Loane DJ, Pocivavsek A, Moussa CE, Thompson R, Matsuoka Y, Faden AI, et al. Amyloid precursor protein secretases as therapeutic targets for traumatic brain injury. Nature Medicine. 2009;**15**(4):377-379

[20] Kenney K, Iacono D, Edlow BL, Katz DI, Diaz-Arrastia R, Dams-O'Connor K, et al. Dementia after moderate-severe traumatic brain injury: Coexistence of multiple proteinopathies. Journal of Neuropathology and Experimental Neurology. 2018;**77**(1):50-63

[21] Zakaria N, Kallakuri S, Bandaru S, Cavanaugh JM. Temporal assessment of traumatic axonal injury in the rat corpus callosum and optic chiasm. Brain Research. 2012;**1467**:81-90

[22] Uryu K, Chen XH, Martinez D, Browne KD, Johnson VE, Graham DI, et al. Multiple proteins implicated in neurodegenerative diseases accumulate in axons after brain trauma in humans. Experimental Neurology. 2007;**208**(2):185-192

[23] Sundman MH, Hall EE, Chen NK. Examining the relationship between head trauma and neurodegenerative disease: A review of epidemiology, pathology and neuroimaging techniques. Journal of Alzheimers Disease & Parkinsonism. 2014;**4**:137. DOI: 10.4172/2161-0460.1000137

[24] Zandi PP, Carlson MC, Plassman BL, Welsh-Bohmer KA, Mayer LS, Steffens DC, et al. Hormone replacement therapy and incidence of Alzheimer disease in older women: The Cache County Study. Journal of the American Medical Association. 2002;**288**(17):2123-2129

[25] O'Meara ES, Kukull WA, Sheppard L, Bowen JD, McCormick WC, Teri L, et al. Head injury and risk of Alzheimer's disease by apolipoprotein E genotype. American Journal of Epidemiology. 1997;**146**(5):373-384

[26] Julien J, Joubert S, Ferland MC, Frenette LC, Boudreau-Duhaime MM, Malo-Veronneau L, et al. Association of traumatic brain injury and Alzheimer disease onset: A systematic review. Annals of Physical and Rehabilitation Medicine. 2017;**60**(5):347-356

[27] Plassman BL, Grafman J. Traumatic brain injury and late-life dementia. Handbook of Clinical Neurology. 2015;**128**:711-722

[28] Lye TC, Shores EA. Traumatic brain injury as a risk factor for Alzheimer's disease: A review. Neuropsychology Review. 2000;**10**(2):115-129

[29] Magnoni S, Brody DL. New perspectives on amyloid-beta dynamics after acute brain injury: Moving between experimental approaches and studies in the human brain. Archives of Neurology. 2010;**67**(9):1068-1073

[30] Plassman BL, Havlik RJ, Steffens DC, Helms MJ, Newman TN, Drosdick D, et al. Documented head injury in early adulthood and risk of Alzheimer's disease and other dementias. Neurology. 2000;**55**(8):1158-1166

[31] Washington PM, Villapol S, Burns MP. Polypathology and dementia after brain trauma: Does brain injury trigger distinct neurodegenerative diseases, or should they be classified together as traumatic encephalopathy? Experimental Neurology. 2016;**275**(Pt 3):381-388

[32] Shively S, Scher AI, Perl DP, Diaz-Arrastia R. Dementia resulting from traumatic brain injury: What is the

pathology? Archives of Neurology. 2012;**69**(10):1245-1251

[33] Blennow K, Hardy J, Zetterberg H. The neuropathology and neurobiology of traumatic brain injury. Neuron. 2012;**76**(5):886-899

[34] Roberts GW, Gentleman SM, Lynch A, Graham DI. Beta A4 amyloid protein deposition in brain after head trauma. Lancet. 1991;**338**(8780):1422-1423

[35] DeKosky ST, Abrahamson EE, Ciallella JR, Paljug WR, Wisniewski SR, Clark RS, et al. Association of increased cortical soluble abeta42 levels with diffuse plaques after severe brain injury in humans. Archives of Neurology. 2007;**64**(4):541-544

[36] Ikonomovic MD, Uryu K, Abrahamson EE, Ciallella JR, Trojanowski JQ, Lee VM, et al. Alzheimer's pathology in human temporal cortex surgically excised after severe brain injury. Experimental Neurology. 2004;**190**(1):192-203

[37] Yu F, Zhang Y, Chuang DM. Lithium reduces BACE1 overexpression, beta amyloid accumulation, and spatial learning deficits in mice with traumatic brain injury. Journal of Neurotrauma. 2012;**29**(13):2342-2351

[38] Su E, Bell MJ, Wisniewski SR, Adelson PD, Janesko-Feldman KL, Salonia R, et al. Alpha-Synuclein levels are elevated in cerebrospinal fluid following traumatic brain injury in infants and children: The effect of therapeutic hypothermia. Developmental Neuroscience. 2010;**32**(5-6):385-395

[39] Surgucheva I, He S, Rich MC, Sharma R, Ninkina NN, Stahel PF, et al. Role of synucleins in traumatic brain injury—An experimental in vitro and in vivo study in mice. Molecular and Cellular Neurosciences. 2014;**63C**:114-123

[40] Laskowitz DT, Song P, Wang H, Mace B, Sullivan PM, Vitek MP, et al. Traumatic brain injury exacerbates neurodegenerative pathology: Improvement with an apolipoprotein E-based therapeutic. Journal of Neurotrauma. 2010;**27**(11):1983-1995

[41] Chauhan NB. Chronic neurodegenerative consequences of traumatic brain injury. Restorative Neurology and Neuroscience. 2014;**32**(2):337-365

[42] Sun XC, Jiang Y. Genetic susceptibility to traumatic brain injury and apolipoprotein E gene. Chinese Journal of Traumatology. 2008;**11**(4):247-252

[43] Abrahamson EE, Ikonomovic MD, Ciallella JR, Hope CE, Paljug WR, Isanski BA, et al. Caspase inhibition therapy abolishes brain trauma-induced increases in Abeta peptide: Implications for clinical outcome. Experimental Neurology. 2006;**197**(2):437-450

[44] Stone JR, Okonkwo DO, Singleton RH, Mutlu LK, Helm GA, Povlishock JT. Caspase-3-mediated cleavage of amyloid precursor protein and formation of amyloid Beta peptide in traumatic axonal injury. Journal of Neurotrauma. 2002;**19**(5):601-614

[45] Hellewell SC, Yan EB, Agyapomaa DA, Bye N, Morganti-Kossmann MC. Post-traumatic hypoxia exacerbates brain tissue damage: Analysis of axonal injury and glial responses. Journal of Neurotrauma. 2010;**27**(11):1997-2010

[46] Chen XH, Johnson VE, Uryu K, Trojanowski JQ, Smith DH. A lack of amyloid beta plaques despite persistent accumulation of amyloid beta in axons of long-term survivors of traumatic brain injury. Brain Pathology. 2009;**19**(2):214-223

[47] Groemer TW, Thiel CS, Holt M, Riedel D, Hua Y, Huve J, et al. Amyloid precursor protein is trafficked and secreted via synaptic vesicles. PLoS One. 2011;**6**(4):e18754

[48] Itoh T, Satou T, Nishida S, Tsubaki M, Hashimoto S, Ito H. Expression of amyloid precursor protein after rat traumatic brain injury. Neurological Research. 2009;**31**(1):103-109

[49] Marklund N, Farrokhnia N, Hanell A, Vanmechelen E, Enblad P, Zetterberg H, et al. Monitoring of beta-amyloid dynamics after human traumatic brain injury. Journal of Neurotrauma. 2014;**31**(1):42-55

[50] Kowalska A. The beta-amyloid cascade hypothesis: A sequence of events leading to neurodegeneration in Alzheimer's disease. Neurologia i Neurochirurgia Polska. 2004;**38**(5):405-411

[51] Kojro E, Fahrenholz F. The non-amyloidogenic pathway: Structure and function of alpha-secretases. Sub-Cellular Biochemistry. 2005;**38**:105-127

[52] Mattson MP, Barger SW, Furukawa K, Bruce AJ, Wyss-Coray T, Mark RJ, et al. Cellular signaling roles of TGF beta, TNF alpha and beta APP in brain injury responses and Alzheimer's disease. Brain Research. Brain Research Reviews. 1997;**23**(1-2):47-61

[53] Smith DH, Chen XH, Iwata A, Graham DI. Amyloid beta accumulation in axons after traumatic brain injury in humans. Journal of Neurosurgery. 2003;**98**(5):1072-1077

[54] Harrison RS, Sharpe PC, Singh Y, Fairlie DP. Amyloid peptides and proteins in review. Reviews of Physiology, Biochemistry and Pharmacology. 2007;**159**:1-77

[55] Muller UC, Deller T, Korte M. Not just amyloid: Physiological functions of the amyloid precursor protein family. Nature Reviews. Neuroscience. 2017;**18**(5):281-298

[56] Hardy J, Selkoe DJ. The amyloid hypothesis of Alzheimer's disease: Progress and problems on the road to therapeutics. Science. 2002;**297**(5580):353-356

[57] Tweedie D, Milman A, Holloway HW, Li Y, Harvey BK, Shen H, et al. Apoptotic and behavioral sequelae of mild brain trauma in mice. Journal of Neuroscience Research. 2007;**85**(4):805-815

[58] Hickman SE, Allison EK, El Khoury J. Microglial dysfunction and defective beta-amyloid clearance pathways in aging Alzheimer's disease mice. The Journal of Neuroscience. 2008;**28**(33):8354-8360

[59] Davies NM, Kehoe PG, Ben-Shlomo Y, Martin RM. Associations of anti-hypertensive treatments with Alzheimer's disease, vascular dementia, and other dementias. Journal of Alzheimer's Disease. 2011;**26**(4):699-708

[60] An J, Nakajima T, Kuba K, Kimura A. Losartan inhibits LPS-induced inflammatory signaling through a PPARgamma-dependent mechanism in human THP-1 macrophages. Hypertension Research. 2010;**33**(8):831-835

[61] Harper JD, Lansbury PT Jr. Models of amyloid seeding in Alzheimer's disease and scrapie: Mechanistic truths and physiological consequences of the time-dependent solubility of amyloid proteins. Annual Review of Biochemistry. 1997;**66**:385-407

[62] Peters PJ, Mironov A Jr, Peretz D, van Donselaar E, Leclerc E, Erpel S, et al. Trafficking of prion proteins through a caveolae-mediated endosomal pathway. The Journal of Cell Biology. 2003;**162**(4):703-717

[63] Olsson A, Csajbok L, Ost M, Hoglund K, Nylen K, Rosengren L, et al. Marked increase of beta-amyloid(1-42) and amyloid precursor protein in ventricular cerebrospinal fluid after severe traumatic brain injury. Journal of Neurology. 2004;**251**(7):870-876

[64] Morishima-Kawashima M. Molecular mechanism of the intramembrane cleavage of the beta-carboxyl terminal fragment of amyloid precursor protein by gamma-secretase. Frontiers in Physiology. 2014;**5**:463

[65] Chen XH, Siman R, Iwata A, Meaney DF, Trojanowski JQ, Smith DH. Long-term accumulation of amyloid-beta, beta-secretase, presenilin-1, and caspase-3 in damaged axons following brain trauma. The American Journal of Pathology. 2004;**165**(2):357-371

[66] von Bernhardi R, Eugenin J. Microglial reactivity to beta-amyloid is modulated by astrocytes and proinflammatory factors. Brain Research. 2004;**1025**(1-2):186-193

[67] Mannix RC, Whalen MJ. Traumatic brain injury, microglia, and beta amyloid. International Journal of Alzheimer's Disease. 2012;**2012**:608732

[68] Ginzburg I. Neuronal polarity: Targeting of microtubule components into axons and dendrites. Trends in Biochemical Sciences. 1991;**16**(7):257-261

[69] Johnson GV, Stoothoff WH. Tau phosphorylation in neuronal cell function and dysfunction. Journal of Cell Science. 2004;**117**(Pt 24):5721-5729

[70] Drewes G. MARKing tau for tangles and toxicity. Trends in Biochemical Sciences. 2004;**29**(10):548-555

[71] Cowan CM, Quraishe S, Mudher A. What is the pathological significance of tau oligomers? Biochemical Society Transactions. 2012;**40**(4):693-697

[72] Lukiw WJ, Bazan NG. Neuroinflammatory signaling upregulation in Alzheimer's disease. Neurochemical Research. 2000;**25**(9-10):1173-1184

[73] Hawkins BE, Krishnamurthy S, Castillo-Carranza DL, Sengupta U, Prough DS, Jackson GR, et al. Rapid accumulation of endogenous tau oligomers in a rat model of traumatic brain injury: Possible link between traumatic brain injury and sporadic tauopathies. The Journal of Biological Chemistry. 2013;**288**(23):17042-17050

[74] Armstrong RA, McKee AC, Alvarez VE, Cairns NJ. Clustering of tau-immunoreactive pathology in chronic traumatic encephalopathy. Journal of Neural Transmission (Vienna). 2017;**124**(2):185-192

[75] Gordon-Krajcer W, Kozniewska E, Lazarewicz JW, Ksiezak-Reding H. Differential changes in phosphorylation of tau at PHF-1 and 12E8 epitopes during brain ischemia and reperfusion in gerbils. Neurochemical Research. 2007;**32**(4-5):729-737

[76] Tran HT, Sanchez L, Esparza TJ, Brody DL. Distinct temporal and anatomical distributions of amyloid-beta and tau abnormalities following controlled cortical impact in transgenic mice. PLoS One. 2011;**6**(9):e25475

[77] Ojo JO, Mouzon B, Greenberg MB, Bachmeier C, Mullan M, Crawford F. Repetitive mild traumatic brain injury augments tau pathology and glial activation in aged hTau mice. Journal of Neuropathology and Experimental Neurology. 2013;**72**(2):137-151

[78] Mitsis EM, Riggio S, Kostakoglu L, Dickstein DL, Machac J, Delman B, et al. Tauopathy PET and amyloid PET in the diagnosis of chronic traumatic

encephalopathies: Studies of a retired NFL player and of a man with FTD and a severe head injury. Translational Psychiatry. 2014;**4**:e441

[79] Kokjohn TA, Maarouf CL, Daugs ID, Hunter JM, Whiteside CM, Malek-Ahmadi M, et al. Neurochemical profile of dementia pugilistica. Journal of Neurotrauma. 2013;**30**(11):981-997

[80] Tartaglia MC, Hazrati LN, Davis KD, Green RE, Wennberg R, Mikulis D, et al. Chronic traumatic encephalopathy and other neurodegenerative proteinopathies. Frontiers in Human Neuroscience. 2014;**8**:30

[81] Tran HT, LaFerla FM, Holtzman DM, Brody DL. Controlled cortical impact traumatic brain injury in 3xTg-AD mice causes acute intra-axonal amyloid-beta accumulation and independently accelerates the development of tau abnormalities. The Journal of Neuroscience. 2011;**31**(26):9513-9525

[82] Neumann M, Sampathu DM, Kwong LK, Truax AC, Micsenyi MC, Chou TT, et al. Ubiquitinated TDP-43 in frontotemporal lobar degeneration and amyotrophic lateral sclerosis. Science. 2006;**314**(5796):130-133

[83] Chen-Plotkin AS, Lee VM, Trojanowski JQ. TAR DNA-binding protein 43 in neurodegenerative disease. Nature Reviews. Neurology. 2010;**6**(4):211-220

[84] McKee AC, Daneshvar DH, Alvarez VE, Stein TD. The neuropathology of sport. Acta Neuropathologica. 2014;**127**(1):29-51

[85] Tan XL, Sun M, Brady RD, Liu S, Llanos R, Cheung S, et al. Transactive response DNA-binding protein 43 abnormalities after traumatic brain injury. Journal of Neurotrauma. 2018. DOI: 10.1089/neu.2017.5491

[86] King A, Sweeney F, Bodi I, Troakes C, Maekawa S, Al-Sarraj S. Abnormal TDP-43 expression is identified in the neocortex in cases of dementia pugilistica, but is mainly confined to the limbic system when identified in high and moderate stages of Alzheimer's disease. Neuropathology. 2010;**30**(4):408-419

[87] McKee AC, Gavett BE, Stern RA, Nowinski CJ, Cantu RC, Kowall NW, et al. TDP-43 proteinopathy and motor neuron disease in chronic traumatic encephalopathy. Journal of Neuropathology and Experimental Neurology. 2010;**69**(9):918-929

[88] Johnson VE, Stewart W, Trojanowski JQ , Smith DH. Acute and chronically increased immunoreactivity to phosphorylation-independent but not pathological TDP-43 after a single traumatic brain injury in humans. Acta Neuropathologica. 2011;**122**(6):715-726

[89] Kwong LK, Neumann M, Sampathu DM, Lee VM, Trojanowski JQ. TDP-43 proteinopathy: The neuropathology underlying major forms of sporadic and familial frontotemporal lobar degeneration and motor neuron disease. Acta Neuropathologica. 2007;**114**(1):63-70

[90] Smith DH, Nakamura M, McIntosh TK, Wang J, Rodriguez A, Chen XH, et al. Brain trauma induces massive hippocampal neuron death linked to a surge in beta-amyloid levels in mice overexpressing mutant amyloid precursor protein. The American Journal of Pathology. 1998;**153**(3):1005-1010

[91] Nakagawa Y, Nakamura M, McIntosh TK, Rodriguez A, Berlin JA, Smith DH, et al. Traumatic brain injury in young, amyloid-beta peptide overexpressing transgenic mice induces marked ipsilateral hippocampal atrophy and diminished Abeta deposition during aging. The Journal of Comparative Neurology. 1999;**411**(3):390-398

[92] Uryu K, Laurer H, McIntosh T, Pratico D, Martinez D, Leight S, et al. Repetitive mild brain trauma accelerates Abeta deposition, lipid peroxidation, and cognitive impairment in a transgenic mouse model of Alzheimer amyloidosis. The Journal of Neuroscience. 2002;**22**(2):446-454

[93] Hu W, Tung YC, Zhang Y, Liu F, Iqbal K. Involvement of activation of asparaginyl endopeptidase in tau hyperphosphorylation in repetitive mild traumatic brain injury. Journal of Alzheimer's Disease. 2018;**64**(3):709-722

[94] Lewen A, Li GL, Nilsson P, Olsson Y, Hillered L. Traumatic brain injury in rat produces changes of beta-amyloid precursor protein immunoreactivity. Neuroreport. 1995;**6**(2):357-360

[95] Pierce JE, Trojanowski JQ, Graham DI, Smith DH, McIntosh TK. Immunohistochemical characterization of alterations in the distribution of amyloid precursor proteins and beta-amyloid peptide after experimental brain injury in the rat. The Journal of Neuroscience. 1996;**16**(3):1083-1090

[96] Roberts GW, Gentleman SM, Lynch A, Murray L, Landon M, Graham DI. Beta amyloid protein deposition in the brain after severe head injury: Implications for the pathogenesis of Alzheimer's disease. Journal of Neurology, Neurosurgery, and Psychiatry. 1994;**57**(4):419-425

[97] Gentleman SM, Greenberg BD, Savage MJ, Noori M, Newman SJ, Roberts GW, et al. A beta 42 is the predominant form of amyloid beta-protein in the brains of short-term survivors of head injury. Neuroreport. 1997;**8**(6):1519-1522

[98] Szczygielski J, Mautes A, Steudel WI, Falkai P, Bayer TA, Wirths O. Traumatic brain injury: Cause or risk of Alzheimer's disease? A review of experimental studies. Journal of Neural Transmission. 2005;**112**(11):1547-1564

[99] Wang H, Durham L, Dawson H, Song P, Warner DS, Sullivan PM, et al. An apolipoprotein E-based therapeutic improves outcome and reduces Alzheimer's disease pathology following closed head injury: Evidence of pharmacogenomic interaction. Neuroscience. 2007;**144**(4):1324-1333

[100] Hartman RE, Laurer H, Longhi L, Bales KR, Paul SM, McIntosh TK, et al. Apolipoprotein E4 influences amyloid deposition but not cell loss after traumatic brain injury in a mouse model of Alzheimer's disease. The Journal of Neuroscience. 2002;**22**(23):10083-10087

[101] Maestre G, Ottman R, Stern Y, Gurland B, Chun M, Tang MX, et al. Apolipoprotein E and Alzheimer's disease: Ethnic variation in genotypic risks. Annals of Neurology. 1995;**37**(2):254-259

[102] Jordan BD, Relkin NR, Ravdin LD, Jacobs AR, Bennett A, Gandy S. Apolipoprotein E epsilon4 associated with chronic traumatic brain injury in boxing. Journal of the American Medical Association. 1997;**278**(2):136-140

[103] Nakagawa Y, Reed L, Nakamura M, McIntosh TK, Smith DH, Saatman KE, et al. Brain trauma in aged transgenic mice induces regression of established abeta deposits. Experimental Neurology. 2000;**163**(1):244-252

[104] Han SD, Suzuki H, Drake AI, Jak AJ, Houston WS, Bondi MW. Clinical, cognitive, and genetic predictors of change in job status following traumatic brain injury in a military population. The Journal of Head Trauma Rehabilitation. 2009;**24**(1):57-64

[105] Han SD, Drake AI, Cessante LM, Jak AJ, Houston WS, Delis DC, et al. Apolipoprotein E and traumatic brain

injury in a military population: Evidence of a neuropsychological compensatory mechanism? Journal of Neurology, Neurosurgery, and Psychiatry. 2007;**78**(10):1103-1108

[106] Raby CA, Morganti-Kossmann MC, Kossmann T, Stahel PF, Watson MD, Evans LM, et al. Traumatic brain injury increases beta-amyloid peptide 1-42 in cerebrospinal fluid. Journal of Neurochemistry. 1998;**71**(6):2505-2509

[107] Irving EA, Nicoll J, Graham DI, Dewar D. Increased tau immunoreactivity in oligodendrocytes following human stroke and head injury. Neuroscience Letters. 1996;**213**(3):189-192

[108] Tran HT, Sanchez L, Brody DL. Inhibition of JNK by a peptide inhibitor reduces traumatic brain injury-induced tauopathy in transgenic mice. Journal of Neuropathology and Experimental Neurology. 2012;**71**(2):116-129

[109] Murai H, Pierce JE, Raghupathi R, Smith DH, Saatman KE, Trojanowski JQ, et al. Twofold overexpression of human beta-amyloid precursor proteins in transgenic mice does not affect the neuromotor, cognitive, or neurodegenerative sequelae following experimental brain injury. The Journal of Comparative Neurology. 1998;**392**(4):428-438

[110] Abrahamson EE, Ikonomovic MD, Dixon CE, DeKosky ST. Simvastatin therapy prevents brain trauma-induced increases in beta-amyloid peptide levels. Annals of Neurology. 2009;**66**(3):407-414

[111] Mannix RC, Zhang J, Park J, Lee C, Whalen MJ. Detrimental effect of genetic inhibition of B-site APP-cleaving enzyme 1 on functional outcome after controlled cortical impact in young adult mice. Journal of Neurotrauma. 2011;**28**(9):1855-1861

[112] Schwetye KE, Cirrito JR, Esparza TJ, Mac Donald CL, Holtzman DM, Brody DL. Traumatic brain injury reduces soluble extracellular amyloid-beta in mice: A methodologically novel combined microdialysis-controlled cortical impact study. Neurobiology of Disease. 2010;**40**(3):555-564

[113] Sabo T, Lomnitski L, Nyska A, Beni S, Maronpot RR, Shohami E, et al. Susceptibility of transgenic mice expressing human apolipoprotein E to closed head injury: The allele E3 is neuroprotective whereas E4 increases fatalities. Neuroscience. 2000;**101**(4):879-884

[114] Iwata A, Chen XH, McIntosh TK, Browne KD, Smith DH. Long-term accumulation of amyloid-beta in axons following brain trauma without persistent upregulation of amyloid precursor protein genes. Journal of Neuropathology and Experimental Neurology. 2002;**61**(12):1056-1068

[115] Hoshino S, Tamaoka A, Takahashi M, Kobayashi S, Furukawa T, Oaki Y, et al. Emergence of immunoreactivities for phosphorylated tau and amyloid-beta protein in chronic stage of fluid percussion injury in rat brain. Neuroreport. 1998;**9**(8):1879-1883

[116] Gabbita SP, Srivastava MK, Eslami P, Johnson MF, Kobritz NK, Tweedie D, et al. Early intervention with a small molecule inhibitor for tumor necrosis factor-alpha prevents cognitive deficits in a triple transgenic mouse model of Alzheimer's disease. Journal of Neuroinflammation. 2012;**9**:99

[117] Smith DH, Chen XH, Nonaka M, Trojanowski JQ, Lee VM, Saatman KE, et al. Accumulation of amyloid beta and tau and the formation of neurofilament inclusions following diffuse brain injury in the pig. Journal of Neuropathology and Experimental Neurology. 1999;**58**(9):982-992

Chapter 9

Inhibition of Protein Fibrillation by Hydrogen Sulfide[1]

Manuel F. Rosario-Alomar, Tatiana Quiñones-Ruiz, Dmitry Kurouski, Valentin Sereda, Eduardo DeBarros-Ferreira, Lorraine De Jesús-Kim, Samuel Hernández-Rivera, Dmitri V. Zagorevski, Leishla M. Cruz-Collazo, Igor K. Lednev and Juan López-Garriga

Abstract

Amyloid fibrils are misfolded proteins, which are often associated with various neurodegenerative diseases such as Alzheimer's. The amount of hydrogen sulfide (H_2S) is known to be reduced in the brain tissue of people diagnosed with Alzheimer's disease relative to that of healthy individuals. Hen Egg-White Lysozyme (HEWL) forms typical β-sheet-rich fibrils during 70 minutes at low pH and high temperatures. These results are consistent with the ThT findings that β-sheets structure is also present in myoglobin (Mb), and hemoglobin (Hb) in the presence of 45% TFE. The addition of H_2S in the process completely inhibits the formation of amyloid fibrils in HEWL, Mb, and Hb as revealed by several spectroscopic techniques. Non-resonance Raman bands corresponding to disulfide (RSSR) vibrational modes in the 550-500 cm^{-1} spectral range decreases in intensity and is accompanied by the appearance of a new 490 cm^{-1} band assigned to the trisulfide group (RSSSR). Intrinsic tryptophan fluorescence shows a partial denaturation of HEWL containing trisulfide bonds. Overall, the Mb and Hb result ties excellent with the HEWL data showing that the presence of H_2S during these proteins fibrillation processes protects the α-helical protein structures, preventing the formation of amyloids in these different proteins moieties.

Keywords: hydrogen sulfide, amyloid fibril, protein aggregates, lysozyme, myoglobin, hemoglobin, Raman spectroscopy, ultraviolet Raman spectroscopy, unordered protein, disulfide, trisulfide

---

[1] Materials in this chapter related to the lysozyme fibrillation and its inhibition by H2S, including text and figures was previously published in Journal of Physical Chemistry. 2015;119:1265-1274. PMID: 2554579. The direct link to the article is https://pubs.acs.org/doi/10.1021/jp508471v. Any further permissions related to the related material should be directed to the ACS.

1. Introduction

Amyloids are large aggregates of misfolded proteins with a highly stable cross β-structure, which are associated with a variety of degenerative illnesses such as Alzheimer's, Parkinson's, and Huntington's diseases [1–3]. Proteins with different functionalities and native structures ranging from α-helical and β-sheet rich to intrinsically unordered are able to form amyloid fibrils *in vitro* with a characteristic cross-β core structure [4–6]. This observation leads to the conclusion that protein fibrillation is a generic property of a polypeptide chain. There are numerous research reports demonstrating that a general fibrillation mechanism involves a partially unfolded protein as the first intermediate state [7, 8]. Steps to follow include the formation of small aggregates and a β-sheet rich nucleus, which generates further protein aggregation and the formation of mature fibrils.

A reduced amount of hydrogen sulfide (H_2S) in the brain tissue of patients with Alzheimer's disease has been recently reported [9]. For centuries, people have been interested in H_2S for its role as a poisonous chemical. At high concentrations, H_2S inhibits cytochrome c and, as a consequence, the electron transport chain [10]. It also binds to hemoglobin forming a sulfhemoglobin complex as detected during sulfhemoglobinemia [11]. More recently, it has been demonstrated that H_2S has gasotransmitter functions, similar to CO and NO [12]. For example, a suspended animation-like state in mice has been achieved by administering ppm-levels of H_2S at low temperatures. The metabolic rate and body core temperature decrease and fully recover after such exposure, a promising medical benefit that reduces physiological damage after trauma [13]. In the last two decades, significant attention has been paid to understand the physiological role of H_2S and its endogenous production. H_2S is biosynthesized in mammalian tissue by non-enzymatic reactions and by the enzymatic degradation of cysteine by cystathionine β synthase (CBS), cystathionine γ lyase (CSE), cysteine aminotransferase (CAT), and cysteine lyase (CL) [14]. Consumption of garlic induces non-enzymatic H_2S production [15]. Moreover, aged garlic extract has been shown to cause a reduction of *in vivo* Aβ fibrils and soluble amyloid, as well as a decrease in tau conformational changes [16]. This indirect evidence concerning the role of H_2S in neurodegenerative diseases has motivated us to investigate the effects of H_2S on the formation of amyloid fibrils.

Small molecules can have a significant effect on the formation of amyloid fibrils. There is extensive literature on the inhibitory activity of various small molecules on protein fibrillation [17]. Recently, Arosio and coauthors have reviewed the development of amyloid inhibitors, such as antibodies and chaperones, small molecules (e.g., Congo red and polyphenols), colloidal inhibitors and organic/inorganic nanoparticles, as possible participants in the various states of protein aggregation [17–19]. These states include the inhibition of primary nucleation (monomer-to-oligomer transition), secondary nucleation (oligomer elongation), and postelongation. However, we have not found any published reports on the role of H_2S in protein aggregation.

It is well documented that H_2S reacts with disulfide bonds, leading one to hypothesize that this reaction could have a significant effect on the mechanism of protein fibrillation. Kumar and co-workers have reported that protecting disulfide bridges with iodoacetamide in an alkaline solution limits the lysozyme fibril growth to 50% [20]. This group has concluded that changing the dynamics of disulfide to *aberrant* disulfide bonds would redirect the process toward the formation of native-like lysozyme aggregates [20]. It has been reported that treating antibodies with H_2S has resulted in SS bond modifications, including the formation of trisulfide bonds (SSS) [21]. Surprisingly, no changes in antibody stability and function have been observed. H_2S can be incorporated as a sulfane sulfur, a divalent sulfur with six valence electrons, and an oxidation number of zero (S^0) that only binds to other sulfur atoms to form polysulfides [22]. Several research groups have also reported that the sulfur atom of

H_2S can be endogenously incorporated into a large amount of proteins by sulfuration, also known as sulfhydration of cysteines. This leads to the formation of protein persulfides (SSH), which could play an intermediary role in protein SSS formation [23].

Here, we have investigated the effect of H_2S on the aggregation of lysozyme, a glycoside hydroxylase responsible for antimicrobial protection in most mammalian species. HEWL is a single chain protein stabilized by four SS bonds in positions cys6-cys127, cys30-cys115, cys64-cys80, and cys76-cys94 [24]. It was found that H_2S inhibits the formation of HEWL fibrils. The effect of H_2S has been investigated under typical fibrillation conditions such as high temperature and acidic pH using DUVRR and non-resonance Raman spectroscopy, fluorescence, and atomic force microscopy (AFM). We have shown that in the presence of H_2S, HEWL forms spherical aggregates of unordered protein under fibrillation conditions. Cytotoxicity tests reveal that these spherical aggregates have no cell toxicity by contrast with typical HEWL fibrils. Our spectroscopic results, buttressed by data that has been published, indicate that H_2S reacts with protein disulfide bonds to form trisulfide bridges. This reaction results in significant lysozyme denaturation and the formation of spherical aggregates of unordered proteins, which prevent protein fibrillation.

However, because myoglobin (Mb) and hemoglobin (Hb) do not have any cysteine chemical bond, we pursued the effect of H_2S on the fibril formation of these vital hemeproteins. Mb and Hb are the most studied hemeproteins, because of their biological significance of oxygen binding. The role of Mb and Hb in the body is so important that the minimal unbalance of normal physiology can lead to toxicity and to cascade of reactions generating harmful products. For example, free radical formation in these hemeproteins unavoidably leads to oxidative damage of the heme and amino acids [25]. Also in certain circumstances, Mb and Hb isolated from their cellular environment may crosslink leading to kidney dysfunction, rhabdomyolysis, coma, and subarachnoid brain hemorrhage [26]. Other maladies include heme loss (hemophilia, hemolytic anemia), hemoglobinopathies (thalassemia [α and β], methemoglobinemia, posttranslational alterations), cardiovascular, and renal diseases [27–31]. Likewise, hemoglobin can protagonist sickle cell anemia where a mutation at the β6 position of Hb (β6Glu → Val) results in the polymerization of deoxy-sickle cell Hb (HbS) and subsequent aggregation into long fibers with amyloid-like structures [32, 33]. Regarding this, it has been shown that Hb under physiological conditions and in the presence of 45% 2,2,2-trifluoethanol (TFE) produces amyloid-like fibril structures. This observation was supported by ThT fluorescence, CD, and FTIR suggesting that Hb β-sheet conformation leads to Hb fibril formation [28]. The mechanism surrounding these fibril events remain almost unknown. Interestingly, our results also show that H_2S inhibits the fibril formation in both myoglobin and hemoglobin under physiological conditions and 45% TFE concentration and that increasing concentration of H_2S inhibits β-sheet formation and predominates the α-helix structure. The findings demonstrate the same H_2S effect on to the fibrillation of Mb monomer and Hb tetramer. Overall, it is very interesting that hydrogen sulfide is able to avoid the formation of fibril derivative in lysozyme and myoglobin and hemoglobin being their structures completely different.

2. Materials and methodology

The following chemicals were purchased from Sigma-Aldrich (St. Louis, MO, USA): 99.7% acetic acid (695092), sodium chloride (NaCl) (S771-3), HEWL (L6876), hemoglobin bovine (H2500), myoglobin from horse skeletal muscle (M0630), 2,2,2-trifluoroethanol 99% (T63002), potassium chloride (P3911), potassium phosphate monobasic (P5655) and potassium phosphate dibasic (1551128), sodium sulfide nonahydrate salt (208043), dipropyl disulfide (149225), and trisulfide (6028-61-1).

2.1 HEWL solution preparation

Lysozyme was dissolved (25 mg/mL) in 20% acetic acid and 100 mM NaCl at pH 2.0 and incubated at 60°C to form fibrils under initial (control) conditions. To study the effect of H_2S, sodium sulfide nonahydrate salt (12 mM) was added to the control solution in a molar ratio of 1:5 (HEWL:H_2S), prior to the temperature elevation.

2.2 Myoglobin and hemoglobin fibril preparation

Myoglobin and hemoglobin were dissolved (15 and 20 mg/mL, respectively) in 20 mM phosphate buffer at pH 7.4; samples of Mb and Hb solutions were mixed with 45% of 2,2,2-trifluoroethanol and incubated at 37°C for 24 hours to form the fibrils (control conditions). Another batch of samples was prepared with sodium sulfide nonahydrate salt (60–300 μM, 12 mM) under the same control conditions, to evaluate H_2S effect [28, 34].

2.3 Non-resonance Raman experiments

Powder samples of native and aggregated HEWL were prepared by drying the solutions under nitrogen at room temperature, which removed the acetic acid. Raman spectra (785-nm excitation) of HEWL powder samples and pure dipropyl di- and trisulfide liquids were recorded using a Renishaw inVia confocal Raman spectrometer equipped with a research grade Leica microscope and 50× objective (numerical aperture, 0.55). Five accumulations of 30 s each were collected for each sample in the range of 400–1800 cm^{-1}. Wire 4.0 software was used for data collection. A laser power of approximately 11.5 mW was used to avoid sample photo-degradation.

2.4 TCEP test for trisulfides

A reaction with tris(2-carboxyethyl)phosphine (TCEP) reducing agent was used as a test for trisulfides [35]. Hen egg white lysozyme (HEWL) in native and aggregated form was incubated at pH 2.0 and room temperature for 90 minutes in the presence of TCEP. The reaction products were analyzed using normal Raman spectroscopy. Powder samples of HEWL-aggregates incubated at different concentrations of TCEP were prepared for non-resonance Raman spectroscopic analysis by drying the corresponding solutions under a nitrogen flow.

2.5 Deep UV resonance Raman spectroscopy (DUVRR)

DUVRR spectra (199.7 nm excitation) of 25 mg/mL HEWL were collected using a home built instrument equipped with a CCD camera (Roper Scientific, Inc.) cooled in liquid nitrogen [36]. A spinning quartz NMR tube with a magnetic stirrer was used for sampling. Each spectrum recorded an average of 20 accumulations with 30 s acquisition time. GRAMS/AI 7.0 software (Thermo Galactic, Salem, NH) was used for data processing.

2.6 Tryptophan and ThT fluorescence

Fluorescence spectra were measured in a JobinYvon Fluoromax-3 spectrofluorometer (JobinYvon, Edison, NJ). Intrinsic tryptophan fluorescence of

25 mg/mL HEWL was measured in a 10-μm path length cell without dilutions. The UV absorption was <0.05 at an excitation wavelength of 295.5 nm. The excitation and emission slits were 0.5 and 5 nm, respectively. Three spectral accumulations were taken, and the spectra were averaged for each sample. HEWL fibrils formed after 90 minutes of incubation were also characterized using intrinsic tryptophan fluorescence. Fibrils were washed in acetic acid solution twice in a procedure which included sonication for 10 minutes, centrifugation for 4 minutes at 13,000 rpm, the removal of supernatant liquid and re-suspension in an acetic acid solution. Fluorescence dye thioflavin T (ThT) is one of the most used probes for identification and analysis in the formation of amyloid fibrils both *in vivo* and *in vitro*. Once ThT binds to β-sheet-rich amyloid fibril structures, there is a characteristic blue shift in the emission spectrum from 510 to 480 nm [37–39]. In the ThT fluorescence assay, aliquots of 25 mg/mL HEWL were diluted in a molar ratio of 1:10 (HEWL:thioflavin T (ThT) dye) to a final concentration of 2.5 mM ThT. The excitation and emission wavelengths were 450 and 480 nm, respectively. The excitation and emission slits were 5 nm. Three recorded spectra were averaged for each measurement. ThT fluorescence intensity of Mb and Hb was monitored during fibrillation experiment: λ_{ex} = 440 nm and λ_{em} = 480 nm. The final protein sample and ThT concentration were 10 and 10 μM, respectively [28]. Fluorescence was measured using Biotek Synergy 4 (multi-mode microplate reader) with a 96 well-plate in a continuous acquisition (kinetics mode), every 5 minutes for 20 hours with gently orbital shake. We examined the time-dependence of Mb and Hb amyloid-like structures by monitoring thioflavin T fluorescence (480 nm) enhancement under a pH = 7.4 and T = 37°.

2.7 Circular dichroism spectroscopy

Far-UV circular dichroism (CD) measurements of Hb and Mb samples were performed on a Jasco-815 spectropolarimeter. Each spectrum was the average of six scans. Three replicates for each time point of the kinetic experiment were analyzed. Spectra were acquired at 0.5-nm intervals with a 4-s integration time and a bandwidth of 1.0 nm. Mb and Hb were analyzed at a final concentration of 0.5 mg/mL. All measurements were performed under nitrogen flow. The results were expressed as the mean residue ellipticity. Data were corrected for buffer contributions [28, 40, 41].

2.8 Atomic force microscope

Aliquots of HEWL incubated at 60°C, pH 2.0, 100 mM NaCl were cooled to room temperature and deposited on freshly cleaved mica. After a few minutes of exposure, the mica surface was rinsed with MQ water and dried. AFM images were collected using the SmartSPM 1000 system (AIST-NT, Novato, CA). Images were acquired in the tapping mode using silicon cantilevers with a 10–25 nm tip curvature radius.

3. Results

3.1 Aggregation and structural rearrangements of lysozyme

To form fibrils, HEWL was incubated at 60°C in 20% acetic acid (pH 2.0) and 100 mM NaCl, from here on referred to as control conditions. The morphology of lysozyme aggregates formed in the course of incubation under the fibrillogenic conditions and in the presence of H_2S was characterized by AFM. The presence of typical long rode-like fibrils was evident after 90 minutes of incubation under control conditions (**Figure 1A**). However, incubation of HEWL in the presence of H_2S resulted in the formation of spherical aggregates instead of fibrils, as evident from AFM images (**Figure 1B**).

ThT fluorescence is used often to monitor the formation of amyloid fibrils. ThT fluorescence intensity increased dramatically after 70 minutes of incubation of lysozyme under control conditions, indicating the formation of amyloid fibrils (**Figure 1C**). However, no increase in ThT fluorescence intensity was observed for the HEWL solution incubated with H_2S within 48 hours. We investigated changes in the lysozyme secondary structure during incubation with and without H_2S using deep UV resonance Raman (DUVRR) spectroscopy. DUVRR has been used to study structural rearrangements of HEWL at all stages of fibrillation [36, 45, 46]. The DUVRR spectrum of HEWL excited at 199.7 nm was mainly composed of the amide chromosphere and the aromatic amino acid (Phe and Tyr) contributions [47]. A noticeable increase in the intensity and sharpness of the Am I band (approximately 1672 cm^{-1}) indicated the appearance of β-sheets due to the formation of fibrils [36, 48–50]. The DUVRR spectrum of fibrillated lysozyme under control conditions confirmed the formation of β-sheets. The spectrum of HEWL after 30 minutes of incubation under control conditions (**Figure 1D**, red) is similar to that reported previously for HEWL fibrils [36]. However, the DUVRR spectrum of lysozyme

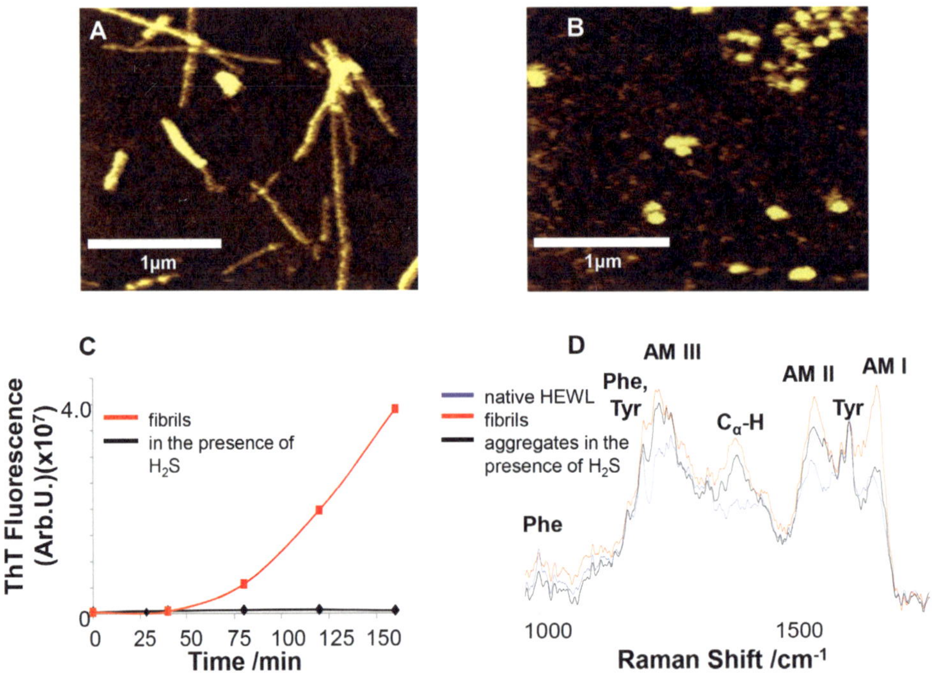

Figure 1.
Lysozyme forms β-sheet-rich fibrils under fibrillogenic control conditions and spherical aggregates of unordered protein under fibrillogenic conditions with H_2S incubation. AFM images of (A) HEWL fibrils formed after incubation of the control solution for 90 minutes and (B) HEWL aggregates formed after incubation of the solution in the presence of H_2S for 48 hours; scale bars are 1 µm. (C) Aggregation kinetics (ThT fluorescence) of HEWL incubated under control conditions (red) and in the presence of H_2S (black). (D) DUVRR spectra of native HEWL (blue), HEWL fibrils (red), and HEWL spherical aggregates (black) formed in the presence of H_2S; all spectra were normalized using the aromatic amino acid Raman band (approximately 1600 cm^{-1}) for comparison. The amide I vibrational mode (Am I) is dominated by C = O stretching, with minor contributions from C—N stretching and N—H bending [42]. Amide II (Am II) and amide III (Am III) bands involve significant C—N stretching, N—H bending, and C—C stretching [43]. The C_α—H bending vibrational mode involves C_α—H symmetric bending and C—C_α stretching [44].

incubated in the presence of H_2S confirmed the lack of β-sheet formation. In this case, the Am I band (approximately 1670 cm^{-1}) did not show a significant intensity change (**Figure 1D**, black). Instead, the Am I band shifted slightly to a higher frequency, signifying the formation of an unordered protein [36, 42]. This was further supported by the increase in C_α—H band intensity at 1390 cm^{-1} that was indicative of α-helix melting [51]. A significant change in Raman bands for Am III (approximately 1250 cm^{-1}) and Am II (approximately 1555 cm^{-1}) was consistent with the transition of α-helix to unordered protein. Therefore, AFM, ThT fluorescence, and DUVRR spectroscopy indicated the formation of unordered spherical aggregates of HEWL by contrast with β-sheet-rich fibrils in the presence of H_2S.

3.2 Intrinsic tryptophan fluorescence marker of the tertiary structural rearrangement

Tryptophan (Trp) fluorescence is an efficient intrinsic marker of local environments, which is often used for monitoring tertiary structural changes in proteins [47]. Native lysozyme at neutral pH shows a maximum Trp emission at 340 nm [52]. At pH 2.0 (20% acetic acid), the Trp fluorescence peak shifts to 345 nm, indicating a partial denaturation of lysozyme. A further minor shift to 347 nm due to HEWL fibril formation under control conditions was observed (**Figure 2B** and **C**). To confirm that the intrinsic Trp fluorescence is dominated by the signal from HEWL fibrils, the solutions (after incubation for 40 and 90 minutes) were sonicated, centrifuged, and re-suspended in 20% acetic acid to remove possible monomeric and oligomeric forms of the protein (**Figure 2B**). A significant shift of the Trp emission maximum, from 345 to 357 nm, was observed after 90 minutes of lysozyme incubation in the presence of H_2S (**Figure 2A** and **C**), with no further changes for at least 48 hours. This significant red shift is consistent with the previously reported maximum emission at 352 nm for fully denatured lysozyme in 6 M guanidinium-HCl at pH 7.0 [53]. Therefore, we conclude that incubation of lysozyme in the presence of H_2S results in a stronger denaturation than that which occurs during control fibrillation conditions.

3.3 Rearrangement of disulfide bonds

Non-resonance Raman spectroscopy of proteins offers a unique opportunity for characterizing the conformation of disulfide bridges [49]. The SS symmetric stretching vibrational mode is typically represented as a strong Raman band in the range of 505–550 cm^{-1} [49, 54]. The Raman spectrum of HEWL was found to change significantly in the SS signature region with incubation time (**Figure 3A**). A strong 507 cm^{-1} peak in the Raman spectrum of native HEWL represents the gauche-gauche-gauche (g-g-g) configuration of three SS bonds, and a small 523 cm^{-1} peak can be attributed to the gauche-gauche-trans (g-g-t) configuration of the fourth SS bond of lysozyme [49, 55]. The amplitudes of these peaks decreased, and a new peak appeared at 490 cm^{-1} as a result of HEWL incubation in the presence of 12 mM H_2S, indicating significant rearrangements of SS bonds (**Figure 3A**). The concentration of 12 mM H_2S corresponded to a 5:1 (H_2S:HEWL) molar ratio, chosen so that a sufficient number of H_2S molecules could react with all four lysozyme SS bonds assuming a 1:1 stoichiometric ratio. We are currently investigating the effect of H_2S concentrations. The 1003 cm^{-1} peak corresponding to phenylalanine was used to normalize Raman spectra in **Figure 3A** (region not shown). **Figure 3C** shows synchronous kinetic change in the area of the 507 and 490 cm^{-1} bands with incubation time up to 90 minutes [56]. No further changes were observed during 48 hours of additional incubation in the presence of H_2S

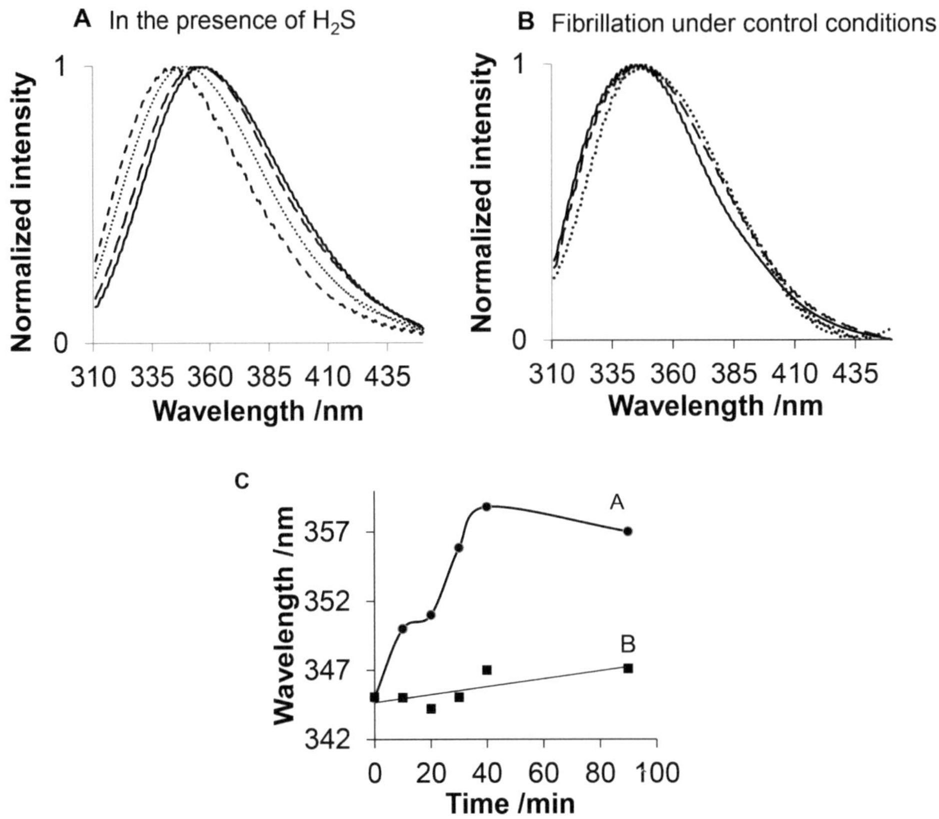

Figure 2.
Time dependent Trp fluorescence changes of lysozyme (A) incubated in the presence of H_2S for 0 minutes (dashes ---), 10 minutes (dots ...), 90 minutes (long dashes ---), 48 hours (solid line ___); (B) incubated with control solution for 0 minutes (solid line ___), 40 minutes (long dashes ---), and 90 minutes (dots ...); (C) Trp maximum emission wavelength of HEWL incubated with H_2S (A circles) and fibrillation under control conditions (B squares).

(data not shown). As discussed in detail below, dipropyl-trisulfide (DPTS) Raman spectrum contains a 485 cm^{-1} band (**Figure 3D**) characteristic to the trisulfide moiety that motivated us to investigate the possibility of assigning 490 cm^{-1} band in HEWL aggregate Raman spectrum to the SSS group. The non-resonance Raman spectroscopy of HEWL fibrillation under control conditions indicate that the 507 cm^{-1} peak does not change significantly during fibril formation (**Figure 3B**). Therefore, in the absence of H_2S, HEWL SS bands remain intact and the g-g-g conformation dominates, in agreement with our previous report [57].

3.4 Reduction of trisulfide bridges by TCEP

To test the hypothesis about the formation of trisulfide groups, we investigated the reaction of HEWL aggregates with TCEP reduction agent by normal Raman spectroscopy. TCEP reaction with SS groups is well known to result in oxidation of TCEP and formation of TCEP(O) and R-SH groups [58]. More recently, Cumnock et al. reported that TCEP reacted preferentially with SSS moieties in the presence of SS bridges until the majority of SSS groups were consumed according to Eqs. (1) and (2) [35]. SS bridges and thiophosphine TCEP(S) species are main products of TCEP-SSS reaction [35]. **Figure 4** shows Raman spectra of HEWL aggregates after incubation with different concentrations of TCEP (0.5, 1, 2.5, and 10 mM). The amount of aggregated HEWL molecules in these samples was kept about 3.0 mM.

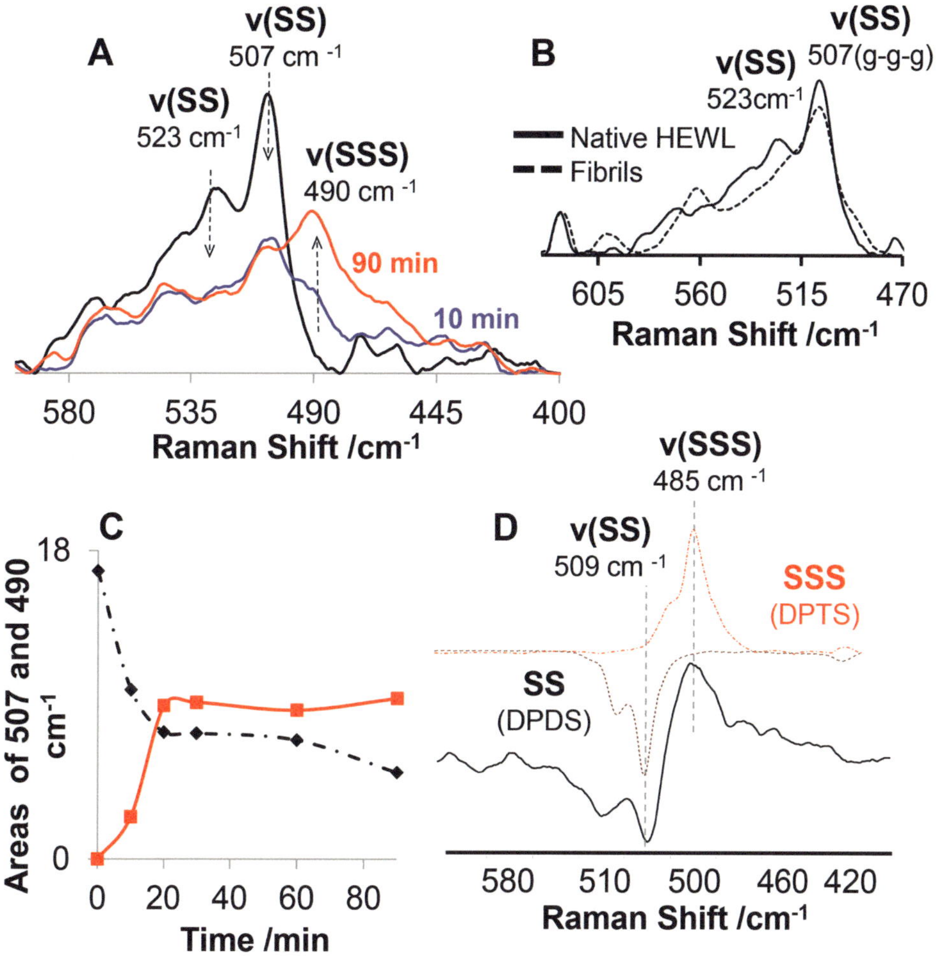

Figure 3.
Evolution of lysozyme disulfide bonds in the presence of H_2S probed by normal Raman spectroscopy. Raman spectra of HEWL incubated (A) in the presence of H_2S and (B) under control conditions, where 507 and 523 cm^{-1} bands correspond to g-g-g and g-g-t SS configurations, respectively. Synchronous kinetic change in the area of the 507 and 490 cm^{-1} bands is assigned to the newly formed RSSSR group. (C) The kinetics of RSSSR formation (490 cm^{-1}) and the decrease in the amount of RSSR (507 cm^{-1}) during the incubation of HEWL in the presence of H_2S. (D) The difference spectrum between normal Raman spectra of HEWL aggregated in the presence of H_2S acquired at 90- and 0-minute incubation [shown in (A), gray solid line]. The latter spectrum is represented by the expected spectral change demonstrating the disulfide-to-trisulfide transition symbolized by the inverted Raman spectrum of dipropyl disulfide (black dots and dash, -.-.-) and dipropyl trisulfide (red dots, ...).

$$TCEP + R - SSS - R \rightarrow TCEP(S) + R - SS - R \quad (1)$$

$$TCEP + R - SS - R \rightarrow TCEP(O) + 2\,R - SH \quad (2)$$

The Raman spectrum of HEWL aggregates was found to change significantly in the SSS/SS vibrational signature region with the addition of TCEP (**Figure 4A**). The SSS band at 490 cm^{-1} decreases after 0.5 mM TCEP addition that is in a good agreement with predominant reaction of TCEP with SSS groups. The amplitudes of both 490 and 507 cm^{-1} bands (SSS and SS, respectively) decreased as a result of HEWL incubation in the presence of higher concentration of TCEP (1–10 mM) indicating significant reduction of SS and SSS groups and formation of R-SH moiety in agreement with an increase in 2575 cm^{-1} band intensity (**Figure 4B**).

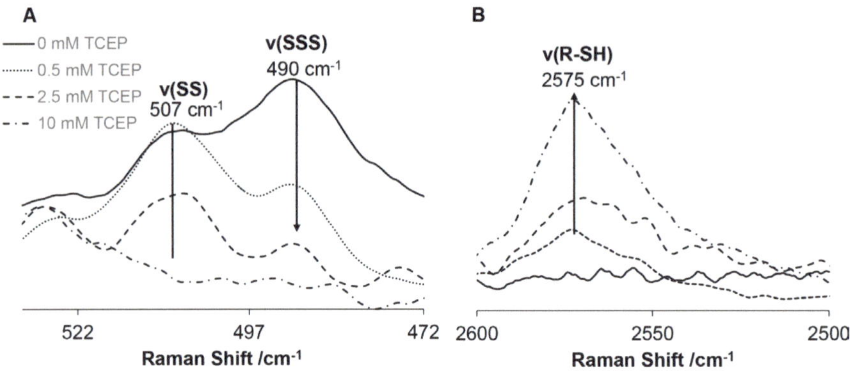

Figure 4.
Normal Raman spectra of HEWL aggregates in the presence of reducing agent TCEP with concentration 0 mM (solid line), 0.5 mM (dotted line), 1 mM (short dashed line), 2.5 mM (dashed line), and 10 mM (dashed dotted line). Selected spectral regions with characteristic Raman bands of disulfide and trisulfide moieties (A) as well as sulfhydryl (—SH) group (B) are shown. Phenylalanine Raman band at 1003 cm^{-1} was used to normalize the spectra (spectral region not shown).

3.5 Hydrogen sulfide inhibition of myoglobin and hemoglobin fibril formation

Figures 5A and **6A** demonstrate the formation of myoglobin and hemoglobin fibrils and its inhibition by hydrogen sulfide, respectively. The ThT fluorescence intensity associated to Mb and Hb amyloid fibrils (black) shows an initial lag process followed by a drastic increase as function of time. ThT fluorescence intensity is descriptive of prefibrillar oligomer intermediate species associated to the lag phase, while the positive slope is representative of fibrils with differing sizes and structures. Thus, the interaction of ThT with amyloid fibrils is highly specific, but neither amorphous aggregates nor soluble proteins in folded, unfolded, or partially folded states enhance ThT fluorescence [37–39]. Therefore, the data clearly show the existence of the myoglobin and hemoglobin amyloid fibril formation under the control condition of 2,2,2-trifluoroethanol (45%) and incubated at 37°C for

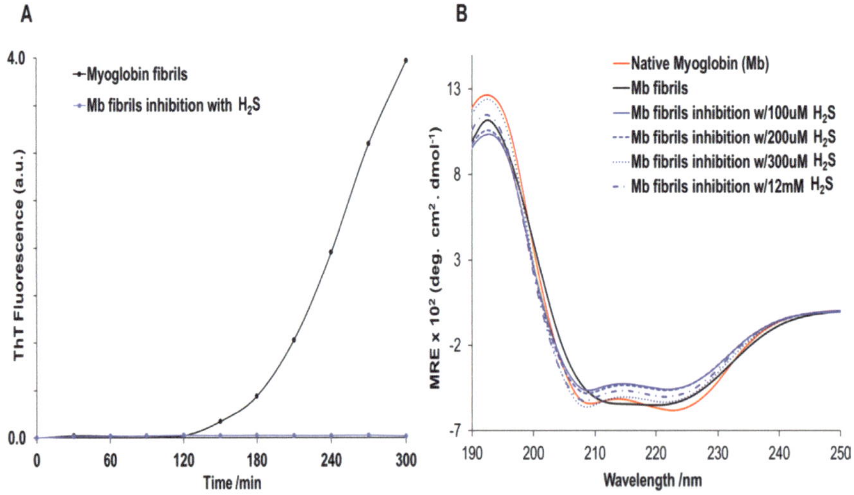

Figure 5.
Myoglobin fibrils and their inhibition by hydrogen sulfide. (A) Kinetics of myoglobin amyloid formation (black) and inhibition of Mb fibril formation (blue) in the presence of H_2S. (B) Far UV CD spectra of native Mb with a characteristic alpha-helical structure, Mb fibrils exhibiting beta-sheet structure, and Mb structures formed under the same condition of fibril formation, but in the presence of various H_2S (blue).

24 hours. There is a slightly difference between Mb and Hb lag phase leading to amyloid formation. However, when hydrogen sulfide is added under the control condition to Mb or Hb to generate fibrils, **Figures 5** and **6**, there is not an increase of ThT fluorescence (blue lines) for the duration of the experiment, independent of the lag phase difference between these hemeproteins. Therefore, the results demonstrate that under the experimental conditions, Mb and Hb fibrils are not observed in the presence of hydrogen sulfide. Curiously, a similar result was reported [34] for hen egg white lysozyme (HEWL), where the addition of H_2S in the fibril process completely inhibits the formation of β-sheet of amyloid fibrils.

Furthermore, **Figures 5B** and **6B** also show CD the spectra of native Mb and Hb with clear minima at 208 and 222 nm characteristic for α-helix conformation of protein (red line). These negative peaks at 208 and 222 nm result from n → π* transition in the peptide bond of α-helical conformation [40, 41, 59, 60]. The presented results also indicate that both Mb and Hb form beta-sheet structures with a characteristic negative band near 218 nm and the positive band at 195 nm in CD spectra, which could be attributed to amyloid fibrils, in the presence of 45% of 2,2,2-trifluoroethanol (TFE) (black line). The data also collaborate analogous results indicating the formation of hemoglobin fibrils [28, 40, 41, 59, 60]. Nevertheless, when hydrogen sulfide is added, the CD spectra of both myoglobin and hemoglobin show 208 and 222 nm negative peaks typical for alpha-helical proteins (blue lines), suggesting the inhibition of fibrils by H_2S.

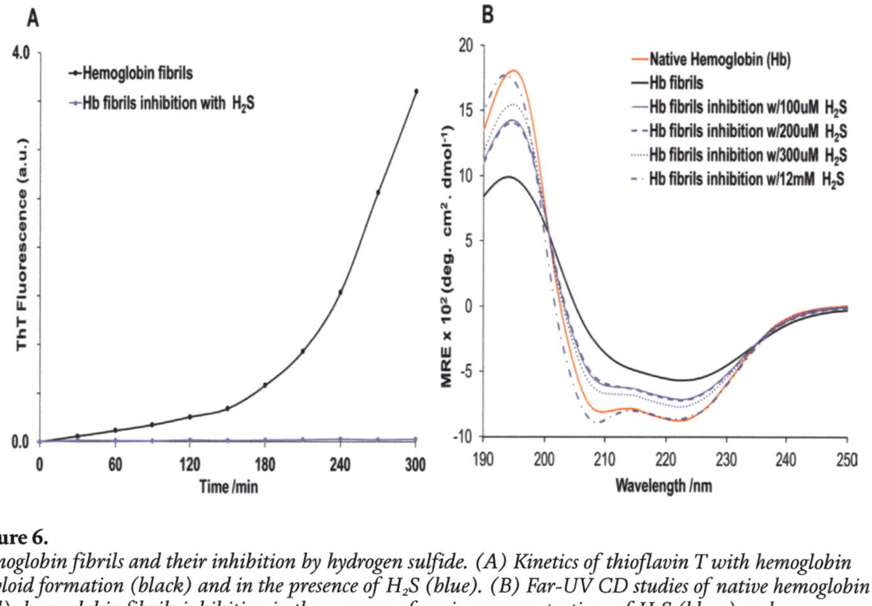

Figure 6.
Hemoglobin fibrils and their inhibition by hydrogen sulfide. (A) Kinetics of thioflavin T with hemoglobin amyloid formation (black) and in the presence of H_2S (blue). (B) Far-UV CD studies of native hemoglobin (red); hemoglobin fibrils inhibition in the presence of various concentrations of H_2S (blues) and hemoglobin fibrils (black).

4. Discussion

4.1 Evaluation of lysozyme secondary and tertiary structure

Lysozyme fibril formation has been extensively studied and characterized [36, 45, 61]. The most common methods used for studying the fibrillation process include AFM, ThT, and Trp fluorescence. DUVRR spectroscopy has been shown to be uniquely suitable for the structural characterization of proteins at all stages of the fibrillation process [51]. We utilized these complementary methods for studying the effect of H_2S on the morphology and structure of lysozyme aggregates. Although fibril formation was not detected by AFM and ThT fluorescence assays, the intrinsic Trp fluorescence marker suggested that significant tertiary structure changes had taken place minutes after H_2S incubation began. The red shift of Trp fluorescence of greater than 10 nm is typical for unfolded lysozyme [36]. Changes were also evident for SS bridges at the same time scale, as discussed in the next section. The changes observed in the tryptophan local environment and in SS bonds indicate substantial changes in HEWL tertiary structure.

DUVRR spectroscopy was utilized to investigate changes in HEWL secondary structure during the incubation with and without H_2S. It was found that H_2S prevented the formation of β-sheet and resulted in a significant transition of α-helix to unordered protein. Moreover, we utilized DUVRR spectra of aggregated lysozyme to evaluate the protein secondary structure composition. Xu et al. have reported on the quantitative analysis of lysozyme DUVRR spectral changes during its denaturation [36]. According to that work, the amount of α-helix melting can be estimated from the intensity of C_α—H bending band. This band is conveniently isolated from other Raman bands. β-Sheet and unordered structures only contribute to C_α—H bending DUVRR band, while the α-helix does not make a noticeable input [51]. It is evident from amide I Raman bands in DUVRR spectra presented in **Figure 1D** that no fibril-type β-sheet is formed in HEWL aggregates since the Am I intensity does not increase. Therefore, the increase in the C_α—H band intensity in the spectrum of HEWL aggregates relative to that of native protein could be assigned to newly formed unordered structures. We normalized the DUVRR spectra of HEWL aggregates and native protein with the denatured-reduced HEWL spectrum reported by Xu et al. and estimated the amount of α-helix in HEWL aggregates as 11% [36]. Assuming that the amount of β-sheet in HEWL aggregates is approximately the same as in the native protein, we estimated the secondary structural composition of HEWL aggregates as 83% unordered, 11% α-helix, and 6% β-sheet.

To summarize the results concerning the significant tertiary structural rearrangements, α-helix melting, and lack of β-sheet formation, we conclude that H_2S causes more significant denaturation of lysozyme than that taking place during the initial stages of protein fibrillation, which is typically reported as *partial* protein denaturation [36]. We hypothesize that this significant lysozyme denaturation results in rapid protein aggregation, the formation of spherical species, and the prevention of the formation of β-sheets and fibrillation. In other words, H_2S redirects the process to "off-pathway" aggregation, preventing fibril formation [8, 62, 63]. This observation is consistent with an earlier report by Wang and colleagues, which demonstrated that fully denatured lysozyme forms amorphous aggregates that prevent fibril formation [64]. The protein has been fully denatured by reducing SS bonds with DTT_{red}. As a result, fully denatured lysozyme may lack the hydrophobic regions which are present in the partially unordered intermediates formed at the early stage of fibril formation. In addition, it is possible that amorphous aggregates decreased the effective concentration of HEWL available for fibril formation [64]. In agreement with Wang's report, our results suggest that lysozyme denatures strongly in the presence of H_2S and forms unordered aggregates that prevent β-sheet formation and fibrillation.

4.2 Formation of trisulfide bridges

According to **Figure 3**, the contributions of both g-g-g (507 cm^{-1} band) and g-g-t (523 cm^{-1} band) conformations of SS bonds to the Raman spectrum of HEWL decreased significantly during its incubation with H_2S. Simultaneously, a new peak appeared at 490 cm^{-1} (**Figure 3A** and **C**). Nielsen and colleagues proposed that SSS bridges can form in proteins in the presence of H_2S via the thiol-disulfide exchange reaction, which is known to occur within cells [23]. We investigated the possibility of assigning a new Raman band at 490 cm^{-1} to the SSS moiety. Initially, we reproduced Raman spectra of two model compounds, dipropyl disulfide (DPDS) and dipropyl trisulfide (DPTS), shown in **Figure 3D**. In agreement with other published studies, these compounds exhibit strong Raman bands at 509 and 485 cm^{-1}, respectively, in agreement with the Raman spectra of native HEWL and HEWL spherical aggregates formed in the presence of H_2S [65, 66]. Furthermore, we obtained the difference spectrum by subtracting HEWL spectra after 0 and 90 minutes of incubation in the presence of H_2S and compared it to the expected spectral change representing the SS to SSS transition. The latter spectral change is depicted as a combination of dipropyl-disulfide and dipropyl-trisulfide spectra (**Figure 3D**). This spectral comparison provides further support for the hypothetical assignment of the 490 cm^{-1} Raman band to the SSS moiety.

Several studies have identified a 490 cm^{-1} Raman band in inorganic compounds and small organic molecules containing sulfur, and we report the appearance of this band in proteins for the first time [66–69]. Wieser and Krueger have assigned the 488 cm^{-1} Raman peak of H-SSS-H to a symmetric SS stretch with a contribution from the SSS bend [69]. Freeman has reported the Raman spectra of organic SS and SSS compounds, found in natural products where a strong 485 cm^{-1} stretching band has been observed in cyclic and acyclic trisulfides [66]. Janz et al. have reported Raman spectra of inorganic SSS from BaS_3 where 458 and 476 cm^{-1} bands were assigned to the symmetric stretching of SSS [68]. It is noteworthy that these frequencies can potentially be shifted in peptides. Kimbaris et al. have reported the Raman spectra of garlic oil, which contains a variety of compounds with SS and SSS groups [70]. We noticed an intense band at 489 cm^{-1} in these spectra that could potentially originate from an SSS moiety, although the assignment of the band was not discussed in the article. Overall, our hypothetical assignment of the 490 cm^{-1} Raman band to the SSS moiety is in agreement with data from the literature [66, 68]. The mechanism of SSS formation in proteins is unclear despite the significant interest that this topic has gained in recent years [21, 23, 35]. There is emerging evidence indicating that sulfane sulfur (S^0), which is generated from H_2S [56], is responsible for sulfuration through the formation of persulfide or trisulfide in proteins [71–73]. It would be interesting to investigate whether these SSS form by intra- or intermolecular processes. We are currently testing this hypothesis. It is noteworthy that the 490 cm^{-1} Raman band cannot be assigned to RSSH groups. These groups could form as a result of disulfide bond reduction in the presence of H_2S by a process known as sulfuration or sulfhydration [74].

4.3 The mechanism of HEWL, Mb, and Hb aggregation vs. fibrillation

Approximately 50% of all extracellular proteins have disulfide bridges [61]. SS bonds preserve the three dimensional structure of proteins and their cleavage typically results in significant disruption of the native conformations of proteins [57]. It is well established that SS bonds play a significant role in amyloid fibrillation [75]. Dobson and colleagues have reported that the reduction of SS bridges significantly accelerated the rate of human lysozyme aggregation [61]. It has also been demonstrated that reduction of four SS bonds to three bonds of apo-α-LA accelerates its fibrillation and leads to the formation of a new fibril polymorph with a different morphology and structure compared to fibrils formed from the wild-type LA [57]. At the same time, SS bonds of insulin remain intact and preserve their conformation during the fibrillation process [75]. Similar to insulin, the conformation of the SS bonds in HEWL remains intact during the fibrillation of HEWL in control solution, as we have described here. It has been suggested that a partial denaturation of lysozyme precedes fibril formation because the native tertiary structure would not allow rearrangement to the cross-β sheet structure due to steric constraints [8, 76]. It has also been reported that partial denaturation, the first step of lysozyme fibrillation, is an irreversible process [46]. At the same time, a fully denatured lysozyme forms amorphous aggregates that prevent fibril formation [64]. It is believed that the fully denatured protein lacks the hydrophobic side chains present in partially unordered intermediates. In addition, amorphous aggregates potentially decrease the effective concentration of HEWL available for fibril formation [64]. In agreement with these observations, our results suggest that lysozyme denatures strongly in the presence of H_2S and forms unordered aggregates that prevent β-sheet formation and fibrillation.

Regarding this, it has been shown that Hb under physiological conditions and in presence of 45% 2,2,2-trifluoethanol (TFE) produces amyloid-like fibril species [28]. The mechanism surrounding these fibril events remains almost unknown. Curiously, myoglobin and hemoglobin do not have any S-S moiety in their chemical structures, and **Figures 5** and **6** show that the fibrillation inhibition effect of H_2S depends on its concentration. Specifically, the Mb and Hb α-helix assemblies are almost preserved at higher H_2S concentrations. Therefore, in these hemeproteins, it is not clear the inhibition mechanism by H_2S, since CD indicates that hydrogen sulfide prevents β-sheet formation and fibrillation without altering significantly the α-helical structure of Mb or Hb. Also similar to HEWL, the addition of H_2S to Mb or Hb fibrils does not revert the β-sheet amyloid fibrils to the native α-structure. These results are consistent with the ThT findings that β-sheets are present in Mb and Hb amyloid-like fibrils in the presence of 45% TFE and that increasing concentration of H_2S inhibits β-sheet formation. The findings demonstrate the same H_2S effect on to the fibrillation of Mb monomer and Hb tetramer, although some quantitative kinetic differences may be evident and need further study.

Acknowledgements

This work was supported in part by the National Science Foundation under Award CHE-1152752 (I.K.L.), NSF PREM: Wisconsin-Puerto Rico Partnership for Research and Education in Materials under Award DMR-0934115 (J.L.G), the National Institute of Health-INBRE PR under Award P20GM103475-13 (J.L.G.), the Alfred P. Sloan NACME Grant No. 2010-3-02, and BioXFEL-National Science Foundation Grant No. 1231306.

Abbreviations

H_2S	hydrogen sulfide
HEWL	hen egg white lysozyme
DUVRR	deep ultraviolet resonance Raman
AFM	atomic force microscopy
ThT	thioflavin T
cys	cysteine
SOD	super oxide dismutase
hGH	human growth hormone
DPDS	dipropyl disulfide
DPTS	dipropyl trisulfide
DTT	dithiothreitol

Mb	myoglobin
Hb	hemoglobin
TFE	2,2,2-trifluoroethanol
CD	circular dichroism spectroscopy

Author details

Manuel F. Rosario-Alomar[1†], Tatiana Quiñones-Ruiz[2†], Dmitry Kurouski[2], Valentin Sereda[2], Eduardo DeBarros-Ferreira[2], Lorraine De Jesús-Kim[3], Samuel Hernández-Rivera[1], Dmitri V. Zagorevski[4], Leishla M. Cruz-Collazo[1†], Igor K. Lednev[2] and Juan López-Garriga[1*]

1 Department of Chemistry, University of Puerto Rico at Mayagüez, Mayagüez, Puerto Rico

2 Department of Chemistry, University at Albany, Albany, NY, USA

3 Department of Biology, University of Puerto Rico at Mayagüez, Mayagüez, Puerto Rico

4 Center for Biotechnology and Interdisciplinary Studies, Rensselaer Polytechnic Institute, Troy, NY, USA

*Address all correspondence to: juan.lopez16@upr.edu

† These authors contributed equally

References

[1] Serpell LC. Alzheimer's amyloid fibrils: Structure and assembly. Biochimica et Biophysica Acta-Molecular Basis of Disease. 2000;**1502**:16-30

[2] Conway KA, Harper JD, Lansbury PT Jr. Fibrils formed in vitro from alpha-synuclein and two mutant forms linked to Parkinson's disease are typical amyloid. The Biochemist. 2000;**39**:2552-2563

[3] Kantcheva RB, Mason R, Giorgini F. Aggregation-prone proteins modulate huntingtin inclusion body formation in yeast. PLoS Currents Huntington Disease. 2014;**6**:1-11

[4] Glenner GG. Amyloid deposits and amyloidosis. The beta-fibrilloses (first of two parts). The New England Journal of Medicine. 1980;**302**:1283-1292

[5] Blake C, Serpell L. Synchrotron X-ray studies suggest that the core of the transthyretin amyloid fibril is a continuous beta-sheet helix. Structure. 1996;**4**:989-998

[6] Lednev IK. Amyloid fibrils: The eighth wonder of the world in protein folding and aggregation. Biophysical Journal. 2014;**106**:1433-1435

[7] Uversky VN, Li J, Fink AL. Evidence for a partially folded intermediate in alpha-synuclein fibril formation. The Journal of Biological Chemistry. 2001;**276**:10737-10744

[8] Uversky VN, Fink AL. Conformational constraints for amyloid fibrillation: The importance of being unfolded. Biochimica et Biophysica Acta-Proteins Proteomics. 2004;**1698**:131-153

[9] Eto K, Asada T, Arima K, Makifuchi T, Kimura H. Brain hydrogen sulfide is severely decreased in Alzheimer's disease. Biochemical and Biophysical Research Communications. 2002;**293**:1485-1488

[10] Wang R. Physiological implications of hydrogen sulfide: A whiff exploration that blossomed. Physiological Reviews. 2012;**92**:791-896

[11] Pietri R, Roman-Morales E, Lopez-Garriga J. Hydrogen sulfide and hemeproteins: Knowledge and mysteries. Antioxidants & Redox Signaling. 2011;**15**:393-404

[12] Fukuto JM, Carrington SJ, Tantillo DJ, Harrison JG, Ignarro LJ, Freeman BA, et al. Small molecule Signaling agents: The integrated chemistry and biochemistry of nitrogen oxides, oxides of carbon, dioxygen, hydrogen sulfide, and their derived species. Chemical Research in Toxicology. 2012;**25**:769-793

[13] Blackstone E, Morrison M, Roth MB. H_2S induces a suspended animation-like state in mice. Science. 2005;**308**:518

[14] Li L, Rose P, Moore PK. Hydrogen sulfide and cell signaling. Annual Review of Pharmacology and Toxicology. 2011;**51**:169-187

[15] Benavides GA, Squadrito GL, Mills RW, Patel HD, Isbell TS, Patel RP, et al. Hydrogen sulfide mediates the vasoactivity of garlic. Proceedings of the National Academy of Sciences of the United States of America. 2007;**104**:17977-17982

[16] Chauhan NB. Effect of aged garlic extract on APP processing and tau phosphorylation in Alzheimer's transgenic model Tg2576. Journal of Ethnopharmacology. 2006;**108**:385-394

[17] Arosio P, Vendruscolo M, Dobson CM, Knowles TPJ. Chemical kinetics for drug discovery to

combat protein aggregation diseases. Trends in Pharmacological Sciences. 2014;**35**:127-135

[18] Kayed R, Head E, Sarsoza F, Saing T, Cotman CW, Necula M, et al. Fibril specific, conformation dependent antibodies recognize a generic epitope common to amyloid fibrils and fibrillar oligomers that is absent in prefibrillar oligomers. Molecular Neurodegeneration. 2007;**2**:18

[19] Kurouski D, Luo H, Sereda V, Robb FT, Lednev IK. Rapid degradation kinetics of amyloid fibrils under mild conditions by an archaeal chaperonin. Biochemical and Biophysical Research Communications. 2012;**422**:97-102

[20] Ravi VK, Goel M, Kotamarthi HC, Ainavarapu SRK, Swaminathan R. Preventing disulfide bond formation weakens non-covalent forces among lysozyme aggregates. PLoS One. 2014;**9**:e87012

[21] Gu S, Wen D, Weinreb PH, Sun Y, Zhang L, Foley SF, et al. Characterization of trisulfide modification in antibodies. Analytical Biochemistry. 2010;**400**:89-98

[22] Ogasawara Y, Isoda S, Tanabe S. Tissue and subcellular distribution of bound and acid-labile sulfur, and the enzymic capacity for sulfide production in the rat. Biological & Pharmaceutical Bulletin. 1994;**17**:1535-1542

[23] Nielsen RW, Tachibana C, Hansen NE, Winther JR. Trisulfides in proteins. Antioxidants & Redox Signaling. 2011;**15**:67-75

[24] David C, Foley S, Enescu M. Protein S-S bridge reduction: A Raman and computational study of lysozyme interaction with TCEP. Physical Chemistry Chemical Physics. 2009;**11**:2532-2542

[25] Reeder B, Sharpe M, Kay A, Kerr M, Moore K, Wilson M. Toxicity of myoglobin and haemoglobin: Oxidative stress in patients with rhabdomyolysis and subarachnoid haemorrhage. Biochemical Society Transactions. 2002;**30**(4):745-748. DOI: 10.1042/bst0300745

[26] Reeder B. The redox activity of hemoglobins: From physiologic functions to pathologic mechanisms. Antioxidants and Redox Signaling. 2010;**13**(7):1087-1123. DOI: 10.1089/ars.2009.2974

[27] Sawicki K, Chang H, Ardehali H. Role of heme in cardiovascular physiology and disease. Journal of the American Heart Association. 2015;**4**(1):e001138. DOI: 10.1161/JAHA.114.001138

[28] Iram A, Naeem A. Detection and analysis of protofibrils and fibrils of hemoglobin: Implications for the pathogenesis and cure of heme loss related maladies. Archives of Biochemistry and Biophysics. 2013;**533**:69-78. DOI: 10.1016/j.abb.2013.02.019

[29] Forget B, Bunn H. Classification of the disorders of hemoglobin. Cold Spring Harbor Perspectives in Medicine. 2013;**3**:a011684. DOI: 10.1101/cshperspect.a011684

[30] Bilska-Wilkosz A, Iciek M, Górny M, Kowalczyk-Pachel D. The role of hemoproteins: Hemoglobin, myoglobin and neuroglobin in endogenous thiosulfate production processes. International Journal of Molecular Sciences. 2017;**18**:1315. DOI: 10.3390/ijms18061315

[31] Alayash A. Hemoglobin-based blood substitutes and the treatment of sickle cell disease: More harm than help? Biomolecules. 2017;7:2. DOI: 10.3390/biom7010002

[32] Garcia-Seisdedos H, Empereur-Mot C, Elad N, Levy E. Proteins evolve

on the edge of supramolecular self-assembly. Nature. 2017;**548**:244-247. DOI: 10.1038/nature23320

[33] Dykes G, Crepeau R, Edelstein S. Three-dimensional reconstruction of the 14-filament fibers of hemoglobin S. Journal of Molecular Biology. 1979;**130**(4):451-472. DOI: 10.1016/0022-2836(79)90434-0

[34] Rosario-Alomar M, Quiñones-Ruiz T, Kurouski D, Sereda V, Ferreira E, De Jesus-Kim L, et al. Hydrogen sulfide inhibits amyloid formation. The Journal of Physical Chemistry B. 2015;**119**: 1265-1274. DOI: 10.1021/jp508471v

[35] Cumnock K, Tully T, Cornell C, Hutchinson M, Gorrell J, Skidmore K, et al. Trisulfide modification impacts the reduction step in antibody-drug conjugation process. Bioconjugate Chemistry. 2013;**24**:1154-1160

[36] Xu M, Ermolenkov VV, Uversky VN, Lednev IK. Hen egg white lysozyme fibrillation: A deep-UV resonance Raman spectroscopic study. Journal of Biophotonics. 2008;**1**:215-229

[37] Gade Malmos K, Blancas-Mejia L, Weber B, Buchner J, Ramirez-Alvarado M, Naiki H, et al. ThT 101: A primer on the use of thioflavin T to investigate amyloid formation. Amyloid. 2017;**24**(1):1-16. DOI: 10.1080/13506129.2017.1304905

[38] Shoffner S, Schnell S. Estimation of the lag time in a subsequent monomer addition model for fibril elongation. Physical Chemistry Chemical Physics. 2016;**18**:21259. DOI: 10.1039/c5cp07845h

[39] Xue C, Lin TY, Chang D, Guo Z. Thioflavin T as an amyloid dye: Fibril quantification, optimal concentration and effect on aggregation. Royal Society Open Science. 2017;**4**:160696. DOI: 10.1098/rsos.160696

[40] Nasreen K, Ahamad S, Ahmad F, Hassan M, Islam A. Macromolecular crowding induces molten globule state in the native myoglobin at physiological pH. International Journal of Biological Macromolecules. 2018;**106**:130-139. DOI: 10.1016/j.ijbiomac.2017.08.014

[41] Grenfield NJ. Using circular dichroism spectra to estimate protein secondary structure. Nature Protocols. 2006;**1**(6):2876-2890. DOI: 10.1038/nprot.2006.202

[42] Copeland RA, Spiro TG. Ultraviolet resonance Raman spectra of cytochrome c conformational states. The Biochemist. 1985;**24**:4960-4968

[43] Myshakina NS, Asher SA. Peptide bond vibrational coupling. The Journal of Physical Chemistry B. 2007;**111**:4271-4279

[44] Wang Y, Purrello R, Jordan T, Spiro TG. UVRR spectroscopy of the peptide bond. 1. Amide S, a nonhelical structure marker, is a C.alpha.H bending mode. Journal of the American Chemical Society. 1991;**113**:6359-6368

[45] Xu M, Ermolenkov VV, He W, Uversky VN, Fredriksen L, Lednev IK. Lysozyme fibrillation: Deep UV Raman spectroscopic characterization of protein structural transformation. Biopolymers. 2005;**79**:58-61

[46] Xu M, Shashilov V, Lednev IK. Probing the cross-β core structure of amyloid fibrils by hydrogen-deuterium exchange deep ultraviolet resonance Raman spectroscopy. Journal of the American Chemical Society. 2007;**129**:11002-11003

[47] Lednev IK. Vibrational spectroscopy: Biological applications of ultraviolet Raman spectroscopy. In: Uversky VN, Permyakov EA, editors. Protein Structures, Methods in Protein Structures and Stability Analysis. New York: Nova Science Publishers, Inc.; 2007

[48] Asher SA, Ianoul A, Mix G, Boyden MN, Karnoup A, Diem M, et al. Dihedral ψ angle dependence of the amide III vibration: A uniquely sensitive UV resonance Raman secondary structural probe. Journal of the American Chemical Society. 2001;**123**:11775-11781

[49] Tu AT. Raman Spectroscopy in Biology: Principles and Applications. Wiley: University of California; 1982

[50] Lednev I, Ermolenkov V, He W, Xu M. Deep-UV Raman spectrometer tunable between 193 and 205 nm for structural characterization of proteins. Analytical and Bioanalytical Chemistry. 2005;**381**:431-437

[51] Oladepo SA, Xiong K, Hong Z, Asher SA, Handen J, Lednev IK. UV resonance Raman investigations of peptide and protein structure and dynamics. Chemical Reviews. 2012;**112**:2604-2628

[52] Imoto T, Forster LS, Rupley JA, Tanaka F. Fluorescence of lysozyme: Emissions from tryptophan residues 62 and 108 and energy migration. Proceedings of the National Academy of Sciences of the United States of America. 1972;**69**:1151-1155

[53] Pajot P. Fluorescence of proteins in 6-M guanidine hydrochloride. The FEBS Journal. 1976;**63**:263-269

[54] Van Wart HE, Lewis a, Scheraga HA, Saeva FD. Disulfide bond dihedral angles from Raman spectroscopy. Proceedings of the National Academy of Sciences of the United States of America. 1973;**70**:2619-2623

[55] Nakanishi M, Takesada H, Tsuboi M. Conformation of the cystine linkages in bovine α-lactalbumin as revealed by its Raman effect. Journal of Molecular Biology. 1974;**89**:241-243

[56] Kocherbitov V, Latynis J, Misiūnas A, Barauskas J, Niaura G. Hydration of lysozyme studied by Raman spectroscopy. Journal of the Chemical Society B. 2013;**117**:4981-4992

[57] Lednev DKAIK. The impact of protein disulfide bonds on the amyloid fibril morphology. International Journal of Nanoscience and Nanotechnology. 2011;**2**:167-176

[58] Burns JA, Butler JC, Moran J, Whitesides GM. Selective reduction of disulfides by tris(2-carboxyethyl) phosphine. The Journal of Organic Chemistry. 1991;**56**:2648-2650

[59] Chen T, Zhu S, Shang Y, Ge C, Jiang G. Binding of dihydromyricetin to human hemoglobin: Fluorescence and circular dichroism studies. Spectrochimica Acta Part A: Molecular and Biomolecular Spectroscopy. 2012;**93**:125-130. DOI: 10.1016/j.saa.2012.02.109

[60] Kelly SM, Jess TJ, Price NC. How to study proteins by circular dichroism. Biochimica et Biophysica Acta (BBA)-Proteins and Proteomics. 2005;**1751**(2):119-139. DOI: 10.1016/j.bbapap.2005.06.005

[61] Mossuto MF, Bolognesi B, Guixer B, Dhulesia A, Agostini F, Kumita JR, et al. Disulfide bonds reduce the toxicity of the amyloid fibrils formed by an extracellular protein. Angewandte Chemie International Edition in English. 2011;**50**:7048-7051

[62] Dobson CM. Protein folding and misfolding. Nature. 2003;**426**:884-890

[63] Powers ET, Powers DL. Mechanisms of protein fibril formation: Nucleated polymerization with competing off-pathway aggregation. Biophysical Journal. 2008;**94**:379-391

[64] Wang SS, Liu K-N, Wang B-W. Effects of dithiothreitol on the amyloid fibrillogenesis of hen egg-white lysozyme. The FBES Journal. 2010;**39**:1229-1242

[65] Sugeta H, Go A, Miyazawa T. Vibrational spectra and molecular conformations of dialkyl disulfides. Bulletin of the Chemical Society of Japan. 1973;**46**:3407-3411

[66] Freeman SK. Applications of laser Raman spectroscopy to natural products research. Journal of Agricultural and Food Chemistry. 1973;**21**:521-525

[67] Rebouças JS, Patrick BO, James BR. Thiol, disulfide, and trisulfide complexes of Ru porphyrins: Potential models for iron-sulfur bonds in heme proteins. Journal of the American Chemical Society. 2012;**134**:3555-3570

[68] Janz GJ, Roduner E, Coutts JW, Downey JR. Raman studies of sulfur-containing anions in inorganic polysulfides. Barium trisulfide. Inorganic Chemistry. 1976;**15**:1751-1754

[69] Wieser H, Krueger PJ, Muller E, Hyne JB. Vibrational spectra and a force field for H_2S3 and H_2S4. Canadian Journal of Chemistry. 1969;**47**:1633-1637

[70] Kimbaris AC, Siatis NG, Pappas CS, Tarantilis PA, Daferera DJ, Polissiou MG. Quantitative analysis of garlic (*Allium sativum*) oil unsaturated acyclic components using FT-Raman spectroscopy. Food Chemistry. 2006;**94**:287-295

[71] Toohey JI. Sulfur signaling: Is the agent sulfide or sulfane? Analytical Biochemistry. 2011;**413**:1-7

[72] Greiner R, Palinkas Z, Basell K, Becher D, Antelmann H, Nagy P, et al. Polysulfides link H_2S to protein thiol oxidation. Antioxidants & Redox Signaling. 2013;**19**:1749-1765

[73] Kimura H. The physiological role of hydrogen sulfide and beyond. Nitric Oxide. 2014;**41**:4-10

[74] Kabil O, Banerjee R. Redox biochemistry of hydrogen sulfide. The Journal of Biological Chemistry. 2010;**285**:21903-21907

[75] Kurouski D, Washington J, Ozbil M, Prabhakar R, Shekhtman A, Lednev IK. Disulfide bridges remain intact while native insulin converts into amyloid fibrils. PLoS One. 2012;**7**:e36989

[76] Booth DR, Sunde M, Bellotti V, Robinson CV, Hutchinson WL, Fraser PE, et al. Instability, unfolding and aggregation of human lysozyme variants underlying amyloid fibrillogenesis. Nature. 1997;**385**:787-793

Chapter 10

Pathophysiology of Amyloid Fibril Formation

George H. Sack Jr.

Abstract

All amyloid comprises fibrillar polymers of tightly associated protein monomers. Central to the fibril structure is a highly ordered β-pleated sheet domain although this interacting region may only be a relatively short stretch of each constituent polypeptide chain. Fibril formation begins as a nucleation event based either on the constituent monomer protein or its proteolytic fragment(s). The resulting fibrils are generally chemically inert and very stable.

Keywords: amyloid, fibril, β-sheet, polymer, nucleation

1. Introduction

The term "amyloid" is intrinsically a misnomer. It was derived in the nineteenth century to describe what was then thought to be amorphous material composed of carbohydrate (*Gk* "amyl," starch) in both plants and pathologic specimens from humans and animals. In human pathology these deposits were identified in the kidney, liver, heart, brain, and elsewhere and were often associated with organ dysfunction. In 1942, Hass [1] showed that the material was largely protein, not carbohydrate. An important observation in 1959 [2] used electron microscopy to show that the material was not amorphous but, rather, consisted of long fibrils. **Figure 1** shows an example of amyloid fibrils.

Subsequent studies have been directed to identifying the constituent proteins and clarifying the process(es) of fibril formation. Treatment for affected individuals depends upon addressing the underlying chemistry and biology. We will review these in turn.

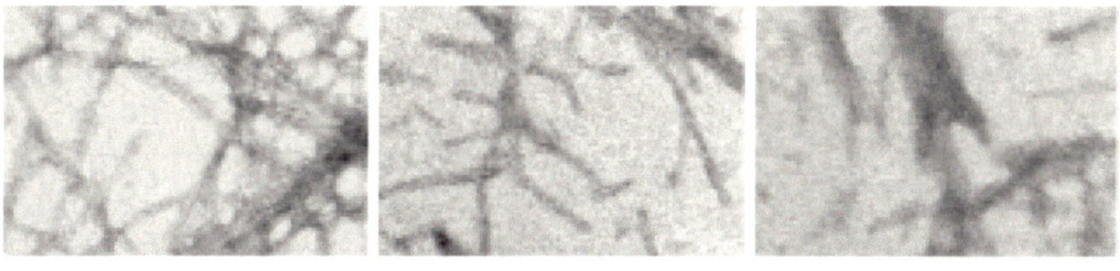

Figure 1.
Electron microscopic images of amyloid fibrils derived from synthetic sequences of Alzheimer β(1-42) polypeptides each containing different amino acid substitutions and yet forming characteristic fibrils, emphasizing the generalizability of amyloid fibril formation [3]. Copyright, 2005. National Academy of Sciences, used by permission.

2. Protein constituent(s) of amyloid fibrils

Many types of disorders are associated with amyloid deposits. Different fibril proteins underlie different pathologic contexts. **Table 1** presents examples of some types of amyloid diseases, the proteins from which their fibril proteins are derived, and their clinical associations. As will be noted below, it has become important to identify the precise molecular constituent(s) of the fibrils in order to establish the correct diagnosis and plan appropriate treatment.

In humans, the most frequently encountered pathologic amyloid fibrils are derived from fragments of immunoglobulin proteins. Some (but not all) immunoglobulin light chains (both κ and λ) have stretches of amino acids that can form the basic unit of amyloid fibrils. These are usually found in association with clonal proliferations of plasma cells which range from "monoclonal gammopathy of unknown significance" (i.e., "MGUS") to disorders such as myeloma. The fibrils themselves can cause distortion of organ microanatomy leading to cell dysfunction, disrupted cell-cell communication and, ultimately, organ failure.

Another well-studied type of amyloid fibril is derived from fragments of a small (104 amino acid) serum protein called "serum amyloid A (SAA)." Deposits of this type of amyloid are characteristic of chronic inflammatory or infectious disorders. It is likely that many of the examples of "amyloid" disease described in the pre-antibiotic era were derived from SAA (examples include tuberculosis and osteomyelitis).

Many genetic variants of transthyretin (TTR), another small, 127 amino acid serum protein, are associated with familial forms of amyloid disease. Affected individuals show progressive neurologic and/or cardiac dysfunction with concomitant amyloid deposition [6]. In addition, some individuals develop TTR amyloid disease (particularly involving the heart) in the absence of an underlying mutation in the protein.

Amyloid fibrils and plaques are characteristic of the neurodegeneration of Alzheimer disease. In this case, the parent protein is a large membrane-spanning protein referred to as β-amyloid. Only a small fragment of the primary protein is found in amyloid fibrils [7]. Specific endoproteases release this fragment from the parent molecule. As **Figure 1** shows, characteristic amyloid fibrils can be formed from Aβ(1-42) polypeptides with individual amino acid variation(s).

Parkinson disease is another disorder of the central nervous system associated with cellular depositions. In this case, α-synuclein accumulates in cells of the basal ganglia associated with loss of function. In neurons, relatively disorganized oligomers of α-synuclein appear first, and there is gradual compaction with β-sheet domains becoming prominent later [8, 9].

Considerable interest has arisen regarding prions. These are alternative conformations of proteins that can self-associate and self-propagate. First determined to be causative agents of "spongiform encephalopathy" in humans (e.g., Creutzfeldt-Jakob disease), prions also have become recognized as responsible for transmissible neuropathies in animals (e.g., "mad cow" disease). Studies of Sup35 prions in yeast have been particularly informative, and multiple strains can be isolated [10].

Another interesting category of disorders associated with amyloid fibril formation includes polypeptide hormones. Many of these are originally stored in relatively concentrated form within membrane-enclosed secretory granules. **Table 1** lists several associated types. In normal physiology dissociation of these organized structures must occur in order to release individual hormones [11]. In certain situations, however, these same hormones (or their precursors) can persist and become detected as fibrils.

Designation	Precursor protein	Clinical example(s)
AL	κ, λ Light chains	Myeloma, MGUS
AA	Serum amyloid A	Secondary
ATTR	Transthyretin	Nerve/heart
Aβ	β-Protein precursor	Alzheimer
APrP	Prion protein	Encephalopathy
Aβ_2M	β_2-Microglobulin	Dialysis related
AIAPP	Amylin	Type II diabetes
ACal	(Pro)calcitonin	Medullary thyroid carcinoma
AANF	Atrial natriuretic factor	Atrial amyloid
AαSyn	α-Synuclein	Parkinson disease

Table 1.
Examples of pathologic human amyloid fibril proteins [4, 5].

3. Fibril structure

All amyloid fibrils share a basic unit comprising a relatively short and (usually) contiguous stretch of amino acids whose three-dimensional contours can be accommodated in a β-pleated sheet conformation (both parallel and antiparallel assemblies are recognized in fibrils). Hydrogen bonds between the amide groups polarize each other. Van der Waals forces also develop between the β-sheets. Water molecules are displaced from between the faces of the sheets. These important features emphasize that protein precursors of amyloid fibrils are not in their native state—the constituent monomer is in an altered conformation, and this state may only be transient prior to nucleation. Thus, there is an array of polypeptide species that may underlie fibril formation; the most (transiently) stable and/or abundant species is most likely to be captured in a stable β-sheet.

As shown by Riek and Eisenberg [12], amyloids derived from different protein constituents may have very different β-sheet domains. In addition, these regions may be rather small in comparison with the length of the parent protein(s). This implies that only a fragment of the parent (i.e., longer) protein may be found in the ultimate amyloid fibril, and this, in turn, implies that cleavage of the parent protein is often part of the process of fibril formation. **Figure 2** presents example details of the particularly well-studied Alzheimer Aβ(1-42) fibril.

The β-pleated sheet topology of the basic interacting region permits individual regions to stack upon one another in a highly ordered manner—thus extending into the long axis of the fibril (see **Figure 2**). The result is stabilization not only between β-sheet domains but also between stacked subunits. Fibrils often show a twist along their long axis.

Once the requisite region for forming β-sheets becomes available, fibril formation begins as a nucleation event. Usually small numbers of monomers interact, but once the primordial oligomeric fibrillary unit is assembled, further extension can occur by aligning new monomers with the growing fibril surface. The kinetics of this process are consistent with this scheme, there generally being a lag in assembling the oligomer followed by more rapid extension as subunits are added.

Most amyloid fibrils share relatively common dimensions although their lengths often vary. Because the fibrils are so tightly associated within their common nuclei of β-sheet domains, they are themselves rather resistant to dissociation (substantial free energy of formation) as well as to attack by proteases (regions susceptible to

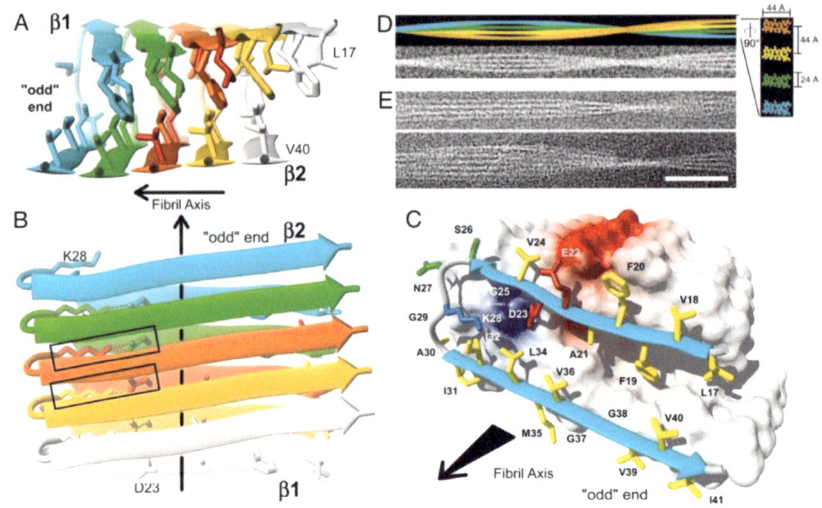

Figure 2.
Details of Alzheimer Aβ(1-42) fibril emphasizing amino acids 17-42. (A) Ribbon diagram of the core. (B) Salt bridges are indicated by the rectangles. (C) View of the "odd" end of the growing fibril showing the van der Waals surface as well as the amino acid side chains. The fibril axis is shown, corresponding to that in A and B. (D) Simulation of a fibril with four filaments (the adjacent figure shows the filament ends and the dimensions). (E) Cryoelectron micrographs of single fibrils [3]. Copyright 2005, National Academy of science, used by permission.

proteolysis may not be accessible). These molecular features help explain both the chronicity and the progressive nature of amyloid disorders.

Amyloid fibrils characteristically bind planar dye molecules. Upon binding to fibrils, these dyes can show birefringence when viewed using polarized light microscopy, providing a widely used method for identifying amyloid deposits in biologic tissues. The dyes Congo Red and Thioflavin T are used most frequently.

Another feature of amyloid fibrils is that they are usually found associated with other molecules. These include glycosaminoglycans (which may be responsible for calcium binding) as well as the pentraxin protein—"serum amyloid P" (SAP) [13]. These common features permit some imaging techniques to identify amyloid fibrils radiographically. For example, it is often possible to scan for SAP in order to localize amyloid deposits of various types [14].

Reference to **Table 1** emphasizes the variety of proteins that can form the β-pleated sheet structural units of amyloid fibrils. The proteins generally do not share common sequences or large-scale features because the region(s) essential for nucleating fibrils is(are) small (recall **Figure 2**). The protein constituent(s) of fibrils can frequently be determined using specific antibodies. The choice of antibodies to use is generally aided by the location of the deposit(s) and the clinical and/or pathologic context.

4. Fibril formation

As noted above, the fundamental event in amyloid formation is highly specific interaction between adjacent (usually) small protein units to form antiparallel (and, in some cases, parallel) β-sheets. The native state of the parent protein is generally thermodynamically more stable than the amyloid state. However, it is important to note that the stability of the amyloid state depends on protein concentration while that of the native precursor is largely independent of protein concentration. There thus arises a concentration above which the stability of the amyloid state can become the same as or even transiently greater than that of the native state. Not surprisingly, the complex topology of long proteins makes them unlikely to nucleate and extend into stable fibrils. This generally limits formation of amyloid fibrils to proteins <150 aa [5].

Once the requisite region for forming the β-sheet becomes accessible, fibril formation begins as a stochastic nucleation event. Usually small numbers of monomers interact, but once the primordial oligomeric fibrillary unit is assembled, further extension can occur by aligning new monomers with the growing fibril surface. The kinetics of this process are consistent with this scheme, there generally being a lag in assembling the oligomer followed by more rapid extension as subunits are added.

Because different types of amyloid fibrils have different protein constituents and may be found in different locations, it is not always possible to identify common features. An important distinction is between fibrils that have soluble, generally blood-based, precursors and those derived from specific intracellular or organ-limited proteins. Among the former are immunoglobulins (usually κ or λ light chains) and serum amyloid A. The latter include hormone precursors such as procalcitonin, prolactin, as well as amylin and the β-protein precursor. Prions generally begin intracellularly.

As noted earlier, the protein precursors of amyloid fibrils are usually complex with multiple domains, and the critical, nucleating region is often small. Thus, many must undergo proteolysis in order to eliminate domains that are topologically incompatible with fibril dimensions and structure. In the best-studied examples, proteolysis occurs within lysosomes or related organelles although not all sites (or responsible proteases) have been determined.

Figure 3 presents a scheme for AA fibril formation from circulating SAA. SAA is usually found in association with high-density lipoprotein in the blood, and it must dissociate and enter the cell, often using clathrin-mediated endocytosis. Within the cell (in lysosomes or related structures), the acidic pH leads to unfolding of the precursor as reactive groups are titrated (steps A–C). This likely exposes region(s) with increased susceptibility to proteolysis. The considerable free energy of anti-parallel (or, for some other fibril precursors, parallel) β-pleated sheet formation and the relatively high local concentrations of appropriate domains leads to nucleation and at least some oligomer formation (steps C, D).

Intracellular oligomeric fibril nucleation ultimately causes organelle disruption followed by loss of cellular integrity (step E). The possibility of exosome participation at this stage has not been excluded. The result is a local mixture of nascent and growing amyloid fibrils and cell debris. Having oligomeric "seeds" already formed intracellularly, fibril elongation can then be extended. The result becomes a mixed,

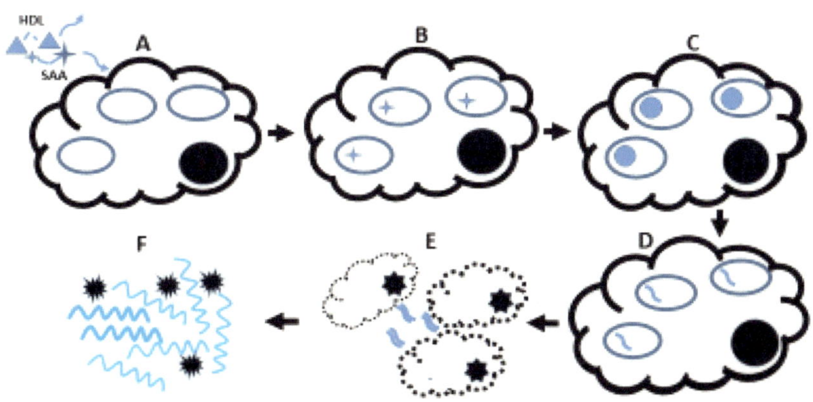

Figure 3.
Scheme for multiple steps in AA fibril formation from circulating SAA (from [16] see text for details).

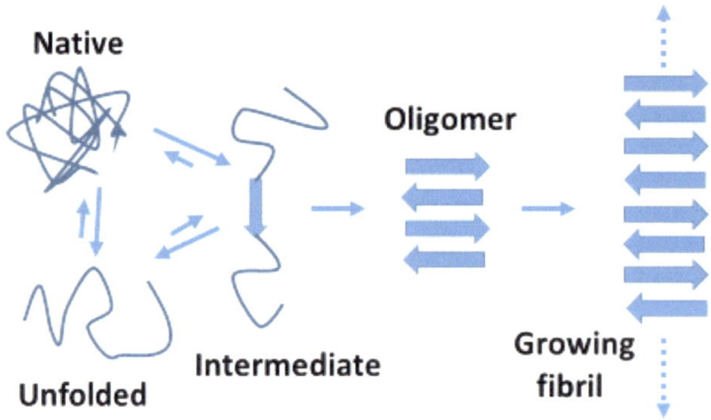

Figure 4.
Scheme for nucleation of TTR amyloid oligomers.

largely acellular, region where amyloid fibrils become the predominant structured species (step F) [15, 16].

A contrasting situation can occur in situations where the fibril precursor is not only soluble but also intrinsically capable of β structure formation without cleavage. **Figure 4** shows events for transthyretin (TTR). TTR is a 127 amino acid protein circulating in the blood as a stable tetramer that binds thyroid hormone and retin A (hence, its name). The TTR monomer itself contains prominent β-sheet domains. If the tetramer dissociates, the free monomers can misfold into various forms. Among these, some can associate as oligomers which then can be extended into fibrils. TTR amyloid fibrils are particularly prone to cause dysfunction in nerves and the heart. Interestingly, over 100 amino acid substitutions (i.e., mutations) have been identified in TTR [17]. Mutations differentially affect tetramer stability—some increase it, while others reduce it. Among the latter are several that are associated with inherited amyloid diseases, and the Val30Met and Val122Ile mutations have been particularly well-studied (affecting nerves and/or the heart). Kinetic and other evidence implicates the oligomer form(s) as directly involved in organ dysfunction. Amyloid fibrils become detectable by microscopy as the disease progresses. One proposed therapeutic strategy involves developing small molecules that stabilize the circulating tetramer, hence reducing (or eliminating) dissociation, oligomer formation, and tissue toxicity [18].

5. Pathologic consequences of amyloid formation

As indicated by **Table 1**, many disorders can be associated with amyloid deposition. In many cases, the precise mechanism of pathologic dysfunction is unknown. Nevertheless, several notions are important.

First, as noted, some polypeptide hormones are apparently stored in amyloid-like conformations. These differ from most of the other types in being reversible upon hormone release. Only in rare situations do these protein accumulations persist as amyloid deposits and become associated with disease.

Second, evolution has often minimized protein sequences that are particularly prone to nucleate amyloid fibrils [19]. Many proteins are located in intracellular regions or are associated with chaperones that reduce their likelihood of assuming alternative conformations. Degradation mechanisms including proteasomes can minimize intracellular aggregation.

In so-called "secondary" amyloid disease, the bulk of accumulated fibrils likely interferes with cellular and organ function. For example, remarkably large quantities of AA protein were isolated from the kidneys, liver, and spleen in earlier studies [20, 21]. Examining affected tissues by light microscopy clearly shows large interruptions in organ structural integrity due to massive amyloid deposits. Similar accumulations often accompany "primary" (i.e., immunoglobulin-derived) amyloid disease where fragments of immunoglobulin light chains may be found in large deposits.

Evidence from other types of amyloid disease indicates that large, microscopically visible deposits of amyloid fibrils may not always be the initial cause of cell/organ dysfunction. While fibrils are often seen later in study of affected tissues (and, hence, appear as classic "amyloid" by staining), they may be late consequences. Earlier, oligomeric forms may be more disruptive and lead to organ dysfunction well before large deposits are detectable by microscopy.

Figure 4 (above) presents a simple scheme for oligomer formation. This is likely to occur as a basic pathway in various types of amyloid-related diseases. As described above, destabilization of the TTR tetramer occurs extracellularly and can lead to oligomers that are relatively small. Various TTR mutations can destabilize the tetramer and accelerate this process although even the normal protein also appears susceptible in some situations. This likely is a problem for various intracellular neurotoxic fibrils and their predecessors (e.g., β-protein and α-synuclein) as well [22]. Thus, finding substantial amounts of extracellular Congo Red staining deposits may be a late feature of the basic disorder rather than the primary cause of dysfunction. As noted above, such material is generally quite stable and often resistant to dissociation. Hence, extracellular deposits (or even substantial accumulations within organelles) may be the end point of the toxic oligomer pathway.

6. Therapeutic approaches to amyloid pathophysiology

As described above, once formed, amyloid fibrils are intrinsically quite stable due to intra- and intermolecular bonds and relative inaccessibility to proteases. Ideally, disrupting the fibrils themselves would be an appropriate approach to treating at least some amyloid disorders. In this regard, chaotropic molecules (e.g., urea, guanidinium, etc.), often used in the laboratory, are not options for treatment due to their toxicity. Alternative agents, compatible with in vivo use have not yet been identified. Thus, successful intervention(s) for amyloid disorders must either prevent formation of the precursor(s) or stabilize the protein predecessors of oligomers (or their proteolytic cleavage). Several approaches have been introduced, and these depend upon the *specific* type of amyloidosis (recall **Table 1**).

Immunoglobulin light chain overproduction ("primary" amyloidosis) is basically a clonal disorder of plasma cell proliferation/overexpression. Here, treatment generally depends on suppression or elimination of the responsible cell population. This falls into the spectrum of treatment of myeloma and related disorders and depends on oncologic approaches.

Amyloid A (SAA) disorders ("secondary" amyloidosis) generally reflect overproduction of the SAA precursor. These usually are related to chronic or periodic and recurrent infection/inflammation. The incidence of these has been reduced by successful treatment of conditions such as tuberculosis and osteomyelitis. However, these and other types of infections and inflammation remain prominent in certain parts of the world and can be accompanied by amyloidosis. Genetic disorders such as familial Mediterranean fever with recurrent, self-limited inflammatory episodes can usually be controlled with agents such as colchicine [23], minimizing SAA synthesis and AA amyloid accumulation.

For TTR-related disorders several approaches are recognized. First, because the liver is the main site for the synthesis of TTR, liver transplantation can eliminate production of the mutant TTR protein. Although this has been used successfully, it is a complex process with its own intrinsic short- and long-term complications [24]. Second, synthesis of the responsible mutant protein can be suppressed. Several approaches based on specifically interrupting stability of TTR messenger RNA through RNAi have been developed. (Carriers of TTR mutations are usually heterozygotes, so these approaches generally reduce levels of both mutant and normal TTR—apparently, a reduced concentration of TTR is well-tolerated.) Third, the circulating tetramer can be stabilized by exogenous agents (e.g., Tafamidis™) to shift the equilibrium away from dissociation (and, hence, minimize oligomer formation). These approaches show promise [25, 26].

For neurologic disorders where the underlying problem is likely intracellular (e.g., α-synuclein and β-protein), the above approaches have not been feasible. It is more likely that clarification of complex intracellular pathways will be required in order to develop approaches to prevent and/or interrupt fibril accumulation in these and related conditions.

7. Conclusions

Amyloid formation and related disorders present examples of situations where there is fundamental dependence on protein structure, its variation(s), abundance, and the consequences of alternative conformation(s). Because the molecules involved are quite different for each type of amyloid disease, different organs may be involved, and stabilizing or eliminating the precursors likely will vary. Successful therapeutic intervention will likely be unique to each type of amyloidosis. The basic concerns are similar, however, and considerable progress has already clarified both the problem(s) and the options.

Acknowledgements

Support for these studies was provided by generous gifts to the author from Stuart Bainum, Mary Nell and George A. Berry, Ethelbert Cooper, Gloria and Edward Felsenthal, Ruth Frey, Shirley Griffin, Ruth and George Harms, Yancey and David Hillegas, Diantha Johnson, Bassem Kudsi, Steven Lazinsky, Judy Lewent and Mark Shapiro, Terrence O'Donnell, Jay Ripley, Israel Vainboim, the Foundation for Greater Good, the Health Network Foundation, and the MetLife Foundation.

Conflict of interest

The author declares no conflict of interest.

Author details

George H. Sack Jr.
Departments of Biological Chemistry and Medicine, Johns Hopkins University School of Medicine, Baltimore, Maryland, USA

*Address all correspondence to: gsack@jhmi.edu

References

[1] Hass G. Studies of amyloid. II. The isolation of a polysaccharide from amyloid-bearing tissues. Archives of Pathology. 1942;**34**:92-105

[2] Cohen AS, Calkins E. Electron microscopic observations on a fibrous component in amyloid of diverse origins. Nature. 1959;**183**:1202

[3] Lührs T, Christiane R, Adrian M, et al. 3D structure of Alzheimer's amyloid-B(1-42) fibrils. Proceedings of the National Academy of Sciences of the United States of America. 2005;**102**:17341-17347

[4] Sack GH Jr. Amyloidosis. In: Stone JH, editor. A Clinician's Pearls and Myths in Rheumatology. Dordrecht Heidelberg London New York: Springer; 2009. pp. 461-466

[5] Knowles TPJ, Vendrusolo M, Dobson CM. The amyloid state and its association with protein misfolding diseases. Nature Reviews. Molecular Cell Biology. 2014;**15**:384-396

[6] Skinner M. Familial amyloidotic cardiomyopathy. The Journal of Laboratory and Clinical Medicine. 1991;**117**:171-172

[7] Sack GH Jr. Chemistry of Alzheimer disease. Encyclopedia of Biological Chemistry. 2013;**2**:473-479

[8] Cremades NC, Samuel IA, Deas E, et al. Direct observation of the interconversion of normal and toxic forms of alpha-Synuclein. Cell. 2012;**149**:1048-1059

[9] Jucker M, Walker LC. Self-propagation of pathogenic protein aggregates in neurodegenerative diseases. Nature. 2013;**501**:45-51

[10] True HL, Lindquist SL. A yeast prion provides a mechanism for genetic variation and phenotypic diversity. Nature. 2000;**407**:477-483

[11] Maji SK, Perrin MH, Sawaya MR, et al. Functional amyloids as natural storage of peptide hormones in pituitary granules. Science. 2009;**325**:328-332

[12] Riek RE, Eisenberg DS. The activities of amyloids from a structural perspective. Nature. 2016;**539**:227-235

[13] Pepys MB. Pathogenesis, diagnosis and treatment of systemic amyloidosis. Philosophical Transactions. Royal Society of London. 2001;**356**:203-211

[14] Bokhari S, Castano A, Posniakoff T, et al. (99m)TC-pyrophosphate scintigraphy for differentiating light-chain cardiac amyloidosis from the transthyretin-related familial and senile cardiac amyloidoses. Circulation. Cardiovascular Imaging. 2013;**6**:195-201

[15] Claus S, Meinhardt K, Aumuller T, et al. Cellular mechanism of fibril formation from serum amyloid A1 protein. EMBO Reports. 2017;**18**:1352-1366

[16] Sack GH Jr. Serum amyloid A—A review. Molecular Medicine. 2018;**24**:46. DOI: 10.1186/s10020-018-0047-0

[17] Saraiva MJM. Transthyretin mutations in health and disease. Human Mutation. 1995;**5**:191-196

[18] Sekijima Y, Dendle MA, Kelly JW. Orally administered diflunisal stabilizes transthyretin against dissociation required for amyloidogenesis. Amyloid. 2006;**13**:236-249

[19] Tartaglia GG. Prediction of aggregation-prone regions in structured proteins. Journal of Molecular Biology. 2008;**380**:425-436

[20] Benditt EP, Eriksen N, Hermodson MA, Ericsson LH. The major proteins or human and monkey amyloid substance: Common properties including unusual N-terminal amino acid sequences. FEBS Letters. 1971;**19**:169-173

[21] Benditt EP, Eriksen N. Chemical similarity among amyloid substances associated with long-standing inflammation. Laboratory Investigation. 1972;**26**:615-625

[22] Caughey BL. Protofibrils, pore fibrils, and neurodegeneration: Separating the responsible protein aggregates from the innocent bystanders. Annual Review of Neuroscience (Palo Alto, CA). 2003;**26**:267-298

[23] Shohat MH, Gabrielle J. Familial mediterranean fever. Genetics in Medicine. 2011;**13**:487-498

[24] Castano A, Drachman BM, Judge D, Maurer MS. Natural history and therapy of TTR-cardiac amyloidosis: Emerging disease-modifying therapies from organ transplantation to stabilizer and silencer drugs. Heart Failure Reviews. 2015;**20**:163-178

[25] Adams D, Gonzales-Duarte A, O'Riordan WD, et al. Patisiran, an RNAi therapeutic, for hereditary transthyretin amyloidosis. The New England Journal of Medicine. 2018;**379**:11-21

[26] Buxbaum JN. Oligonucleotide drugs for transthyretin amyloidosis. The New England Journal of Medicine. 2018;**379**:82-85

Chapter 11

Neuroprotective Function of Non-Proteolytic Amyloid-β Chaperones in Alzheimer's Disease

Bhargy Sharma and Konstantin Pervushin

Abstract

This chapter attempts to explore protective role of chaperone proteins in the neurodegenerative diseases caused by amyloidosis. These chaperones prevent amyloid pathology either directly, through chemical interactions with amyloidogenic species to mediate their refolding, solubilization and degradation, or indirectly, by scavenging reactive oxygen species produced as by-products of amyloid aggregation. Here we focus on structural and morphological changes during aggregation of amyloids which have been identified using Nuclear magnetic resonance spectroscopy, X-ray crystallography, Electron microscopy, Atomic force microscopy and other biophysical techniques as well as interactions between chaperone proteins and amyloid moieties. Non-proteolytic chaperones mediate amyloid clearance and metabolism through conformational changes due to proximity binding. In this chapter, we delineate these interactions as well as the molecular mechanism of chaperones used to sequester ROS products of amyloidosis with focus on amyloid-β peptides associated with the Alzheimer's disease.

Keywords: amyloid-β, structural biology, aggregation, chaperone, neuroprotection, Alzheimer's disease

1. Introduction

Abnormal deposition of amyloids or "Amyloidosis" is hallmark of several chronic cerebrovascular diseases including neurodegeneration culminating into dementia. Efforts to develop targeted drugs against amyloids have been hindered since there is no universal mechanism that leads to protein misfolding or aggregation, and the aggregates usually do not correspond directly to clinical symptoms of the diseases. A clearer understanding of molecular interactions of amyloids can drive the ongoing therapeutic efforts to prevent aggregation of nascent amyloids into pathological species and to design timely interventions. In addition to aging, precursor mutations in genes and proteins, gene multiplication, expansion of amyloidogenic sequences, and xenobiotics such as air pollutants are risk factors usually associated with amyloidosis disorders [1]. There are different amyloidogenic species causing a variety of neuropathic diseases such as Alzheimer's disease (AD), Parkinson's disease (PD), Poly-glutamine disorders like Huntington disease (HD), Prion diseases including Creutzfeldt-Jakob disease, Lewy body disease, Amyotrophic Lateral Sclerosis (ALS) as well as metabolic diseases such as type II diabetes (T2D) and corneal dystrophy to name a few [2]. AD is a pandemic form of dementia caused due to improper aggregation of amyloidogenic proteins-amyloid-β (Aβ), which is a cleavage product of amyloid precursor protein (APP) and tau, stabilizes microtubules in neurons [3]. Prognosis is also closely associated with aggregation of α-Synuclein (αS) protein into Lewy bodies usually concentrated in presynaptic terminals [4]. Human islet amyloid polypeptide (IAPP), also known as amylin, is secreted along with insulin from pancreatic β-islet cells. IAPP rich amyloid plaques, facilitated by insulin resistance, are hallmarks of T2D [5]. β-sheeted infectious isoform of cellular prion protein (PrP) causes transmissible spongiform encephalopathy (TSE), broadly known as prion disease [2].

In this chapter, we review various structures and conformations attained by Aβ peptides during the process of aggregation. We begin with introducing different morphologies and conformations attained by amyloids during this process. We outline mechanisms of amyloid pathology, either directly mediated by aggregates or indirectly through generation of oxidative stress. We have briefly alluded to chaperone functions of Heat shock protein (Hsp) family and their interactions to different amyloid structures as well as intracellular protease mechanisms. It is important to note that such intracellular proteases are almost entirely inefficient in dealing with large insoluble plaques. Here we emphasize on additional endogenous proteins which show potential as chaperones, albeit through different mechanisms. Towards the end, we discuss the role of oxidative stress in accelerating AD pathology and the effect of Aβ interactions with metal species. Mechanisms to alleviate oxidative stress and their possible protective role in AD have been discussed.

2. Structural and biophysical basis of amyloid aggregation

Membrane glycoprotein APP is cleaved by β-secretase and γ-secretase enzymes generating 36–49 residue long peptides, among which amyloidogenic Aβ(1–40) and Aβ(1–42) are well-known culprits in AD [6]. Unstructured monomeric amyloids polymerize to form fibrillar structures with characteristic cross-β morphology formed by in-register β-sheets which align parallel to the fibrillar axis whereas perpendicularly extended side-chains pack closely to form tight steric zippers [2]. Nuclear magnetic resonance (NMR) spectroscopy studies on amyloid monomers or fibrillar structures to identify characteristic dynamic structural features. X-ray crystallographic studies have helped in identifying structural motifs through fiber diffraction and mass-per-length studies through EM provide information regarding specific symmetries identified in filaments. NMR models of Aβ monomeric peptides show predominantly α-helices with propensity to convert into β-sheets [6]. The α-helical conformation is also observed among on-pathway transient intermediates, possibly mediated by interactions of hydrophilic N-terminal residues [7]. These intermediates then give way to β-sheet conformation in higher oligomeric species which eventually transition into mature fibrils. *In vitro* aggregation of Aβ monomers into fibrils can be carefully curated to obtained different fibril morphology. In solid state nuclear magnetic resonance (ssNMR) spectra, cross-peaks originating from hydrophobic core and C-terminal regions within amyloid fibrils, prepared without seeding indicate presence of polymorphs. Formation of homogenous fibrils from Aβ(1–42) seeds precludes aggregation of Aβ(1–40) [8].

αS binds to neuronal membranes in a highly α-helical state as opposed to the unfolded monomeric conformation [7]. The antipathic N-terminal sequence has tendency to form α-helical conformation, central region from aa 61–95 is highly hydrophobic and amyloidogenic, and the C-terminal domain provides flexibility to the protein without attaining any specific structure [7]. Prefibrillar αS shows conformational plasticity and the soluble monomers combine to form unstable dimeric molecules which further aggregate into higher oligomers and fibrils. IAPP structure in detergent micelles shows a helical conformation kinked around residue His18 at neutral pH and an extended α-helix in acidic conditions; thus the ability to attain specific conformation also depends on its chemical environment [5].

2.1 Morphological differences in amyloid aggregates

Disordered or misfolded monomers can convert into a range of amyloid species, e.g., spherical oligomers, amorphous aggregates, annular oligomers, protofibrils, inclusion bodies or insoluble fibrils, based on the pathological pathways (**Table 1**). Dynamic intermediate oligomers form transient structures facilitating on-pathway conversion from misfolded monomers to fibrils. The spherical and annular aggregates get generated off-pathway and contribute highly to amyloid mediated neurotoxicity [2, 9]. The Lewy bodies formed by αS are example of intracellular amyloid inclusions [10]. Formation of a specific aggregated form is usually controlled by process of nucleation. In primary nucleation, seeds are formed by spontaneous aggregation of monomers followed by fibril elongation, whereas fragments from mature fibrils recruit monomers to facilitate the polymerization in secondary nucleation process. However, this process is specific to monomeric species; seeding with Aβ(1–42) fibrils does not contribute to aggregation of Aβ(1–40) [8]. Comparison between kinetic profiles of seeded and non-seeded Aβ(1–40) suggest that aggregation follows the seeded fibrils template [8]. Monomeric Aβ(1–40) samples form striated ribbons under constant agitation, and twisted fibrils under undisturbed conditions [11]. NMR can also be used to study kinetics of oligomer interactions by utilizing the constant exchange of detectable monomers with other invisible oligomeric species, through saturation transfer difference (STD) experiments [12]. Amyloid fibrils show protease resistance and are insoluble in detergents. However, their affinity to small lipophilic molecules is amenable for detection through biophysical assays using Congo red and thioflavin dyes [13]. These fluorescent dyes can be used to quantify β-sheet rich amyloid fibrils under laboratory conditions where fluorescent intensity linearly correlates with fibril formation [14]. Morphology of amyloid fibrils can be studied using transmission electron microscopy (TEM) by observing diffraction patterns. Whether fibrils form a ribbon-like or a striated pattern, can be calculated by mass-per-length constraints [15]. Different amyloid structures can be categorized

Amyloid structure	Structure/symmetry	Toxicity	Relevance	Refs.
Monomer	Disordered, random coil	Non-toxic	On pathway*	[20]
Small oligomers	Rich in β-sheet (spherical, annular, ADDLs)	Toxic	On pathway	[21, 22]
Amyloid inclusions	Amorphous aggregates	Non-toxic	Off pathway	[2, 23]
Protofilaments	Homogenous, up to 200 nm long	Toxic	On pathway	[24]
Fibrils	Cross-β	Non-toxic	On pathway	[25]
Plaque	Amorphous meshworks, fibril bundles, amyloid stars	Non-toxic	—	[26]

**On-pathway structures are intermediates involved in aggregation of amyloids into fibrils.*

Table 1.
Summary of amyloid structures observed in AD.

based on symmetry and periodicity with these methods [16]. Aβ40 fibrils structure have either 2-fold (2A) or 3-fold (3Q) rotational symmetry with a twisted morphology with periodicity of 120 ± 20 nm, and roughly 8 nm width [2, 11]. IAPP fibrils also lead to formation of striated and twisted ribbons [11].

2.2 Structural properties of amyloid aggregates

Basic structural architecture of amyloid fibrils consists of a characteristic 4.7 Å repeat through the cross-β structure [2]. Still, there exist some variations in morphology of different Aβ fibrils; the C-terminus in Aβ(1–40) is hidden within the core, while the corresponding residues are exposed on the surface of Aβ(1–42) [10]. Solid state NMR studies of amyloid fibril structures employ 2D dipolar-assisted rotation resonance (DARR) experiments and frequency selective rotational-echo double resonance (REDOR) experiments along with distance measurements between ^{13}C-^{13}C and ^{13}C-^{15}N nuclei [8]. Studies of Aβ(1–42) fibrils using ssNMR suggested unidirectional protofibril growth with two molecules coming together to form parallel intermolecular β-sheets. The ssNMR structure of homogeneous Aβ(1–42) fibrils (PDB ID: 2MXU) exhibits triple-β-strands encompassing residues 12–18, 24–33 and 36–40 respectively, connected by coil-and-turns at residues 19–23 and 34–42 [8]. The other structure of Aβ(1–42) fibrils with oxidized Met35 (PDB:2BEG), suggests structural inhomogeneity in N-terminal residues from 1 to 17 and presence of two β-strands in residues 18–26 and 31–42, respectively [17]. The AD related Aβ(1–42) polymorph shows double-horseshoe like cross-β structure where N terminus of monomeric Aβ(1–42) has L shape and the C terminus takes an S-shape. The structure comprises five in-register parallel strands with each fibril layer comprising of two molecules with hydrophobic side chains buried maximally [16]. In addition to hydrophobic core, parallel β-sheets also show polar zipper interactions through intermolecular hydrogen bonds. A recent 4.0 Å resolution ssNMR-cryoEM hybrid structure (PDB ID: 5OQV) of intertwined Aβ(1–42) protofilaments showed an approximate 21 screw helical symmetry with 4.67 Å rise [18]. This implicated step-wise shift between the subunits is similar to tau dimers. Three hydrophobic clusters involving Ala, Val, Phe, Leu, Ile, and Met residues expand along the fibril axis and contribute to overall stability of fibrils [18]. Tertiary interactions in Aβ(1–42) fibrils are different compared to Aβ(1–40) fibrils owing to differences in side-chain packaging in hydrophobic core of protofilaments [17]. The N-terminus of Aβ(1–40) peptides is disordered and highly prone to proteolysis whereas the ordered region from tyrosine residue onwards acquires a double-layered structure with a "β-arch" motif where two β-strands are separated by a short loop [19]. This motif is stabilized by formation of a salt bridge between Asp23 and Lys28 across the bend. Interactions between Lys28 and Ala42 observed in these fibrils differ to those found in Aβ(1–40) [8]. Similarly, salt bridges between Asp1 and Lys28, Asp7 and Arg5, Glu11 and His6 and His13, and Asn-Gln ladders further contribute to stability of the Aβ(1–42) fibril structure [16, 18]. Point mutations introduced in basic amino acid sequences lead to varied fibril architecture compared to the wild-type Aβ40 fibrils [2].

NMR structure of tau monomers shows detectable propensity to β-sheet, poly-proline helices and transient α-helical conformations. Aggregation of the R3 fragment consisting of 26 amino acid residues is strongly associated with formation of fibrils in the presence of polyanions as well as during self-assembly of pristine tau [7]. Phosphorylation of serine and threonine residues stabilize the α-helical conformation. αS fibrils acquire an overall assembly that mimics a Greek key as seen in atomic resolution structure of purified protein [7].

2.3 Role of amyloidosis in AD pathology

Amyloidosis in cerebrovascular system is mediated through aggregation of wild type proteins as the consequence of multivalent interactions in intrinsically disordered proteins or regions of proteins, mutations in amyloidogenic precursors, expansion of repeats in the amyloidogenic sequences, actions of proteases or chemical modifications on the precursor sequences, overexpression of the precursor, liquid–liquid phase separation, actions of small metabolites or age-related cell death [27–31]. The number of human proteins capable of causing amyloidosis has exceeded 50 and are associated with many neurological disorders based of variations in the disease precursors [2]. Different oligomeric and morphologically distinct species affect cells and tissues in different manner. Amyloid oligomers can be cytotoxic with the long-term potentiation disrupting membranes to cause ion permeability and homeostasis imbalance [2]. Fully matured fibrils contribute to the disease by disturbing lipid membranes and thus interfere with the general membrane bound cellular organelles, or by forming physical barriers which disrupt inter-cellular communications [2]. Structural inhomogeneity was observed in fibrils from the different clinical variants of amyloids in AD. Differences in morphology of Aβ aggregates can change the phenotype observed in different forms of AD. While a single Aβ structure is found in brain cortex in the cases of typical prolonged duration AD, different polymorphs are found in the cases of rapidly progressive form of AD [32]. There are six isoforms of tau protein in brain and CNS, longest one containing a stretch of 441 amino acids, with high tendency for phosphorylation and self-assembly. Tau filaments cause different tauopathies, including neurofibrillary tangles in AD [7]. Neurofibrillary tangles and neuropil threads are predominantly tau aggregates localized in neuronal cell bodies and processes, respectively, whereas the mature Aβ plaques are present extracellularly [33].

2.4 Toxicity of amyloid aggregates

Aβ(1–42) is more potent fibrillogenic Aβ variant in human brain, yet its concentration accounts for only about 5–10% of Aβ(1–40) concentration produced [33]. Accumulation of Aβ(1–42) in brain and cerebrovascular system due to its aggregation propensity, and by extension, the relative ratio of Aβ(1–42): Aβ(1–40) is a biomarker for AD [33]. Aβ(1–40) fibrils are less toxic compared to Aβ(1–42) fibrils which show differential toxicity and Aβ(1–43) fibrils are most cytotoxic [10]. Soluble Aβ in the form of low-n oligomers, Aβ-derived diffusible ligands and protofibrils are among major toxic contributors towards AD pathology [34]. Interactions of oligomeric species with other molecular complexes, metal ions and cellular membranes also impact the extent of their toxic effects in brain. N-terminus truncated Aβ peptides (Aβ(n–42), where n can vary from 2 to 11) are highly toxic and are usually present in Aβ deposits in AD brain [7]. Peptides cleaved at positions 3 or 11 are prone to pyroglutamylation and prominent components of Aβ deposits, likely owing to their resistance to proteolytic degradation [35]. αS is a major component of Lewy bodies and neurites causing neurotoxicity through dopaminergic mechanism and these aggregates are key identifiers for PD and Lewy body dementia [7]. Detection of αS aggregates early in peripheral nervous system can serve as early biomarkers before motor disabilities develop in PD patients [36]. Horizontal transfer of amyloid aggregates and oligomers between cells also contributes to propagation of disease pathology [37]. IAPP oligomers can impair insulin secretion in pancreatic cells and cause cell death and cellular uncoupling [7].

3. β-Amyloid chaperones

The main function of molecular chaperones is to facilitate their protein targets acquire proper functional conformation or fold into correct oligomeric assemblies [38]. Several proteins have been shown to bind misfolded amyloids and inhibit amyloid aggregation or promote refolding of polymorphs. They usually play other physiological roles, yet show tendency to prevent amyloidosis under specific stimuli. We will discuss some of these non-proteolytic chaperones in more detail below. Additionally, albumin binding to polymeric Aβ, α1-antitrypsin, immunoglobulins A and G are endogenous human cerebrospinal fluid (CSF) proteins with capability to control amyloid formation, although the inhibitory activity is lesser by two orders of magnitude compared to plasma [39].

3.1 Heat shock proteins

Heat shock proteins (Hsp) are the most commonly known chaperones in human body, divided into five classes Hsp70, Hsp90, Hsp60, Hsp40, and small Hsps, differing in protein size. Chaperones in Hsp60 and Hsp70 family mediate folding, Hsp33 family hold partially folded proteins till other chaperones or degradation system can act, and Hsp104 promotes solubilization of aggregated proteins [38]. Mutations in αA- or αB-crystallin and other small heat shock proteins have been linked to increased risk of certain amyloidosis conditions [40]. Hsp70 and Hsp90 are capable of utilizing ATP molecules to perform energy costly unfolding of stable misfolded aggregates and then convert them into properly folded conformations. Similarly other members like Hsp110 can act as disaggregases to forcibly solubilize preformed fibrillar aggregates [41]. Hsp70 recognizes KFERQ motif in proteins to mediate degradation by transporting them to lysosomal compartments inside the cell, a typical example of chaperone mediated autophagy [41]. Disaggregation machinery in humans mainly involves proteins from Hsp family namely, Hsp110, Hsp105, Hsp100, and Hsp70/40 co-chaperone cognates [41]. Proteins in Hsp40 co-chaperone family, mainly DnaJB6 and B8, can decrease the aggregation of polyglutamine peptides in HD in addition to modulating Hsp70 activity [41]. Binding of misfolded proteins and interaction with ATPase domain of Hsp70 are achieved via the highly conserved J domain. Anti-aggregation activity of Hsps, especially Hsp70, is at least partially dependent on presence of ATP [42]. ADP-bound forms of Hsp70 is generated as a result of the ATP hydrolysis by its co-chaperones. This form has high affinity for the hydrophobic residues in misfolded peptides and holds the unfolded ensemble till it spontaneously achieved proper conformational populations. Small Hsps (12–42 KDa) do not require ATP since they usually function as holdases and assist other proteins in Hsp chaperone complex [41]. Hsp104 is part of proteostasis network which regulates prion assembly in yeast, Hsp110 is its human counterpart which facilitates chaperone function of Hsp70 and Hsp40 [43]. Hsp90 and its co-chaperones interact with tau and a close control on their interaction can cause the oligomers to turn into benign species instead of toxic aggregates [44]. Free Hsp90 binds and releases substrates in its monomeric extended form, and attains a dimeric ATP-bound closed conformation mediate by co-chaperones p23/Sba1, Hsp70/90 organizing protein (HOP), Cdc37 and other proteins [41, 45]. Hsp60 chaperonins are mainly located in mitochondria and form heptameric, double ring complexes which provide isolated environment for protein folding with co-chaperonins Hsp10 forming the lid of this cavity. Unlike Hsp60, the cytosolic chaperonins in neurons such as TCP-1 Ring Complex (TRiC or CCT), do not require co-chaperones for their function and form a double ring complex with each ring consisting of eight subunits. Hsp60 can interact with mutant αS in PD brain [41]. B-chain of monomeric or dimeric insulin can bind to IAPP monomers, thus preventing their aggregation [7]. Presence of chaperone proteins such as Hsp27 (HSPB1), αB-crystallin (HSPB5) and Hsp70 (HSPA1A) can decrease cell toxicity, possibly by binding Aβ oligomers and converting them to larger less toxic aggregates, however it not clear whether they bring about any change in secondary or tertiary structure [44]. HSPA6 is induced in neurons post heat shock, unlike other members of this family HSPA1A and HSP8, thus has a unique probable role as a human neuronal chaperone [46]. Hsp70 and Hsp90 have differential roles in case of inflammation and macrophage recruitment. Hsp90 can also stabilize neurotoxic proteins and should be carefully controlled to achieve required therapeutic outcomes.

3.2 Intracellular degradation machinery

Molecular chaperones are capable of binding and folding intracellular soluble amyloid aggregates, however solubilization of amyloid plaques is out of scope for these proteins. While these chaperones may not be able to completely reverse neurodegenerative symptoms, they play crucial anti-apoptotic functions through protein folding and degradation of unfolded or misfolded proteins. There are fundamental mechanisms underlying a chaperone function, namely, unfolded protein response (UPR), protein compartmentalization, heat shock response, chaperone-mediated autophagy and lysosome system, ER associated degradation (ERAD) and ubiquitin-proteasome system (UPS) [46]. Extracellular chaperones mediate proper protein folding and refolding by providing isolated environment or through intermolecular interactions. If proper folding cannot be achieved, they may play a role in mediating intracellular proteasomal degradation or microglial digestion of unfolded protein fragments. Cytosolic chaperone systems like Hsp70 and Hsp40, comprising heat shock cognate 70 (Hsc70), and their interacting proteins like C-terminus of Hsc70-interacting protein (CHIP) can mediate targeting of misfolded proteins to proteasome machinery [38]. Intracellular pathways for degradation of misfolded proteins include the UPS, 26S proteasome and lysosome-mediated phagocytosis [9]. Hsp70 recruits misfolded proteins, especially αS, for degradation by directing them to proteasomes or autophagy-lysosomal pathway [44]. UPS comprises of a cascade of enzymes E1 (Ub activating enzyme), E2 (Ub conjugating enzyme) and E3 (Ub ligase) facilitating binding of ubiquitin (Ub) to target proteins. Ligase enzymes in this cascade can employ chaperone proteins such as Hsc70 for recognition of exposed hydrophobic regions misfolded peptides and together mediate proteolysis of misfolded intracellular proteins. E4 enzyme from UPS can recruit additional Ub molecules to the protein substrate which can be either directed for degradation or other protein interactions based on their topology [41]. 26S proteasome particles degrades polyUb-conjugated proteins with the help of its two 19S regulatory particles responsible for recognition and de-ubiquitination and a 20S core particle through which proteolysis of these substrates into short peptides is mediated [41]. ERAD withholds misfolded proteins from continuing with on-going cargo to golgi apparatus for further downstream processes. UPR is initiated by migration of transcription factors to the nucleus causing upregulation of ER chaperones-encoding gene expression in response to increasing in unfolded proteins, such as Aβ aggregates in neuronal ER, which require assistance of chaperones present in the ER [47, 48]. Reduction in UPS proteolytic activity is linked with disease pathology in AD, PD, ALS, HD as well as TSEs.

3.3 Non-proteolytic amyloid chaperones

Aging is a major risk factor for many neurodegenerative diseases. The UPS system is known to get deregulated with increase in neuronal age and therefore offers less resistance to pathological protein aggregates. Proteins such as Human serum albumin show competitive binding towards Aβ oligomers, with its different domains binding to many oligomeric molecules [12]. It binds almost 90% of plasma Aβ peptides potentially through dual binding mechanism involving Aβ(1-40) monomers and protofibrils likely utilizing residues involved in fibril formation.

Here we suggest non-proteolytic endogenous proteins which show potential as AD therapeutics directed against Aβ, namely, Lipocalin-type prostaglandin D synthase (L-PGDS, also known as β-trace), apolipoprotein E (ApoE), α2 macroglobulin (α2M), haptoglobin and clusterin as alternatives to intracellular Aβ degradation machinery. These proteins have been sporadically studied for their holdase or transporter activity, yet their Aβ chaperone function is still unexplored. L-PGDS is the second most abundant protein in human CSF after albumin [49]. It exhibits dual functions, as a lipophilic ligand transporter in cells and as isomerase in arachidonic acid pathway to convert prostaglandin H2 to prostaglandin D2 [50]. L-PGDS plays protective roles in different neurological diseases including genetic demyelinating disease, brain injuries and multiple sclerosis [51]. It plays protective role against cerebral ischemia as well [52]. It promotes recruitment of astrocytes and glial cells to the source of injury [53]. Early stress stimulus can upregulate L-PGDS suggesting its unknown, yet novel stress protection mechanism. L-PGDS deficient mice showed additional neuronal apoptosis strongly indicating its important protective function in neurons and surrounding oligodendrocytes [51]. L-PGDS binds to various Aβ peptides including fibrils and is colocalized in Aβ plaques [54]. Furthermore, Aβ is physiologically secreted to CSF under normal conditions where L-PGDS is abundant. L-PGDS ratio in CSF:serum is already identified as early biomarker for detection of potential damage to blood–brain barrier and quantifying its complex with transthyretin in CSF is also suggested to be a possible diagnostic marker [55]. L-PGDS colocalizes with amyloid plaques and mediates inhibition of aggregates through cysteine residue [54]. Based on previous studies and our own findings, we posit that secreted L-PGDS binds to monomeric and prefibrillar Aβ and inhibits amyloid aggregation in synergy with its ability to break down mature fibrils.

α2M is also an extracellular glycoprotein showing potential chaperone properties. It can prevent proteases from hydrolyzing proteins and mediates Aβ clearance through formation of α2M/protease complexes [56]. It protects cells from apoptosis through receptor interactions. α2M selectively binds proteins in non-native conformations and in process prevents their aggregation [56]. α2M decreases with age and its clearance mechanisms for Aβ get impaired [57]. A2M gene polymorphisms are associated with sporadic AD in some populations and α2M is also present in amyloid plaques [58]. ApoE isoforms E2, E3 and E4 can delay amyloid aggregation through differential activity as extracellular chaperones [59]. The suggested role of apoE4 as pathological chaperone is partly due to its role in delaying fibril formation from Aβ monomers leading to increase in toxic oligomeric species [60]. Isoform E3 and E2 show binding affinity to oligomeric Aβ as well, thus decreasing their neurotoxic effects [61]. Clusterin, or apolipoprotein J, is also extracellularly secreted and moonlights as a chaperone upon cellular stress stimulus [62]. Very similar to sHsps in its chaperone activity, clusterin preferentially interacts with off-pathway aggregates which are highly toxic and prone to precipitation [63]. Haptoglobin is very similar to α2M as an extracellular chaperone glycoprotein, though is activated in acidic

Chaperone	Function	Amyloid species	Chromosomal and cellular location	Brain expression levels (HPA) [66]	Refs.
Hsp70 (DnaK)	Holdase	Nascent amyloids and oligomers	6p21; intracellular	66.3 TPM	[42, 67, 68]
Hsp90	Holdase	Nascent amyloids and oligomers	14q32; intracellular	1021.5 TPM	[69, 70]
Hsp40 (DnaJ)	Holdase; disaggregase in ternary complex	Higher order aggregates	19p13; intracellular	110.5 TPM	[71]
αB crystallin (Hsp27)	Holdase	Amyloid fibrils	11q23; intracellular, membrane	1888.7 TPM	[72]
Hsp110	Disaggregase; holdase	Prefibrillar oligomers	13q12; intracellular	109.4 TPM	[73]
Hsp28 (sHsp)	Holdase	Unfolded or misfolded proteins	7q11; intracellular	98.7 TPM	[74]
Hsc70 (HSPA8)	Chaperone mediate autophagy	Nascent polypeptides	11q24; intracellular	1119.0 TPM	[75]
Hsp60	Chaperonin	Early oligomeric species	2q33; intracellular	141.6 TPM	[76, 77]
STUB1 (CHIP)	Ubiquitin-mediated protein degradation	Misfolded protein aggregated	16p13; intracellular	137.7 TPM	[78]
L-PGDS (β-trace)	Aggregation inhibitor	Monomers, fibrils	9q34; secreted	1224.7 TPM	[54]
Clusterin (ApoJ)	Stabilizer	Senile plaques/ diffusible aggregates	8p21; secreted	10875.4 TPM	[79]
α2-Macroglobulin	Inhibitor	Prefibrillar species	12p13; extracellular	172.0 TPM	[80]

Table 2.
Mode of function of endogenous amyloid chaperones.

environment and interacts with prefibrillar amyloids to prevent further aggregation [64]. These endogenous proteins and many others may play very important yet undiscovered role to maintain proteostasis in physiological environment.

Ig antibodies such as aducanumab, targeting specific oligomeric forms of Aβ have already reached clinical trials, showing promising therapeutic effects focusing on delaying cognitive decline. However recent withdrawals of some of these antibodies like bapineuzumab and solanezumab, have forced scientists to look for more robust options [65]. Enzymes such as insulin degrading enzymes, neprilysin, cathepsin B are capable of degrading amyloidogenic peptides. Enzymes belonging to peptidyl-prolyl cis/trans isomerase (PPIase) family, e.g., CypB, can convert proline containing peptides from cis to trans conformational isomers thereby facilitating their folding process [47]. Some inherently amyloidogenic proteins such as PrP, hTTR and BRICHOS-domain containing proteins can paradoxically also inhibit aggregation of other amyloids. BRICHOS-domain containing protein ITM2B (Bri2) is a CNS membrane protein which shows chaperone functions for amyloids by binding to tyrosine and other charged residues [43]. Tetrameric form of Transthyretin (TTR) can also prevent aggregation of amyloid oligomers [44]. In recent years, some small molecules have also been put forward as possible inhibitors of amyloid aggregation—such as polyphenols, e.g., epigallocatechin gallate (EGCG), curcumin, resveratrol, etc. [7, 12]. Understanding inhibition mechanisms of non-proteolytic endogenous chaperone proteins and other molecules is very crucial to develop therapies targeting amyloid aggregates in AD (**Table 2**).

4. Oxidative stress

Oxidative stress in human body is mainly mediated by reactive oxygen species (ROS) including hydrogen peroxide (H_2O_2), hydroxyl free radical (•OH), superoxide ($O_2^{\bullet-}$), peroxyl (•OOR), hypochlorous acid (HOCl), nitric oxide (NO), peroxynitrite ($ONOO^-$) and other reactive nitrogen species. Increase in concentration of these reactive species can trigger downregulation of antioxidant enzymes such as superoxide dismutase (SOD), glutathione peroxidase, catalase, thioredoxin and small molecules such as melatonin and coumarin [81]. Endogenous sources of ROS include components in mitochondrial electron transport chain and NADPH oxidase, which can trigger pathological responses leading to lipid peroxidation, DNA damage and cell death mediated by toxic products. Amyloid plaques have been shown to contain multi-fold concentrations of metals like iron (Fe), copper (Cu) and zinc (Zn) [81]. Intracellular Aβ can also trigger production of highly toxic molecules such as 4-hydroxyl-2,3-nonenal (HNE) and malandialdehyde through interactions with Fe or Cu which can catalyze Fenton reactions to generate more OH^- ions. Hydroxyl radicals can also be generated from other brain ROS through Haber-Weiss reaction, particularly within mitochondria which are most prone to such oxidative damage [82]. Such ROS are generated as by-products of amyloid aggregation and are involved with metallobiology of dementia. High concentrations of Fe in brain have drastic effects in cases of dementia leading to cognitive decline through interactions with brain amyloids [83]. Metal ions are crucial for many brain functions and Fe and Cu even possess active sites for binding antioxidant SOD. However, increase in concentrations of some of these metals can cause high levels of toxicity. Twenty percent of cases in familial ALS is affected by mutation in a single enzyme SOD1 functionally affected by Cu/Zn [83]. Metal ions have propensity to bind high affinity, well-protected and redox-shielded binding sites of proteins, and in higher concentrations they can bind to other putative active sites in proteins involved in pathology of various degenerative diseases [84]. While zinc compounds have been tested for their probable therapeutic role in overcoming cognitive degeneration, Zn^{2+} ion has also been implicated as a contributor to formation of amyloid plaques which act as metal sinks [84]. Such mitochondrial damage and mutations have been associated with age related late-onset, non-autosomal dominant AD pathology [85].

4.1 Amyloid-β and oxidative stress

Aβ binds and reduces Fe^{3+} and Cu^{2+} in presence of endogenous reducing agents to generate H_2O_2 further producing other partially ROS [86, 87]. Studies have revealed the role of metal ions such as Fe, Cu and Zn in inducing Aβ aggregation and oligomerization [88–90]. Brain regions rich in Aβ(1–42) show increased oxidative stress, possibly mediated through redox interactions with the only methionine (Met35) present in peptide sequence [91]. Amyloids oligomers can also trigger ROS generation [2]. The three histidine residues-His6, His13 and His14, facilitate Aβ coordination with transition metal ions. These residues get protonated in acidic environment and may increasingly contribute to aggregation at low pH. Cu^{2+} interacts with Aβ and oxidizes sulfur of Met35 to activate formation of disulfide bonds leading to dimerization and other oligomeric formations. Soluble oxidized aggregates avoid clearance causing enrichment of brain regions with these agglomerates. Aβ peptides can successfully recruit ions of metals like Fe, Cu and Zn through sulfide group of Met35 and a chelating domain which involves Asp1 and all three histidines, in a bid to induce redox complexes capable of bringing about oxidative insults [7]. Dityrosine cross-linked Aβ dimers along with nitrotyrosine cross-linked proteins are also associated with oxidative stress [92]. Cell death from oxidative stress is a cumulative result of alteration in proteostasis, protein phosphorylation and glucose metabolism as downstream consequences of increase in Aβ42 concentration [91].

4.2 Pathophysiology of ROS

Excessive free radical production as a result of oxidative stress at cellular levels causes protein oxidation and lipid peroxidation [91]. Lipid peroxidation leads to break down of unsaturated fatty acids among other components of membrane phospholipids, leading to accumulation of isoprostanes, acrolein, thiobarbiturate-reactive substances, etc. [84, 92]. Glutamate receptors overstimulation can trigger downstream cell death cascades through increased calcium influx and generation of nitric oxide species [48]. 8-hydroxy-2′-deoxyguanosine (OHDG) is one of the oxidative markers for DNA, found in PD patients [36]. These products impair glucose transport and glutamate uptake, hence contributing to cell apoptosis. ROS cause imbalance in metal and ion homeostasis, for example Ca^{2+}, which can trigger imbalance in downstream signaling cascades. Oxidative damage can lead to hydroxylation of nucleic acids and carbonylation of proteins. Carbonyls are markers of protein oxidation and have been found concentrated in frontal brain regions of AD patients [92]. Free radicals generated as result of amyloid oligomerization or aggregation can directly mediate mitochondrial damage which triggers neuronal death through downstream pathways, one of them being cytochrome C reduction [48]. OS in PD cases may be a result of deregulation of dopamine-iron redox pathway, since αS can alter expression of enzymes indirectly regulating dopamine synthesis [84]. αS is also known to directly interact with metal ions causing protein aggregation. ALS is mainly characterized by loss of motor neurons, which combined with SOD mutations diminishing its free radical scavenging abilities can exacerbate the impacts to oxidative injury [84]. Oxidative markers localized in plaques and NFTs are toxic products such as 3-nitrotyrosine, HNE, pyrraline and pentosidine, while metal enriched protein carbonyls including ferritin, catalyst, Cu/Zn-SOD and Mn-SOD [93].

4.3 Protective mechanisms from ROS

Chaperones can bind ROS generated as by-product of amyloids and thus prevent triggering breakdown of homeostasis. α2-Macroglobulin can directly bind Aβ and potentially act as a chaperone in addition to its zinc-binding capabilities which can help mitigate redox activity of Aβ [94]. Zn^{2+} is redox-inert and may be helpful in mitigating metal mediated Aβ redox activity. ApoE can mediate Aβ clearance as a chaperone depending on specific isoform interactions; ε4 may potentially increase

Aβ pathology [95]. ApoE interaction with Aβ is modulated by metals [93]. There are two key requirements for metal interactions in dementia-either supplementation or chelation [83]. Metal chelators can help solubilization of Aβ plaques. Effects of chaperones on metal ions need to be carefully curated to maintain metal homeostasis in brain and other organs of nervous system. Several endogenous brain proteins show potential protective response against ROS in diseased brain, including β-trace protein, which is the second most abundant protein in CSF. Competitive binding of metal ions by chaperone proteins may be advantageous in decreasing generation of ROS by-products. Overexpression of metal-affinity proteins have been shown, as example of iron-binding ferritin. Antioxidant alpha-tocopherol has been reported to potentially slow AD progression in addition to action of metal chelators such as clioquinol and desferrioxamine [92]. L-PGDS scavenges ROS and in process protects against neuronal cell death with its ligand binding function intact [96]. It also reduces cytotoxicity mediated by oxidation of heme metabolites such as bilirubin [97]. We have found that L-PGDS can directly interact with Aβ-heme complex and lower its peroxidase activity (to be published). Other non-proteolytic chaperones such as α2M, clusterin and haptoglobin, also show neuroprotective potential in similar manner as L-PGDS and are good candidates for more comprehensive oxidative stress related studies.

5. Conclusions

Alzheimer's disease is a debilitating neurodegenerative condition and is projected to be a major risk factor for global population by the year 2050 [98]. One of the key theories, known as "amyloid cascade hypothesis" postulates that oligomerization of amyloid-β (Aβ) in brain is the key pathological event in AD [99]. Although complete explanation of causation in AD is yet to be established, it has been universally accepted that amyloidosis (perhaps provoked by environmental factors) plays a crucial role in AD progression [99–101]. Conformational alterations in Aβ which lead to its conversion from soluble peptide to insoluble aggregates are considered as a key mechanism in pathogenesis of neurodegenerative diseases such as AD [102]. Early amyloid aggregates can act as biomarkers in most dementia related maladies and associate observed clinical symptoms to underlying pathophysiological mechanisms. Till date, we do not have any therapeutic solution for aggregation of amyloids. Current gold-standard biomarkers in neurodegeneration are neuroimaging systems of degeneration and detectable clinical symptoms represent pathological changes causing irreversible damage to nervous system [33, 36]. Success of theranostic efforts will rely on rational drug design based on a proper understanding of molecular structures and mechanisms involved in aggregation. Aβ mediates AD pathology through direct inhibition of neuronal interactions and signaling cascades, and triggers oxidative stress in the process. Here we have discussed mechanisms of action of amyloid chaperones with focus on Aβ chaperones to better understand their modus operandi. Apart from the protein quality control machinery and housekeeping complexes responsible for maintaining general proteostasis, we have discussed importance of other endogenous chaperones which step up in time of crisis, often as response to stress stimuli. Proteins such as L-PGDS, clusterin, α2M have are involved in many physiological processes, with elusive function as amyloid chaperones. These proteins can provide alternative mechanisms to control amyloid aggregates in events of failure of intracellular Hsp complexes and proteasome machinery. Additionally, their affinity to redox active components may provide additional protective mechanisms against Aβ mediated oxidative stress.

Conflict of interest

Authors declare no conflict of interest.

Abbreviations

Aa	amino acid
AD	Alzheimer's disease
ALS	amyotrophic lateral sclerosis
APP	amyloid precursor protein
Aβ	amyloid-β
CNS	central nervous system
CSF	cerebrospinal fluid
DARR	dipolar assisted rotation resonance
EM	electron microscopy
HD	Huntington disease
HNE	hydroxy-2,3-nonenal
Hsc	heat shock cognate
Hsp	heat shock protein
HSR	heat shock response
IAPP	islet amyloid polypeptide
NMDA	N-methyl-D-aspartate
NMR	nuclear magnetic resonance
OHDG	8-hydroxy-2′-deoxyguanosine
PD	Parkinson's disease
PDB	protein data bank
PrP	prion protein
REDOR	rotational echo double resonance
ROS	reactive oxygen species
SOD	superoxide dismutase
ssNMR	solid state nuclear magnetic resonance
T2D	type II diabetes
TEM	transmission electron microscopy
TSE	transmissible spongiform encephalopathy
Ub	ubiquitin
UPR	unfolded protein response
UPS	ubiquitin proteasome system
αS	α synuclein

Author details

Bhargy Sharma and Konstantin Pervushin*
School of Biological Sciences, Nanyang Technological University, Singapore

*Address all correspondence to: kpervushin@ntu.edu.sg

References

[1] Herguedas B, Garcia-Nafria J, Cais O, Fernandez-Leiro R, Krieger J, Ho H, et al. Structure and organization of heteromeric AMPA-type glutamate receptors. Science. 2016;**352**(6285):aad3873

[2] Iadanza MG, Jackson MP, Hewitt EW, Ranson NA, Radford SE. A new era for understanding amyloid structures and disease. Nature reviews Molecular Cell Biology. 2018;**19**(12):755-773

[3] Dubois B, Hampel H, Feldman HH, Scheltens P, Aisen P, Andrieu S, et al. Preclinical Alzheimer's disease: Definition, natural history, and diagnostic criteria. Alzheimer's & Dementia. 2016;**12**(3):292-323

[4] Benjamin Dehay MB, Gorry P, Przedborski S, Vila M, Hunot S, Singleton A, et al. Targeting α-synuclein for treatment of Parkinson's disease: Mechanistic and therapeutic considerations. Lancet Neurology. 2015;**14**:855-866

[5] Wei L, Jiang P, Xu W, Li H, Zhang H, Yan L, et al. The molecular basis of distinct aggregation pathways of islet amyloid polypeptide. The Journal of Biological Chemistry. 2011;**286**(8):6291-6300

[6] Chen GF, Xu TH, Yan Y, Zhou YR, Jiang Y, Melcher K, et al. Amyloid beta: Structure, biology and structure-based therapeutic development. 2017;**38**(9):1205-1235

[7] Ke PC, Sani MA, Ding F, Kakinen A, Javed I, Separovic F, et al. Implications of peptide assemblies in amyloid diseases. Chemical Society Reviews. 2017;**46**(21):6492-6531

[8] Xiao Y, Ma B, McElheny D, Parthasarathy S, Long F, Hoshi M, et al. Abeta(1-42) fibril structure illuminates self-recognition and replication of amyloid in Alzheimer's disease. Nature Structural & Molecular Biology. 2015;**22**(6):499-505

[9] Muchowski PJ, Wacker JL. Modulation of neurodegeneration by molecular chaperones. Nature Reviews. Neuroscience. 2005;**6**(1):11-22

[10] Chuang E, Hori AM, Hesketh CD, Shorter J. Amyloid assembly and disassembly. Journal of Cell Science. 2018;**131**(8):jcs189928

[11] Anant K, Paravastu RDL, Yau W-M, Tycko R. Molecular structural basis for polymorphism in Alzheimer's β-amyloid fibrils. Proceedings of the National Academy of Sciences. 2008;**105**(47):18349-18354

[12] Ahmed R, Melacini G. A solution NMR toolset to probe the molecular mechanisms of amyloid inhibitors. Chemical Communications (Camb). 2018;**54**(37):4644-4652

[13] Rajamohamedsait HB, Sigurdsson EM. Histological staining of amyloid and pre-amyloid peptides and proteins in mouse tissue. Methods in Molecular Biology. 2012;**849**:411-424

[14] Xue C, Lin TY, Chang D, Guo Z. Thioflavin T as an amyloid dye: Fibril quantification, optimal concentration and effect on aggregation. Royal Society Open Science. 2017;**4**(1):160696

[15] Chen B, Thurber KR, Shewmaker F, Wickner RB, Tycko R. Measurement of amyloid fibril mass-per-length by tilted-beam transmission electron microscopy. Proceedings of the National Academy of Sciences of the United States of America. 2009;**106**(34):14339-14344

[16] Wälti MA, Ravotti F, Arai H, Glabe CG, Wall JS, Böckmann A, et al. Atomic-resolution structure of a disease-relevant Aβ(1-42) amyloid fibril.

Proceedings of the National Academy of Sciences of the United States of America. 2016;**113**(34):E4976-E4984

[17] Lührs T, Ritter C, Adrian M, Riek-Loher D, Bohrmann B, Döbeli H, et al. 3D structure of Alzheimer's amyloid-β(1-42) fibrils. Proceedings of the National Academy of Sciences of the United States of America. 2005;**102**(48):17342-17347

[18] Gremer LSD, Schenk C, Reinartz E, Labahn J, Ravelli RBG, Tusche M, et al. Fibril structure of amyloid-β(1-42) by cryo-electron microscopy. Science. 2017;**358**(6359):116-119

[19] Petkova AT, Ishii Y, Balbach JJ, Antzutkin ON, Leapman RD, Delaglio F, et al. A structural model for Alzheimer's beta-amyloid fibrils based on experimental constraints from solid state NMR. Proceedings of the National Academy of Sciences of the United States of America. 2002;**99**(26):16742-16747

[20] Roche J, Shen Y, Lee JH, Ying J, Bax A. Monomeric Abeta(1-40) and Abeta(1-42) peptides in solution adopt very similar Ramachandran map distributions that closely resemble random coil. Biochemistry. 2016;**55**(5):762-775

[21] Laganowsky A, Liu C, Sawaya MR, Whitelegge JP, Zhao M, Pensalfini A, et al. Atomic view of a toxic amyloid small oligomer. Science. 2012;**335**:1228-1231

[22] Kayed R, Pensalfini A, Margol L, Sokolov Y, Sarsoza F, Head E, et al. Annular protofibrils are a structurally and functionally distinct type of amyloid oligomer. The Journal of Biological Chemistry. 2009;**284**(7):4230-4237

[23] Mainz A, Peschek J, Stavropoulou M, Back KC, Bardiaux B, Asami S, et al. The chaperone alphaB-crystallin uses different interfaces to capture an amorphous and an amyloid client. Nature Structural & Molecular Biology. 2015;**22**(11):898-905

[24] Kotler SA, Ramamoorthy A. Preparation of stable amyloid-beta oligomers without perturbative methods. Methods in molecular biology. 1777;**2018**:331-338

[25] Rambaran RN, Serpell LC. Amyloid fibrils: Abnormal protein assembly. Prion. 2008;**2**(3):112-117

[26] Han S, Kollmer M, Markx D, Claus S, Walther P, Fandrich M. Amyloid plaque structure and cell surface interactions of beta-amyloid fibrils revealed by electron tomography. Scientific Reports. 2017;**7**:43577

[27] Lakshmanan A, Cheong DW, Accardo A, Di Fabrizio E, Riekel C, Hauser CA. Aliphatic peptides show similar self-assembly to amyloid core sequences, challenging the importance of aromatic interactions in amyloidosis. Proceedings of the National Academy of Sciences of the United States of America. 2013;**110**(2):519-524

[28] Hardy J, Selkoe DJ. The amyloid hypothesis of Alzheimer's disease: Progress and problems on the road to therapeutics. Science. 2002;**297**(5580):353-356

[29] Cohen SIA, Linse S, Luheshi LM, Hellstrand E, White DA, Rajah L, et al. Proliferation of amyloid-β42 aggregates occurs through a secondary nucleation mechanism. Proceedings of the National Academy of Sciences of the United States of America. 2013;**110**(24):9758-9763

[30] Kumar EK, Haque N, Prabhu NP. Kinetics of protein fibril formation: Methods and mechanisms. International Journal of Biological Macromolecules. 2016;**100**:3-10

[31] Wegmann S, Eftekharzadeh B, Tepper K, Zoltowska KM, Bennett RE, Dujardin S, et al. Tau protein liquid-liquid phase separation can initiate tau aggregation. EMBO Journal. 2018;**37**(7):e98049

[32] Qiang W, Yau WM, Lu JX, Collinge J, Tycko R. Structural variation in amyloid-beta fibrils from Alzheimer's disease clinical subtypes. Nature. 2017;**541**(7636):217-221

[33] Holtzman DM, Morris JC, Goate AM. Alzheimer's disease: The challenge of the second century. Science Translational Medicine. 2011;**3**(77):77sr1

[34] Walsh DM, Selkoe DJ. A beta oligomers—A decade of discovery. Journal of Neurochemistry. 2007;**101**(5):1172-1184

[35] Perez-Garmendia R, Gevorkian G. Pyroglutamate-modified amyloid Beta peptides: Emerging targets for Alzheimer's disease immunotherapy. Current Neuropharmacology. 2013;**11**:491-498

[36] Sherer TB. Biomarkers for Parkinson's disease. Science Translational Medicine. 2011;**3**(79):79ps14

[37] Lazarev VF, Mikhaylova ER, Guzhova IV, Margulis BA. Possible function of molecular chaperones in diseases caused by propagating amyloid aggregates. Frontiers in Neuroscience. 2017;**11**:277

[38] Uversky VN. Flexible nets of malleable guardians: Intrinsically disordered chaperones in neurodegenerative diseases. Chemical Reviews. 2011;**111**(2):1134-1166

[39] Bohrmann B, Tjernberg L, Kuner P, Poli S, Levet-Trafit B, Näslund J, et al. Endogenous proteins controlling amyloid b-peptide polymerization. The Journal of Biological Chemistry. 1999;**274**(23):15990-15995

[40] Hishiya A, Takayama S. Molecular chaperones as regulators of cell death. Oncogene. 2008;**27**(50):6489-6506

[41] Ciechanover A, Kwon YT. Protein quality control by molecular chaperones in neurodegeneration. Frontiers in Neuroscience. 2017;**11**:185

[42] Evans CG, Wisen S, Gestwicki JE. Heat shock proteins 70 and 90 inhibit early stages of amyloid beta-(1-42) aggregation in vitro. The Journal of Biological Chemistry. 2006;**281**(44):33182-33191

[43] Landreh M, Rising A, Presto J, Jornvall H, Johansson J. Specific chaperones and regulatory domains in control of amyloid formation. The Journal of Biological Chemistry. 2015;**290**(44):26430-26436

[44] Lindberg I, Shorter J, Wiseman RL, Chiti F, Dickey CA, McLean PJ. Chaperones in neurodegeneration. The Journal of Neuroscience. 2015;**35**(41):13853-13859

[45] Hutt D, Balch WE. The proteome in balance. Science. 2010;**329**(5993):766-767

[46] Roodveldt C, Outeiro TF, Braun JEA. Editorial: Molecular chaperones and neurodegeneration. Frontiers in Neuroscience. 2017;**11**:565

[47] Dubnikov T, Cohen E. The emerging roles of early protein folding events in the secretory pathway in the development of neurodegenerative maladies. Frontiers in Neuroscience. 2017;**11**:48

[48] Shen Y, He P, Zhong Z, McAllister C, Lindholm K. Distinct destructive signal pathways of neuronal death in Alzheimer's disease. Trends in Molecular Medicine. 2006;**12**(12):574-579

[49] Mase M, Yamada K, Shimazu N, Seiki K, Oda H, Nakau H, et al.

Lipocalin-type prostaglandin D synthase (beta-trace) in cerebrospinal fluid: A useful marker for the diagnosis of normal pressure hydrocephalus. Neuroscience Research. 2003;**47**(4):455-459

[50] Yoshihiro Urade OH. Biochemical, structural, genetic, physiological, and pathophysiological features of lipocalin-type prostaglandin D synthase. Biochimica et Biophysica Acta. 2000;**1482**(1-2):259-271

[51] Taniguchi H, Mohri I, Okabe-Arahori H, Kanekiyo T, Kagitani-Shimono K, Wada K, et al. Early induction of neuronal lipocalin-type prostaglandin D synthase after hypoxic-ischemic injury in developing brains. Neuroscience Letters. 2007;**420**(1):39-44

[52] Saleem S, Shah ZA, Urade Y, Doré S. Lipocalin-prostaglandin D synthase is a critical beneficial factor in transient and permanent focal cerebral ischemia. Neuroscience. 2009;**160**(1):248-254

[53] Lee S, Jang E, Kim JH, Kim JH, Lee WH, Suk K. Lipocalin-type prostaglandin D2 synthase protein regulates glial cell migration and morphology through myristoylated alanine-rich C-kinase substrate: Prostaglandin D2-independent effects. The Journal of Biological Chemistry. 2012;**287**(12):9414-9428

[54] Kanekiyo T, Ban T, Aritake K, Huang ZL, Qu WM, Okazaki I, et al. Lipocalin-type prostaglandin D synthase/beta-trace is a major amyloid beta-chaperone in human cerebrospinal fluid. Proceedings of the National Academy of Sciences of the United States of America. 2007;**104**(15):6412-6417

[55] Lovell MA, Lynn BC, Xiong S, Quinn JF, Kaye J, Markesbery WR. An aberrant protein complex in CSF as a biomarker of Alzheimer disease. Neurology 2008;**70**(23):2212-2218

[56] French K, Yerbury JJ, Wilson MR. Protease activation of R2-macroglobulin modulates a chaperone-like action with broad specificity. Biochemistry. 2008;**47**:1176-1185

[57] Birkenmeier G, Müller R, Huse K, Forberg J, Gläser C, Hedrich H, et al. Human alpha2-macroglobulin: Genotype-phenotype relation. Experimental Neurology. 2003;**184**:153-161

[58] Michałowska-Wender G, Wawrzynek A, Rossa G, Kozubski W, Wender M. On the lack of a clear-cut association between alpha-2-macroglobulin deletion and the risk of Alzheimer disease in Poland. Folia Neuropathologica. 2014;**52**(4):417-420

[59] Fagan AM, Watson M, Parsadanian M, Bales KR, Paul SM, Holtzman DM. Human and murine ApoE markedly alters A beta metabolism before and after plaque formation in a mouse model of Alzheimer's disease. Neurobiology of Disease. 2002;**9**(3):305-318

[60] Deroo S, Stengel F, Mohammadi A, Henry N, Hubin E, Krammer EM, et al. Chemical cross-linking/mass spectrometry maps the amyloid beta peptide binding region on both apolipoprotein E domains. ACS Chemical Biology. 2015;**10**(4):1010-1016

[61] Ly S, Altman R, Petrlova J, Lin Y, Hilt S, Huser T, et al. Binding of apolipoprotein E inhibits the oligomer growth of amyloid-beta peptide in solution as determined by fluorescence cross-correlation spectroscopy. The Journal of Biological Chemistry. 2013;**288**(17):11628-11635

[62] Humphreys DT, Carver JA, Easterbrook-Smith SB, Wilson MR. Clusterin has chaperone-like activity similar to that of small heat shock proteins. The Journal of Biological Chemistry. 1999;**274**(11):6875-6881

[63] Poon S, Treweek TM, Wilson MR, Easterbrook-Smith SB, Carver JA. Clusterin is an extracellular chaperone that specifically interacts with slowly aggregating proteins on their off-folding pathway. FEBS Letters. 2002;**513**:259-266

[64] Yerbury JJ, Kumita JR, Meehan S, Dobson CM, Wilson MR. Alpha2-macroglobulin and haptoglobin suppress amyloid formation by interacting with prefibrillar protein species. The Journal of Biological Chemistry. 2009;**284**(7):4246-4254

[65] Behl C. Amyloid in Alzheimer's disease: Guilty beyond reasonable doubt? Trends in Pharmacological Sciences. 2017;**38**(10):849-851

[66] Uhlen M, Fagerberg L, Hallstrom BM, Lindskog C, Oksvold P, Mardinoglu A, et al. Proteomics. Tissue-based map of the human proteome. Science. 2015;**347**(6220):1260419

[67] Fernandez-Funez P, Sanchez-Garcia J, de Mena L, Zhang Y, Levites Y, Khare S, et al. Holdase activity of secreted Hsp70 masks amyloid-β42 neurotoxicity in Drosophila. Proceedings of the National Academy of Sciences of the United States of America. 2016;**113**(35):E5212-E5221

[68] Cummings CJ, Sun Y, Opal P, Antalffy N, Mestril R, Orr HT, et al. Over-expression of inducible HSP70 chaperone suppresses neuropathology and improves motor function in SCA1 mice. Human Molecular Genetics. 2001;**10**(14):1511-1518

[69] Martinez-Ruiz A, Villanueva L, Gonzalez de Orduna C, Lopez-Ferrer D, Higueras MA, Tarin C, et al. S-nitrosylation of Hsp90 promotes the inhibition of its ATPase and endothelial nitric oxide synthase regulatory activities. Proceedings of the National Academy of Sciences of the United States of America. 2005;**102**(24):8525-8530

[70] Orenstein SJ, Cuervo AM. Chaperone-mediated autophagy: Molecular mechanisms and physiological relevance. Seminars in Cell & Developmental Biology. 2010;**21**(7):719-726

[71] Chan HYE, Warrick JM, Gray-Board GL, Paulson HL, Bonini NM. Mechanisms of chaperone suppression of polyglutamine disease: Selectivity, synergy and modulation o protein solubility in Drosophila. Human Molecular Genetics. 2000;**9**(19):2811-2820

[72] Raman B, Ban T, Sakai M, Pasta SY, Ramakrishna T, Naiki H, et al. AlphaB-crystallin, a small heat-shock protein, prevents the amyloid fibril growth of an amyloid beta-peptide and beta2-microglobulin. The Biochemical Journal. 2005;**392**(Pt 3):573-581

[73] Nillegoda NB, Kirstein J, Szlachcic A, Berynskyy M, Stank A, Stengel F, et al. Crucial HSP70 co-chaperone complex unlocks metazoan protein disaggregation. Nature. 2015;**524**(7564):247-251

[74] Haruo Shinohara YI, Goto S, Inagaki T, Kato K. Alpha B crystallin and HSP28 are enhanced in the cerebral cortex of patients with Alzheimer's disease. Journal of the neurological sciences. 1993;**119**(04122):203-208

[75] Gao X, Carroni M, Nussbaum-Krammer C, Mogk A, Nillegoda NB, Szlachcic A, et al. Human Hsp70 Disaggregase reverses Parkinson's-linked alpha-synuclein amyloid fibrils. Molecular Cell. 2015;**59**(5):781-793

[76] Mangione MR, Vilasi S, Marino C, Librizzi F, Canale C, Spigolon D, et al. Hsp60, amateur chaperone in amyloid-beta fibrillogenesis. Biochimica et Biophysica Acta. 2016;**1860**(11 Pt A):2474-2483

[77] Walls KC, Coskun P, Gallegos-Perez JL, Zadourian N, Freude K, Rasool S, et al. Swedish Alzheimer mutation

induces mitochondrial dysfunction mediated by HSP60 mislocalization of amyloid precursor protein (APP) and beta-amyloid. The Journal of Biological Chemistry. 2012;**287**(36):30317-30327

[78] Urushitani M, Kurisu J, Tateno M, Hatakeyama S, Nakayama K, Kato S, et al. CHIP promotes proteasomal degradation of familial ALS-linked mutant SOD1 by ubiquitinating Hsp/Hsc70. Journal of Neurochemistry. 2004;**90**(1):231-244

[79] Narayan P, Orte A, Clarke RW, Bolognesi B, Hook S, Ganzinger KA, et al. The extracellular chaperone clusterin sequesters oligomeric forms of the amyloid-beta(1-40) peptide. Nature Structural & Molecular Biology. 2011;**19**(1):79-83

[80] Hughes SR, Khorkova O, Goyal S, Knaeblein J, Heroux J, Riedel NG, et al. a2-macroglobulin associates with b-amyloid peptide and prevents fibril formation. Proceedings of the National Academy of Sciences of the United States of America. 1998;**95**:3275-3280

[81] Poprac P, Jomova K, Simunkova M, Kollar V, Rhodes CJ, Valko M. Targeting free radicals in oxidative stress-related human diseases. Trends in Pharmacological Sciences. 2017;**38**(7):592-607

[82] Mecocci P, Boccardi V, Cecchetti R, Bastiani P, Scamosci M, Ruggiero C, et al. A long journey into aging, brain aging, and Alzheimer's disease following the oxidative stress tracks. Journal of Alzheimer's Disease. 2018;**62**(3):1319-1335

[83] Adlard PA, Bush AI. Metals and Alzheimer's disease: How far have we come in the clinic? Journal of Alzheimer's Disease. 2018;**62**(3):1369-1379

[84] Barnham KJ, Masters CL, Bush AI. Neurodegenerative diseases and oxidative stress. Nature Reviews Drug Discovery. 2004;**3**(3):205-214

[85] Carmichael G. Mitochondrial mutations may underlie late-onset AD. Lancet Neurology. 2004;**3**:513

[86] Pramanik D, Ghosh C, Dey SG. Heme-Cu bound abeta peptides: Spectroscopic characterization, reactivity, and relevance to Alzheimer's disease. Journal of the American Chemical Society. 2011;**133**(39):15545-15552

[87] Pramanik D, Ghosh C, Mukherjee S, Dey SG. Interaction of amyloid β peptides with redox active heme cofactor: Relevance to Alzheimer's disease. Coordination Chemistry Reviews. 2013;**257**(1):81-92

[88] Atwood CS, Moir RD, Huang X, Scarpa RC, Bacarra NM, Romano DM, et al. Dramatic aggregation of Alzheimer Aβ by Cu(II) is induced by conditions representing physiological acidosis. Journal of Biological Chemistry. 1998;**273**(21):12817-12826

[89] Xudong Huang CSA, Hartshorn MA, Multhaup G, Goldstein LE, Scarpa RC, Cuajungco MP, et al. The Aβ peptide of alzheimer's disease directly produces hydrogen peroxide through metal ion reduction. Biochemistry. 1997;**38**(24):7609-7616

[90] Curtain CC, Ali F, Volitakis I, Cherny RA, Norton RS, Beyreuther K, et al. Alzheimer's disease amyloid-beta binds copper and zinc to generate an allosterically ordered membrane-penetrating structure containing superoxide dismutase-like subunits. The Journal of Biological Chemistry. 2001;**276**(23):20466-20473

[91] Butterfield DA, Boyd-Kimball D. Oxidative stress, amyloid-beta peptide, and altered key molecular pathways in the pathogenesis and

progression of Alzheimer's disease. Journal of Alzheimer's Disease. 2018;**62**(3):1345-1367

[92] Smith DG, Cappai R, Barnham KJ. The redox chemistry of the Alzheimer's disease amyloid beta peptide. Biochimica et Biophysica Acta. 2007;**1768**(8):1976-1990

[93] Xudong Huang RDM, Tanzi RE, Bush AI, Rogers JT. Redox-active metals, oxidative stress, and Alzheimer's disease pathology. Annals of the New York Academy of Sciences. 2004;**1012**:153-164

[94] Wyatt AR, Constantinescu P, Ecroyd H, Dobson CM, Wilson MR, Kumita JR, et al. Protease-activated alpha-2-macroglobulin can inhibit amyloid formation via two distinct mechanisms. FEBS Letters. 2013;**587**(5):398-403

[95] Cedazo-Minguez A. Apolipoprotein E and Alzheimer's disease: Molecular mechanisms and therapeutic opportunities. Journal of Cellular and Molecular Medicine. 2007;**11**(6):1227-1238

[96] Fukuhara A, Yamada M, Fujimori K, Miyamoto Y, Kusumoto T, Nakajima H, et al. Lipocalin-type prostaglandin D synthase protects against oxidative stress-induced neuronal cell death. The Biochemical Journal. 2012;**443**(1):75-84

[97] Inui T, Mase M, Shirota R, Nagashima M, Okada T, Urade Y. Lipocalin-type prostaglandin D synthase scavenges biliverdin in the cerebrospinal fluid of patients with aneurysmal subarachnoid hemorrhage. Journal of Cerebral Blood Flow and Metabolism. 2014;**34**(9):1558-1567

[98] Hebert LE, Weuve J, Scherr PA, Evans DA. Alzheimer disease in the United States (2010-2050) estimated using the 2010 census. Neurology. 2013;**80**(19):1778-1783

[99] Hardy JA, Higgins GA. Alzheimer's disease: The amyloid cascade hypothesis. Science. 1992;**256**(5054):184-185

[100] Skaper SD. Alzheimer's disease and amyloid: Culprit or coincidence? International Review of Neurobiology. 2012;**102**:277-316

[101] Gong Y, Chang L, Viola KL, Lacor PN, Lambert MP, Finch CE, et al. Alzheimer's disease-affected brain: Presence of oligomeric A beta ligands (ADDLs) suggests a molecular basis for reversible memory loss. Proceedings of the National Academy of Sciences of the United States of America. 2003;**100**(18):10417-10422

[102] Ru-Jing Ren EBD, Wang G, Seyfried NT, Levey AI. Proteomics of protein post-translational modifications implicated in neurodegeneration. Translational Neurodegeneration. 2014;**3**(1):23

Chapter 12

Diabetes Mellitus and Amyloid Beta Protein Pathology in Dementia

Teresa Ponce-López, Andrew Michael Sorsby-Vargas, Alma Patricia Bocanegra-López, José Luna-Muñoz, Miguel Angel Ontiveros-Torres, Ignacio Villanueva-Fierro, Parménides Guadarrama-Ortiz and Alejandra Martínez-Maldonado

Abstract

Amyloidosis is a pathological condition which consists on the accumulation of fibrillar proteins. This disease is characterized by extracellular amyloid deposits with a clinical variability depending on the affected tissue. Histopathological evidence indicates that diabetes mellitus type 2 (DM2) induces dementia development, specifically Alzheimer's disease (AD). It has been demonstrated in animal subjects that there is a possibility that aberrant signaling of insulin is a key factor in the induction of the pathology of AD. Recently, there has been newly emerged evidence regarding the relationship between the pathogenesis of Parkinson's disease (PD) and insulin resistance. On another note, the importance of the amyloid deposits in the patients' pancreas with DM2 was evidenced by the discovery of islets of amyloid polypeptide. This has generated interest in the search of the etiopathogenic role of DM2 in the carbohydrates' metabolism. Finally, it is important to consider DM2 as a risk factor essential for the formation of deposits of amyloid-β in patients' brains with dementia.

Keywords: diabetes mellitus, insulin resistance, β-amyloid, dementia, Alzheimer's disease, Parkinson's disease

1. Introduction

Dementia has become a worldwide public health issue that currently affects 50 million people. The impact of this disease not only affects the patient himself but also the family and caretaker. This neurodegenerative disorder is characterized by the loss of mental faculties in a progressive and irreversible way which includes language alterations, learning and memory, as well as loss of ethical judgment and social behavior.

Alzheimer's disease is the main cause of dementia, following vascular dementia, senil dementia, frontotemporal dementia, and even Parkinson's disease (P). Age is still the main risk factor to suffer from dementia, even though it is a multifactorial disorder. Smoking, alcoholism, lack of interest in education, and obesity are factors that can increase the risk of developing dementia in an old age [1].

Currently, obesity is another worldwide public health issue. According to the World Health Organization (WHO), the majority of the population lives in countries where overweight and obesity are the cause of more deaths than malnutrition. At the same time, obesity is one of the causes of diabetes mellitus (DM) which is a chronic disease derived from a failure in the pancreas to produce insulin, necessary hormone to process glucose [2].

Studies suggest that insulin is related with the formation of amyloid plaques which are histopathological structures, characteristics of some dementias such as Alzheimer's disease (AD) [3]. For this reason, in recent years, DM has been considered, specifically diabetes mellitus type 2 (DM2, in which the organism is unable to use insulin), as an important risk factor for the development of dementia. In this chapter, general data about DM and dementias, as well as the importance of DM in the formation of amyloid aggregates which converts it in a risk factor for AD and Parkinson's disease (PD), will be discussed.

2. Amyloidosis

Amyloidosis is a chronic disease that is characterized by the extracellular deposits of insoluble proteins in one or many organs (systematic amyloidosis). Such disease is due to the alteration in the metabolism of various proteins which is the origin of extracellular accumulation of material resistant to the digestion protein called amyloid fibrillar protein [4]. Generally, amyloid deposits are located in a systematic way. Amyloidosis can arise by itself (primary amyloidosis) or be a secondary effect of many infections, inflammatory disorders, or malignancies in diseases (secondary amyloidosis) (**Table 1**).

One of the most studied amyloid proteins is amyloid-β peptide (Aβ), which arises from the proteolictic processing (via amyloidogenic) of the precursor amyloid protein (APP) [5]. This peptide is added in an extracellular way and forms highly insoluble fibrils that give rise to the amyloid plaques which are found in patients' brains with neurodegenerative diseases such as Alzheimer's disease. Existing evidence has been suggested that monomers of Aβ do not generate a toxic environment in the brain parenchyma [6]; however, the oligomers of this peptide prevent the synapse and neuronal environment and generate an exacerbated inflammation associated with the glia and microgery favoring the production of

Primary Amyloidosis	*No alternate disease. Occurs by itself*		
Secondary Amyloidosis	*Originate in the bosom of another disease*	*Inflammatory diseases*	*Example: Rheumatoid arthritis*
		Infectious diseases	*Example: Tuberculosis*
		Neoplasias	*Example: Hodgkin's disease*

Table 1.
Amyloidosis classification.

interleukins triggering the formation of reactive oxygen species that have been shown to be toxic, causing neuronal death [7].

3. Definition, clinical characteristics, and epidemiology of diabetes mellitus

DM is a chronic metabolic disease characterized by hyperglycemia caused by a deficit of pancreas insulin production known as diabetes mellitus type 1 (DM1) or by insulin receptor dysfunction known as diabetes mellitus type 2 (DM2) [2]. DM is characterized by the presence of polyuria, polyphagia, and polydipsia. Patients present an unexplained weight loss; paresthesia of the extremities and foot pain may occur, as well as asthenia and recurrent or complicated infections. If the patients are not adequately treated, it can be associated with renal, visual, cardiac, intestinal, diabetic ketoacidosis, or diabetic coma complications, and it can lead to brain damage [8]. DM is currently considered a risk factor for the development of Alzheimer's disease (AD) and Parkinson's disease (PD) [3].

In recent years, the prevalence of this disease has increased in a progressive and alarming way, becoming a public health problem. The National Center for Chronic Disease Prevention and Health Promotion estimates that in 2017, 9.4% of the United States population suffers from diabetes, that is, 30.3 million people, of which 21.1 million people are diagnosed and 7.2 million people who have diabetes have not been diagnosed. On the other hand, the last report of the World Health Organization on the profiles of countries for diabetes in 2016 reports that in the United States, 3% of the population dies from this disease. **Table 2** highlights the figures on the number of deaths caused by this disease in the five countries with the highest number of patients according to the statistics portal Statista.

Year / Country	2016*					2017**
	Population (millions)	Age Range	DM cases		Deaths by DM	DM cases
			Men	Women		
China	1,376	30 – 69 years	16,000	10,600	3% of the population	114,441
		> 40 years	20,400	23,400		
India	1,311	30 – 69 years	75,900	51,700	2 % of the population	73,074
		> 40 years	46,800	45,000		
United States	322	30 – 69 years	16,600	10,600	3% of the population	30,357
		> 40 years	20,400	23,400		
Brazil	208	30 – 69 years	15,000	14,900	6% of the population	12,554
		> 40 years	16,900	25,900		
Mexico	127	30 – 69 years	23,100	22,000	14% of the population	12,056
		> 40 years	17,600	24,300		

Data according to WHO 2016
***Data according to Statista 2017*

Table 2.
Cases and deaths due to diabetes mellitus in the countries with the highest prevalence.

4. Amyloidosis' association with diabetes mellitus

Case studies have shown a deep connection in patients who suffer from amyloidosis and type 2 diabetes, especially in those with pancreatic damage [9, 10]. Studies have focused on a neuro pancreatic hormone called islet amyloid polypeptide (IAPP) or amylin, secreted along with insulin by β pancreatic cells, and its possible etiology in type 2 diabetes [11]. IAPP functions as a glucose homeostatic regulator, but once it suffers synthetic alterations, it starts to accumulate inside and outside the pancreatic cells resulting in apoptosis [12]. Although the specific etiology has remained unknown, there have been many hypotheses on what causes these pancreatic amyloid deposits. One of the most accepted hypotheses consists of a malfunctioning β pancreatic cell which is unable to correctly process amylin, resulting in the installment of amyloid proteins inside and outside the cells [13]. Another accepted theory indicates the genetic overexpression of amylin, which causes amyloid deposits, although there has not been a proven correlation (in humans) between high IAPP circulating levels and glucose intolerance [14]. It has been proved that the amino acids within the 26–29 sequence are a determinant factor proved in the development of amyloid deposits only in humans, simians, and felines, which are presumed to be the only three species to suffer from an amyloid deposit diabetes [9, 10, 15, 16]. It has been proved that in 9% of the diabetic population, there has been an identified mutation within the promoter region in the amyloid gene, increasing its transcription [17–19]. For years it has been proven that high blood glucose is not only toxic to β pancreatic cells, but it also generates an overexpression on the IAPP gene which contributes to pancreatic amyloid deposits, inducting cellular apoptosis [12]. It was never clear whether IAPP was the cause or the consequence of diabetes, but once the genetic mutation in the promoter region was finally identified, there is still more research to be done in order to be completely certain.

5. Definition and epidemiology of dementias

Dementia is a syndrome of generalized deterioration, since it involves cognitive-behavioral damage; is acquired, degenerative in most cases, and multi-etiological; and will have repercussions on the family, work, and social life of the person. Dementia is also characterized by a decrease in mental faculties of the individual, and clinical characteristics may vary depending on the neuropathological process of the disease and even the specific characteristics of each person. Symptoms may include short-term memory loss, temporary and spatial disorientation, and difficulty in communication and behavior alterations [20]. The most frequent types of dementia include vascular dementia, AD, and PD, although there are other forms of dementia such as frontotemporal dementia and dementia caused by Lewy body deposits. It usually affects older adults; however, it is not the result of normal aging.

Currently dementia is not considered a social priority in most countries, despite the increase in incidence. It is estimated that there are at least 50 million people in the world suffering from dementia, with 10 million new cases registered every year. WHO statistics indicates that it is expected that by the year 2030 and 2050, the figures will, respectively, increase to 76 million and 145 million cases. AD is the main cause of dementia, representing at least 60% of cases, with a prevalence of 10–30% in the population over 65 years of age [21–23]. On the other hand, PD is the second most common neurodegenerative disease after AD which frequently goes through a process of dementia. PD has a prevalence between 100 and 300/100,000 of the population [24], and it is expected that by 2030 the number of patients duplicates [25–27].

These numbers are alarming, and they represent a really serious situation that has not been given the attention and follow-up that is required, because as already mentioned, it has not been a social priority for most countries yet has a great economic impact.

6. Diabetes mellitus as a risk factor for dementias

Dementia is a complex disorder of multifactorial etiology that results in alterations in health status changes in lifestyle. It is important to identify the risk factors, at an early age, to prevent this disease. There are several factors related to dementia such as age [28], ethnic group [29], gender [30], genetic factors [31], physical activity [32], smoking, alcoholism [33], education level [34], environmental factors, and obesity [35, 36]. In addition, in the last decade, DM has been associated as a risk factor for dementia, especially DM2, which is also related to obesity.

Damage to cognitive functions has been observed in patients with DM2 compared to healthy patients [37, 38]. Individuals with DM2 present alterations in their attention capacity, execution, processing speed, work memory, and verbal memory [39, 40]. Studies report a reduction of the gray matter in the frontotemporal cortex, as well as the decrease in glucose metabolism in patients with alterations in executive and memory functions [41], but it also has been associated to a white matter reduction [38]. On the other hand, the damages in verbal memory correlate with the integrity of the parahippocampal gyrus [42]. In other words, DM2 represents an important risk factor for dementia. Interestingly, in the five main countries with a high DM prevalence (see **Table 2**), there is also a significant prevalence of dementia (**Figure 1**).

DM2 is the most common type of diabetes in which autoimmune antibodies appear to be the cause. In this type of diabetes, insulin resistance is observed, which limits the ability to respond to hormones, both endogenous and exogenous [43]. In some cases, insulin resistance is a result of a lower number or a mutation of insulin receptors (IR). These receptors are expressed in the central nervous system (CNS), in the hypothalamus, olfactory bulb, cerebral cortex, cerebellum, and hippocampus [44–46]. Insulin can cross the blood-brain barrier and reach its target, generating anorexic effects by activating the satiety center. This happens because insulin and the insulin-like growth factor-1 (IGF-1) activate PI3K causing the opening of ATP-dependent potassium channels (ChK^{*}_{ATP}), thus hyperpolarizing the neuron which causes it to disrupt its activity, and thus, it stimulates the secretion of the

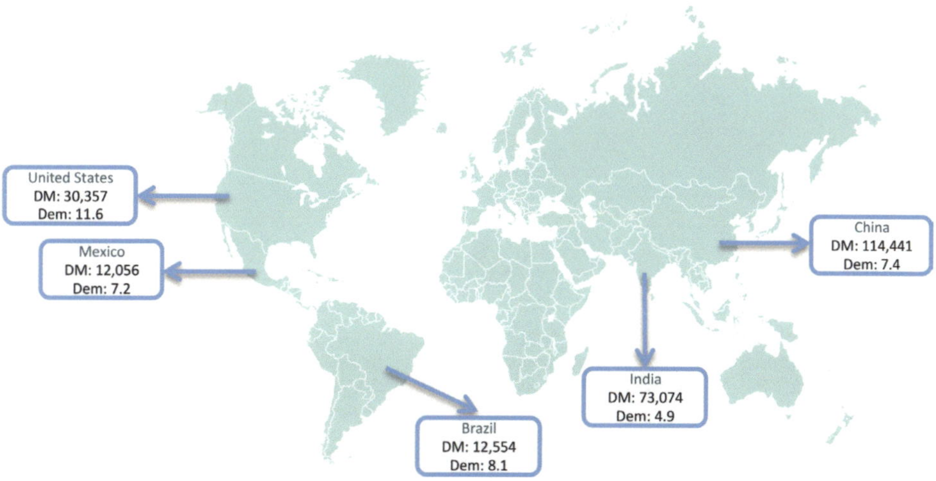

Figure 1.
Dementia prevalence in the five countries with the highest diabetes mellitus prevalence in 2017. DM, diabetes mellitus (thousands); Dem, dementia (for every 1000).

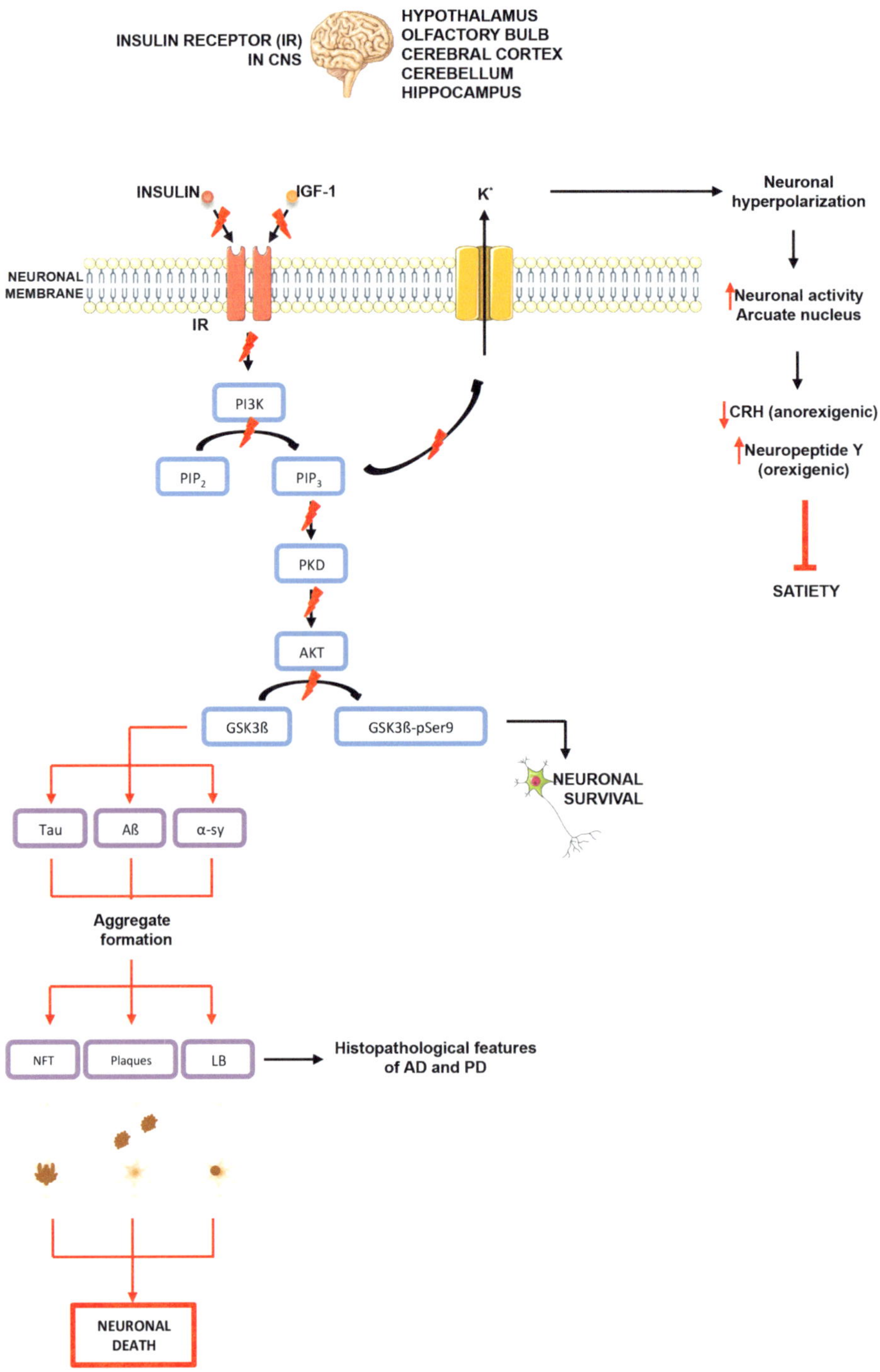

Figure 2.

Pathway of insulin/IGF-1/PI3K/AKT/GSK3β in respect to the neuronal function and its effect on satiety. Normally, this pathway of insulin/IGF-1 begins when it activates IR and it phosphorylates to begin the pathway for PI3K. Once PKD activates AKT, it will inhibit the activity of GSK3β by phosphorylating in Ser9, which is associated to neuronal survival. On another note, PI3K provokes the opening of potassium canals, via PIP2, hyperpolarizing the neuron which is what conducts the activation of the satiety center. When there is no suitable recognition of insulin, GSK3β will not inhibit; therefore, it will act upon proteins [tau, amyloid-β (Aβ) y α-synuclein (α-syn)] related to the formation of aggregates [neurofibrillary tangles (NFT), amyloid plaques, and Lewy bodies (LB), respectively] which lead to neuronal death and are histopathological characteristics of diseases such as AD and PD. Also, the opening of potassium canals will not be taken care of, inhibiting the satiety (in the presence of insulin, back arrows; lack of insulin, red arrows).

corticotropin-releasing hormone (CRH), which is anorexigenic and inhibits the secretion of neuropeptide Y, which is orexigenic. As mentioned above, insulin activates the PI3K/AKT/GSK3β pathway, where GSK3β is phosphorylated in Ser9 (GSK3β-pSer9) by means of AKT; being phosphorylated at this site inactivates it, resulting in neuronal survival. However, when there is insulin resistance as in the case of DM2 or there is no insulin production (DM1), this pathway does not activate; therefore GSK3β will not be inhibited and will act upon proteins involved in neuronal death such as tau, amyloid-β, and α-synuclein. These proteins will form intracellular (tau) and extracellular (tau, amyloid-β, and α-synuclein) deposits, which are histopathological features (neurofibrillary tangles, plaques, and Lewy bodies) of dementias such as AD and PD (**Figure 2**). Neuronal death caused by the lack of insulin is one of the reasons why DM is a risk factor for dementia.

7. Diabetes mellitus and amyloid-β protein pathology in Parkinson's disease

Clinically, Parkinson's disease is defined as a progressive disorder characterized by resting tremor, rigidity, and bradykinesia; however, there may be other manifestations less constant such as postural instability, propulsive gait, dysphagia, autonomic disorders, sebaceous sweating, salivation, and deteriorating superior functions that can lead up to dementia. This disease was described in 1817 by James Parkinson, who described the deficiency of dopamine in the brain of his patients in late 1950 and also described the treatment of this disease with L-dopa in the 1960s. Parkinson's disease is the second most frequent neurodegenerative disorder. It is a motor disease related with the disorder of the basal ganglia specifically via nigrostriatal which is formed by the axons of the dopaminergic neurons of the substance compact nigra which innervate the corpus striatum. This structure is considered the main target of dopaminergic innervation due to the high density of axons it receives and its large size. The main symptoms of Parkinson's disease are caused by the degeneration of dopaminergic neurons via nigrostriatal [47, 48]. A pathological hallmark of Parkinson's disease is the Lewy bodies (LB), eosinophilic inclusions of α-synuclein (α-syn) located in the neuronal soma especially in nigra substance [49]. Besides the (LB) there can be deposits of the protein tau (MNF) and of β-amyloid (plaques).

There is existing evidence that α-syn, tau and Aβ act in a synergistic way in the pathology of AD and PD [50, 51] accelerating the aggregation of each [52]. The presence of tau and Aβ was found in patients with PD, and the cognitive function was lower than healthy patients' [53]. It has also been demonstrated that when these three proteins are found in high concentrations, as in PD, it generates changes in CFS tau levels [54], and if these patients are obese as well, they present insulin resistance [55, 56] even though they do not suffer from DM. These patients have deficits of cognitive functions. It is possible that the resistance to insulin accelerates the demential process in patients with PD, and it can lead to more serious motor symptoms.

As described before, insulin/IGF-1 activates the route PI3K/AKT/GSK3β, which, besides being involved in the glucose metabolism and the ingestion of food, also plays an important role in the learning and memory process associated with long-term potential (LTP) in the hippocampus [57]. Apparently, insulin stabilizes the production of dopamine and decreases the alterations in movement in a PD model [58–61]. When insulin acts over IR in a suitable way, the result is neuronal survival; however, the lack of insulin provokes that the GSK3β will not be inactivated (when it is phosphorylated in Ser9 by AKT), which leads to the favoring of the formation of MNF, LB, and amyloid plaques (see **Figure 2**). These pathological structures are found frequently coexisting in the hippocampus and cerebral cortex in patients

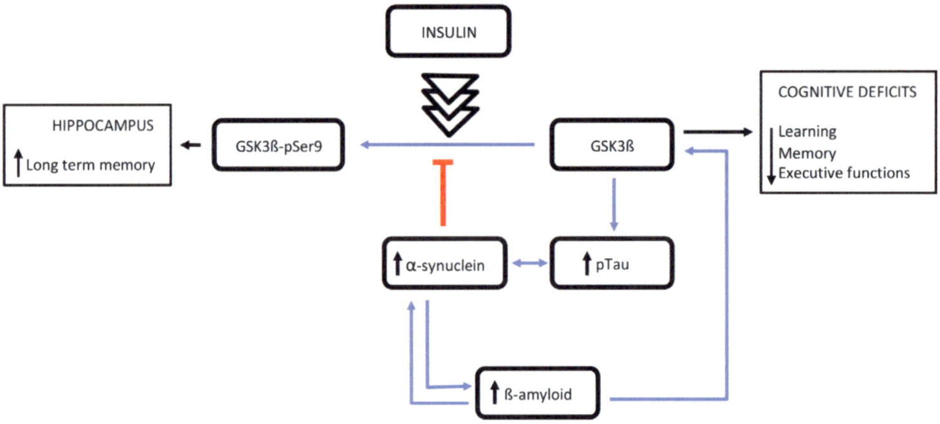

Figure 3.
GSK3β activation regulated by synergistic action of α-synuclein (α-syn), phosphorylated tau (pTau), and β-amyloid (Aβ). In the presence of insulin, a GSK3β inhibition occurs that has as a result, the improvement of long-term memory in the hippocampus. When there are alterations in the recognition of the insulin or there is simply no production, no GSK3β inhibitions occur which promoted the augmentation of α-sy, pTau, and Aβ aggregates which at the same time act synergistically, augmenting GSK3β activity. Therefore, cognitive deficits that include alterations in the learning and memory processes as well as executive functions are favored.

with PD [62]. The negative regulation of GSK3β is extremely important in the neurodegenerative disorders such as PD [63] and even more in the function of α-syn, having as consequences cognitive deficits [64, 65] which include learning and memory alterations as well as executive functions. If this negative regulation of GSK3β does not happen due to the lack of insulin, then there will be a tau phosphorylation increase which will favor the accumulation of α-syn amyloid. These aggregates of α-syn have a positive feedback over the accumulation of phosphorylated tau and facilitate the formation of Aβ deposits. The accumulation of aβ and α-syn (amyloid) activates GSK3β, even though α-syn does so by inhibiting the formation of GSK3β-pSer9 (**Figure 3**).

It is possible that patients with DM-PD deteriorate rapidly due to the favoring of the accumulation of Aβ due to the lack of insulin, since this could generate more oxidative stress and thereby damage dopaminergic neurons. However, more studies are needed regarding the interaction between Aβ and α-syn in the demential process of PD caused by the failure in recognition of insulin such as in DM2.

8. Diabetes mellitus and amylin and amyloid-β protein pathologies in Alzheimer's disease

AD is one of the most prevalent dementias in older people and is characterized by the progressive loss of memory and deterioration of cognitive functions such as judgment and behavior [66]. AD develops through mutations in the chromosomes (presenilin 2), chromosome 14 (presenilin 1) and chromosome 21 (PPA) [67]. Only 5% of patients with AD associate to this genetic factor. It has an early appearance in people around 45 years old; however, the most common form of appearance of this neurodegenerative disease is "sporadic" where there are no mutations and it develops in people around 65 years [68]. There is still doubt regarding the genesis of sporadic AD; risk factors that can lead to the development of AD have been described. One of these risk factors is aging and poor eating habits where it involves ingesting large quantities of fat and sugar. Therefore, obesity is a risk factor for diabetes mellitus type 2.

Histopathologically, the brains of these patients present in great abundance neuritic plaques (NP) and neurofibrillary tangles. (NFT) [69, 70]. Neuritic plaques are constituted by extracellular deposits of the fibrillar beta-amyloid peptide, and associated to these, dystrophic neurites (DN), neuritic plaques bordered by astroglial cells and associated with the amyloid peptide, the tight microglial cells can be observed (**Figure 4**). Together, they unleash the inflammatory cell process observed in a brain with AD [71]. NFT are constituted by highly soluble filaments (paired helical filaments, PHF) inside the neuronal soma. The PHF are constituted by tau protein; in normal conditions, tau protein favors the stability to the microtubules and the organelles and vesicles along the axon. The genesis of PHF has been associated with posttranslational mechanisms of tau protein as in hyperphosphorylation and truncation. Recent studies have suggested that the tau protein plays a dual role in protection and toxicity upon the neurodegenerative process and neuronal death. The phosphorylation of the tau protein could be involved in processes of neuronal protection to degeneration

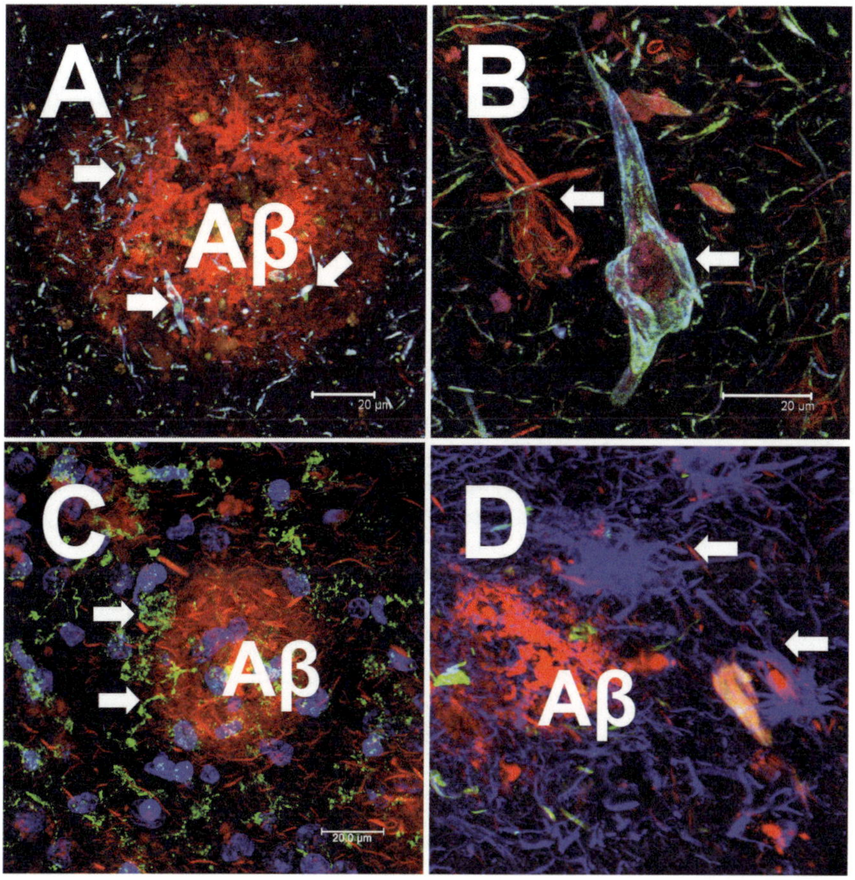

Figure 4.
Characteristic lesions of a brain with Alzheimer's disease. (A) Neuritic plaque. Dystrophic neuritis (green and blue channels) are observed in the periphery of the Aβ deposit (red channel). (B) Neurofibrillary tangles recognized by antibodies directed against phosphorylated tau protein, in the vicinity there is a neurofibrillary tangle evidenced only in the red channel, the dystrophic neuritis in the periphery show different degrees of co-localization. (C) Neuritic plaque evidenced in the red channel, the nuclei are observed in blue color. The microglial cells are closely associated with the Aβ deposit (green channel). (D) Neuritic plaque in the periphery glial cells (blue channel) are observed. And in the channel see observed neuritic dystrophic positive tau protein. Double immunostaining with antibodies directed against the phosphorylated tau protein (A, B), IBA1 (C), and GFAP (D), counterstained with triazine red dye A-D and ToPro (C). Images taken with confocal microscope (SP8, Leica).

upon the fragment of the minimal filament (92–95 amino acids culminating in Glu391). The process of proteolysis in the asp-421 of tau favors in the beginning its polymerization, and the truncation in glu391 favors the stability and insolubility of the PHF [72].

8.1 Amyloid formation is the pathological hallmark of T2D and AD

The incidence of both AD and T2D is increasing at an alarming rate at present and has become a major public health concern in many industrialized countries [73]. Many epidemiological studies have shown that diabetic individuals have a significantly higher risk of developing AD [74]. Recently, it has become increasingly recognized that there is an overlap between the pathology of AD and vascular dementia and cerebrovascular dysfunction plays a role not only in vascular dementia but also in AD [75]. Nevertheless, clinical observations suggest that the association is independent of vascular factors [76], which raises the possibility that diabetic conditions such as insulin resistance and hyperglycemia may affect the fundamental pathogenesis of AD. Many neuronal functions are affected by changes in the insulin signaling pathway; therefore diabetes mellitus may have an important role in the progression of AD ([77]; see **Figure 2**).

Another possible mechanism that has been involved is the **amyloid deposition** in islets composed primarily of islet amyloid polypeptide (IAPP or amylin) that is a common feature in T2D. IAPP amyloid deposition has been correlated with disease severity, reduced β-cell mass, the development of hyperglycemia, and islet inflammation. Similarly, Aβ plays a central role in synaptic dysfunction and in the cognitive deficiencies associated with AD pathogenesis [78]. Evidences from clinical and animal studies associate the pancreatic amyloid, amylin in mediating neuronal loss in AD, suggesting its role as a potential link between AD and T2D pathogenesis [79–81]. The presence of amyloid deposits in pancreas and brain has been demonstrated in patients with T2D, which can serve as seed to increase the aggregation of these deposits. This suggests that pancreatic IAPP can potentiate amyloid beta misfolding in patients with AD [81]. Previously, de la Monte and colleges, 2008, reported that IAPP enters the brain, augments Aβ misfolding, and associates with Aβ plaques, and plasma levels correlate with AD diagnosis [82]. Interestingly, amylin has been identified in human cerebrospinal fluid and brains of diabetic patients with vascular dementia or AD and nondiabetic patients with AD. Furthermore, co-localization of amylin and Aβ deposits was also observed in postmortem human brains [81]. Likewise, amylin deposits were observed in the temporal lobe gray matter in diabetic patients [79]. Therefore, the co-existence of Aβ and amylin in the brain suggests the potential ability of amylin to infiltrate the brain and induce amyloid deposition in the brain [81].

8.2 Potential mechanisms of amylin-Aβ-induced toxicity in neurons and pancreatic β cells

Several studies have showed that amyloid aggregates have been found to be associated with disruption of several cellular functions, including mitochondrial activity [83, 84], oxidative stress [85], receptor mediated functions [86, 87], disruption of Ca^{2+} homeostasis [88], and membrane depolarization and disorder [89]. Possibly there is a toxic interaction between Aβ and tau that together with insulin resistance participate in the progression of AD. Similarly, the accumulation of amylin in the brain and its ability to induce neurotoxicity and form "cross-seeding" aggregates with Aβ provide a role for this pancreatic amyloidogenic protein in neurodegeneration [89].

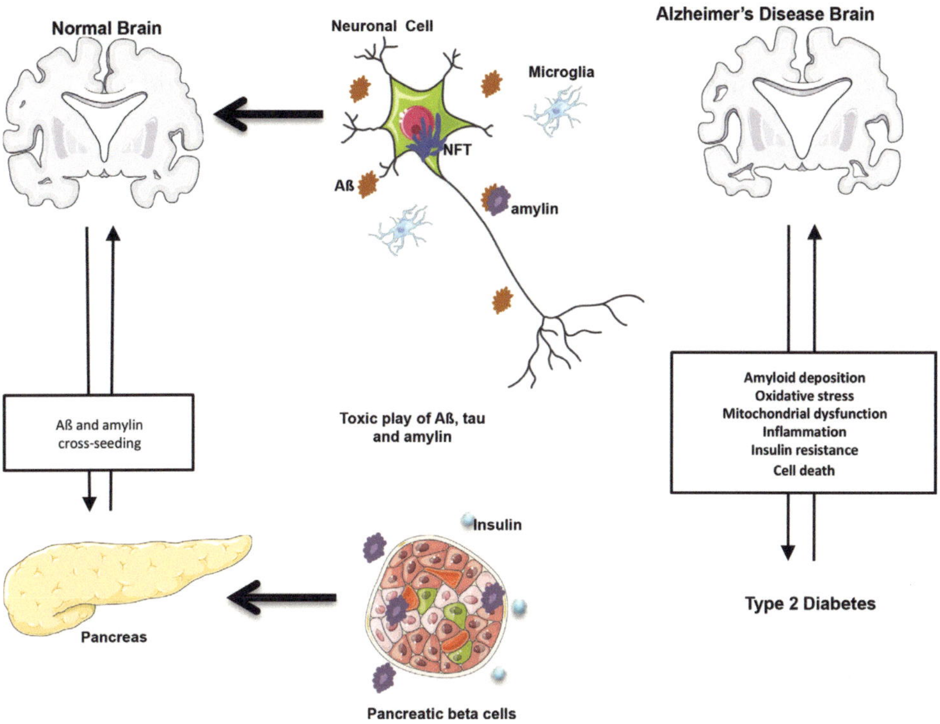

Figure 5.
Association between AD and T2D. Both AD and T2D present cellular loss and abnormal deposition of Aβ, tau, and amylin. These aggregates have the ability to promote the accumulation of amyloid by cross-seeding in neurons and pancreatic cells. The aggregation of amyloid deposits is favored by the presence of aggregates of tau and amylin, which in turn leads to oxidative stress, mitochondrial dysfunction, inflammation, insulin resistances, and finally cell death.

On the other hand, it is likely that there is also a synergistic interaction between the accumulation of amylin in the pancreas and the insulin secretion decrease, which will lead to abnormalities in glucose metabolism, promoting the development of neurodegenerative diseases (**Figure 5**). It is suggested that amylin mediates neurotoxicity by crossing the blood-brain barrier and binding to its receptors [90–92]. This leads to the hyperamulinemia of insulin resistance and to the accumulation of amyloid deposits in the brain.

Both in the animal models and in the clinical trials of AD, those drugs related to production of insulin have been observed or have focused on improving the mechanisms of insulin and improving the condition of patients with cognitive impairment [93]. Analogues of amylin, for example, pramlintide, have been used as adjunctive therapy with insulin for diabetes [94] and are also being evaluated for their ability to prevent neurodegeneration [90, 95, 96].

9. Conclusions

The advantages of studying therapies for T2D in diseases that occur with an insane process are evident. However, no one has questioned whether targeted therapies for dementias could be useful in the treatment of T2D. Immunotherapy targeting Aβ has been shown to improve blood glucose by increasing sensitivity to insulin [97, 98]. Thus, we believe that amyloid deposits as therapeutic targets could be key in the treatment of dementias and alterations in glucose metabolism. But more studies about this issue are needed.

Acknowledgements

Authors want to express their gratitude to Oskar Soto for his support with microglial confocal images and to Ashley Rose Sorsby Vargas for her assistance. We also want to express our gratitude to the Mexican families who donated the brain of their loved ones affected with Alzheimer's disease and made possible our research.

Conflict of interest

The authors declare no conflict of interest.

Author details

Teresa Ponce-López[1], Andrew Michael Sorsby-Vargas[1], Alma Patricia Bocanegra-López[1], José Luna-Muñoz[2], Miguel Angel Ontiveros-Torres[3], Ignacio Villanueva-Fierro[4], Parménides Guadarrama-Ortiz[5] and Alejandra Martínez-Maldonado[1,2]*

1 Anahuac University North Mexico, Mexico City, Mexico

2 National Brain Bank, Laboratorio Nacional de Servicios Experimentales (LaNSE), Centro de Investigación y Estudios Avanzados del IPN (CINVESTAV-IPN), Mexico City, Mexico

3 Bioengineering Department, Engineering and Sciences School, Tecnológico de Monterrey, Mexico

4 Instituto Politécnico Nacional, Becario COFAA, CIIDIR Durango, Mexico

5 Neurosurgery, Specialized Center in Neurology and Neurosciences, México City, México

*Address all correspondence to: alemartinez13@gmail.com

References

[1] Chen JH, Lin KP, Chen YC. Risk factors for dementia. Journal of the Formosan Medical Association. 2009;**108**(10):754-764

[2] Alberti KGMM, Zimmet PZ. Definition, diagnosis and classification of diabetes mellitus and its complications. Part 1: Diagnosis and classification of diabetes mellitus. Provisional report of a WHO consultation. Diabetic Medicine. 1998;**15**(7):539-553

[3] Moran C, Beare R, Phan TG, Bruce DG, Callisaya ML, Srikanth V. Type 2 diabetes mellitus and biomarkers of neurodegeneration. Neurology. 2015;**85**(13):1123-1130

[4] Wechalekar AD, Gillmore JD, Hawkins PN. Systemic amyloidosis. Lancet. 2016;**387**(10038):2641-2654

[5] Geddes JW, Tekirian TL, Mattson MP. N-terminus truncated beta-amyloid peptides and C-terminus truncated secreted forms of amyloid precursor protein: Distinct roles in the pathogenesis of Alzheimer's disease. Neurobiology of Aging. 1999;**20**(1):75-79. Discussion 87

[6] Kontush A. Alzheimer's amyloid-β as a preventive antioxidant for brain lipoproteins. Cellular and Molecular Neurobiology. 2001;**21**(4):299-315

[7] Kelvin WL. Aβ toxicity in Alzheimer's disease globular oligomers ADDLs as new vaccine and drug targets. Neurochemistry International. 2002;**41**:345-352

[8] Alam U, Asghar O, Azmi S, Malik RA. General aspects of diabetes mellitus. In: Handbook of Clinical Neurology. 1st ed. Vol. 126. Netherlands: Elsevier B.V.; 2014. pp. 211-222

[9] Westermark P. Amyloid and polypeptide hormones: What is their interrelationship? Amyloid. 1994;**1**(1):47-60

[10] Zhao HL, Lai FMM, Tong PCY, Zhong DR, Yang D, Tomlinson B, et al. Prevalence and clinicopathological characteristics of islet amyloid in Chinese patients with type 2 diabetes. Diabetes. 2003;**52**(11):2759-2766

[11] Gulli G, Rossetti L, DeFronzo RA. Hyperamylinemia is associated with hyperinsulinemia in the glucose-tolerant, insulin-resistant offspring of two Mexican-American non-insulin-dependent diabetic parents. Metabolism. 1997;**46**(10):1157-1161

[12] Zhang S, Liu J, Dragunow M, Cooper GJS. Fibrillogenic amylin evokes islet β-cell apoptosis through linked activation of a caspase cascade and JNK1. The Journal of Biological Chemistry. 2003;**278**(52):52810-52819

[13] Höppener JWM, Verbeek JS, de Koning EJP, Oosterwijk C, van Hulst KL, Visser-Vernooy HJ, et al. Chronic overproduction of islet amyloid polypeptide/amylin in transgenic mice: Lysosomal localization of human islet amyloid polypeptide and lack of marked hyperglycaemia or hyperinsulinaemia. Diabetologia. 1993;**36**(12):1258-1265

[14] Cadavez L, Montane J, Alcarraz-Vizán G, Visa M, Vidal-Fàbrega L, Servitja JM, et al. Chaperones ameliorate beta cell dysfunction associated with human islet amyloid polypeptide overexpression. PLoS One. 2014;**9**(7):1-11

[15] O'Brien TD, Wagner JD, Litwak KN, Carlson CS, Cefalu WT, Jordan K, et al. Islet amyloid and islet amyloid polypeptide in cynomolgus macaques (*Macaca fascicularis*): An animal model of human non-insulin-dependent diabetes mellitus. Veterinary Pathology. 1996;**33**(5):479-485

[16] Rand J. Current understanding of feline diabetes. Part 1: Pathogenesis. Journal of Feline Medicine and Surgery. 1999;**1**(3):143-153

[17] Mosselman S, Höppener JWM, Zandberg J, van Mansfeld ADM, van Kessel AHMG, Lips CJM, et al. Islet amyloid polypeptide: Identification and chromosomal localization of the human gene. FEBS Letters. 1988;**239**(2):227-232

[18] McCarthy MI, Hitman GA, Mohan V, Ramachandran A, Snehalatha C, Viswanathan M. The islet amyloid polypeptide gene and non-insulin-dependent diabetes mellitus in south Indians. Diabetes Research and Clinical Practice. 1992;**18**(1):31-34

[19] Kajio H, Kobayashi T, Hara M, Nakanishi K, Sugimoto T, Murase T, et al. Islet amyloid polypeptide (IAPP) gene analysis in a Japanese diabetic with marked islet amyloid deposition. Diabetes Research and Clinical Practice. 1992;**15**(1):45-48

[20] Wei K, Liu H, Ma H, Yang X, Zhang Y, Sun Y, et al. Feasible attack on detector-device-independent quantum key distribution. Scientific Reports. 2017;**7**(1):79-87

[21] Hebert LE. Age-specific incidence of Alzheimer's disease in a community population. The Journal of the American Medical Association. 1995;**273**(17):1354

[22] Kawas C, Gray S, Brookmeyer R, Fozard J, Zonderman A. Age-specific incidence rates of Alzheimer's disease: The Baltimore longitudinal study of aging. Neurology. 2000;**54**(11):2072-2077

[23] Evans DA, Bennett DA, Wilson RS, Bienias JL, Morris MC, Scherr PA, et al. Incidence of Alzheimer disease in a biracial urban community. Archives of Neurology. 2003;**60**(2):185

[24] Brookmeyer R, Johnson E, Ziegler-Graham K, Arrighi HM. Forecasting the global burden of Alzheimer's disease. Alzheimer's & Dementia. 2007;**3**(3):186-191

[25] Von Campenhausen S, Bornschein B, Wick R, Bötzel K, Sampaio C, Poewe W, et al. Prevalence and incidence of Parkinson's disease in Europe. European Neuropsychopharmacology. 2005;**15**(4):473-490

[26] Broen MPG, Narayen NE, Kuijf ML, Dissanayaka NNW, Leentjens AFG. Prevalence of anxiety in Parkinson's disease: A systematic review and meta-analysis. Movement Disorders. 2016;**31**(8):1125-1133

[27] Calabrese VP, Dorsey ER, Constantinescu R, Thompson JP, Biglan KM, Holloway RG, et al. Projected number of people with Parkinson disease in the most populous nations, 2005 through 2030. Neurology. 2007;**69**(2):223-224

[28] Kukull WA, Higdon R, Bowen JD, McCormick WC, Teri L, Schellenberg GD, et al. Dementia and Alzheimer disease incidence. Archives of Neurology. 2002;**59**(11):1737

[29] Chen C, Zissimopoulos JM. Racial and ethnic differences in trends in dementia prevalence and risk factors in the United States. Alzheimer's & Dementia: Translational Research & Clinical Interventions. 2018;**4**:510-520

[30] Gannon OJ, Robison LS, Custozzo AJ, Zuloaga KL. Sex differences in risk factors for vascular contributions to cognitive impairment & dementia. Neurochemistry International. 2018;**pii**:S0197-0186(18)30511-4

[31] Corder EH, Saunders AM, Strittmatter WJ, Schmechel DE, Gaskell PC, Small GW, Roses AD, Haines JL, Pericak-Vance MA. Gene

dose of apolipoprotein E type 4 allele and the risk of Alzheimer's disease in late onset families. Science. 1993;**261**(5123):921-923

[32] Yaffe K, Barnes D, Nevitt M, Lui LY, Covinsky K. A prospective study of physical activity and cognitive decline in elderly women women who walk. Archives of Internal Medicine. 2001;**161**(14):1703-1708

[33] Peters R, Peters J, Warner J, Beckett N, Bulpitt C. Alcohol, dementia and cognitive decline in the elderly: A systematic review. Age and Ageing. 2008;**37**(5):505-512

[34] Cobb JL, Wolf PA, Au R, White R, D'Agostino RB. The effect of education on the incidence of dementia and Alzheimer's disease in the Framingham study. Neurology. 1995;**45**(9):1707-1712

[35] Solfrizzi V, Colacicco AM, D'Introno A, et al. Macronutrients, aluminium from drinking water and foods, and other metals in cognitive decline and dementia. Journal of Alzheimer's Disease. 2006;**10**(2-3):303-330

[36] Frith E, Loprinzi PD. Fitness fatness index and Alzheimer-specific mortality. European Journal of Internal Medicine. 2017;**42**:51-53

[37] Smolina K, Wotton CJ, Goldacre MJ. Risk of dementia in patients hospitalised with type 1 and type 2 diabetes in England, 1998-2011: A retrospective national record linkage cohort study. Diabetologia. 2015;**58**(5):942-950

[38] Cheng C, Lin CH, Tsai YW, Tsai CJ, Chou PH, Lan TH. Type 2 diabetes and antidiabetic medications in relation to dementia diagnosis. The Journals of Gerontology. Series A, Biological Sciences and Medical Sciences. 2014;**69**(10):1299-1305

[39] Zhang J, Wang Y, Wang J, Zhou X, Shu N, Wang Y, et al. White matter integrity disruptions associated with cognitive impairments in type 2 diabetic patients. Diabetes. 2014;**63**(11):3596-3605

[40] Mehrabian S, Raycheva M, Gateva A, Todorova G, Angelova P, Traykova M, et al. Cognitive dysfunction profile and arterial stiffness in type 2 diabetes. Journal of the Neurological Sciences. 2012;**322**(1-2):152-156

[41] García-Casares N, Jorge RE, García-Arnés JA, Acion L, Berthier ML, Gonzalez-Alegre P, et al. Cognitive dysfunctions in middle-aged type 2 diabetic patients and neuroimaging correlations: A cross-sectional study. Journal of Alzheimer's Disease. 2014;**42**(4):1337-1346

[42] Nelson EE, Guyer AE. The development of the ventral prefrontal cortex and social flexibility. Dev Cogn Neurosci. 2011;**1**(3):233-245

[43] Sah SP, Singh B, Choudhary S, Kumar A. Animal models of insulin resistance: A review. Pharmacological Reports. 2016;**68**(6):1165-1177

[44] Havrankova J, Roth J. Insulin receptors are widely distributed in the central nervous system of the rat. Nature. 1978;**272**:827-829

[45] Unger J, McNeill TH, Moxley RT, White M, Moss A, Livingston JN. Distribution of insulin receptor-like immunoreactivity in the rat forebrain. Neuroscience. 1989;**31**(1):143-157

[46] Wozniak M, Rydzewski B, Baker S, Raizadai MK. Commentary the cellular and physiological actions of insulin in the central nervous system. Neurochemistry International. 1993;**22**(I):1-10

[47] Damier P, Hirsch EC, Agid Y, Graybiel AM. The substantia nigra

of the human brain. II. Patterns of loss of dopamine-containing neurons in Parkinson's disease. Brain. 1999;**122**(pt8):1437-1448

[48] Fearnley JM, Lees AJ. Ageing and Parkinson's disease: Substantia nigra regional selectivity. Brain. 1991;**114**(5):2283-2301

[49] Braak H, Del K, Rüb U, De Vos RAI, Jansen ENH, Braak E. Staging of brain pathology related to sporadic Parkinson's disease. Neurobiology of Aging. 2003;**24**:197-211

[50] Lee VM-Y, Giasson BI, Trojanowski JQ. More than just two peas in a pod: Common amyloidogenic properties of tau and alpha-synuclein in neurodegenerative diseases. Trends in Neurosciences. 2004;**27**(3):129-134

[51] Giasson BI, Forman MS, Higuchi M, Golbe LI, Graves CL, Kotzbauer PT, et al. Initiation and synergistic fibrillization of tau and alpha-synuclein. Science. 2003;**300**(5619):636-640

[52] Horvath I, Wittung-Stafshede P. Cross-talk between amyloidogenic proteins in type-2 diabetes and Parkinson's disease. Proceedings of the National Academy of Sciences. 2016;**113**(44):12473-12477

[53] Winer JR, Maass A, Pressman P, Stiver J, Schonhaut DR, Baker SL, et al. Associations between tau, β-amyloid, and cognition in Parkinson disease. JAMA Neurology. 2018;**75**(2):227-235

[54] Dolatshahi M, Pourmirbabaei S, Kamalian A, Ashraf-Ganjouei A, Yaseri M, Aarabi MH. Longitudinal alterations of alpha-synuclein, amyloid beta, total, and phosphorylated tau in cerebrospinal fluid and correlations between their changes in Parkinson's disease. Frontiers in Neurology. 2018;**9**:1-12

[55] Bosco D, Plastino M, Cristiano D, Colica C, Ermio C, De Bartolo M, et al. Dementia is associated with insulin resistance in patients with Parkinson's disease. Journal of the Neurological Sciences. 2012;**315**(1-2):39-43

[56] Ashragi MR, Pagano G, Sotirios P, Niccolini F, Politis M. Parkinson's disease, diabetes and cognitive impairment. Recent Patents on Endocrine, Metabolic & Immune Drug Discovery. 2016;**10**(1):11-21

[57] Lee CC, Huang CC, Wu MY, Hsu KS. Insulin stimulates postsynaptic density-95 protein translation via the phosphoinositide 3-kinase-Akt-mammalian target of rapamycin signaling pathway. The Journal of Biological Chemistry. 2005;**280**(18):18543-18550

[58] Hölscher C. Insulin, incretins and other growth factors as potential novel treatments for Alzheimer's and Parkinson's diseases. Biochemical Society Transactions. 2014;**42**(2):593-599

[59] Pang Y, Lin S, Wright C, Shen J, Carter K, Bhatt A, et al. Intranasal insulin protects against substantia nigra dopaminergic neuronal loss and alleviates motor deficits induced by 6-OHDA in rats. Neuroscience. 2016;**318**:157-165

[60] Offen D, Shtaif B, Hadad D, Weizman A, Melamed E, Gil-Ad I. Protective effect of insulin-like-growth-factor-1 against dopamine-induced neurotoxicity in human and rodent neuronal cultures: Possible implications for Parkinson's disease. Neuroscience Letters. 2001;**316**(3):129-132

[61] Kao SY. Rescue of α-synuclein cytotoxicity by insulin-like growth factors. Biochemical and Biophysical Research Communications. 2009;**385**(3):434-438

[62] Majd S, Chegini F, Chataway T, Zhou XF, Gai W. Reciprocal induction between α-synuclein and β-amyloid in adult rat neurons. Neurotoxicity Research. 2013;**23**(1):69-78

[63] Wang Y, Liu W, He X, Zhou F. Parkinson's disease-associated Dj-1 mutations increase abnormal phosphorylation of tau protein through Akt/Gsk-3β pathways. Journal of Molecular Neuroscience. 2013;**51**(3):911-918

[64] Lucas ÂJ, Herna Â, Mora ÂA. Decreased nuclear-catenin, tau hyperphosphorylation and neurodegeneration in GSK-3 conditional transgenic mice. The EMBO Journal. 2010;**20**(1):1-13

[65] King MK, Pardo M, Cheng Y, Downey K, Jope RS, Beurel E. Glycogen synthase kinase-3 inhibitors: Rescuers of cognitive impairments. Pharmacology & Therapeutics. 2014;**141**(1):1-12

[66] Most I, Creutzfeldt J. Alzheimer's disease, Pick's disease and Jakob-Creutzfeldt's disease. In this study the term "presenile dementia" is used in the first, less restricted, sense. Dementia has been defined as a "deterioration in intellectual capacity"; 1969

[67] Terry RD. The pathogenesis of Alzheimer disease: An alternative to the amyloid hypothesis. Journal of Neuropathology and Experimental Neurology. 2017;**91**:399-404

[68] Riedel BC, Thompson PM, Brinton RD. Age, APOE and sex: Triad of risk of Alzheimer's disease. The Journal of Steroid Biochemistry and Molecular Biology. 2016;**160**:134-147

[69] Daniel P. Perl. Neuropathology of Alzheimer's disease. Mount Sinai Journal of Medicine. 2010;**77**(1):32-42

[70] Iqbal K, Grundke-Iqbal I. Discoveries of tau, abnormally hyperphosphorylated tau and others of neurofibrillary degeneration: A personal historical perspective. Journal of Alzheimer's Disease. 2006;**9** (3 Suppl):219-242

[71] Liu L, Chan C. The role of inflammasome in Alzheimer's disease. Ageing Research Reviews. 2014;**15**(1):6-15

[72] Flores-Rodríguez P, Ontiveros-Torres MA, Cárdenas-Aguayo MC, Luna-Arias JP, Meraz-Ríos MA, Viramontes-Pintos A, et al. The relationship between truncation and phosphorylation at the C-terminus of tau protein in the paired helical filaments of Alzheimer's disease. Frontiers in Neuroscience. 2015;**9**:1-10

[73] Després JP, Lemieux I. Abdominal obesity and metabolic syndrome. Nature. 2006;**444**(7121):881-887

[74] Maher PA, Schubert DR. Metabolic links between diabetes and Alzheimer's disease. Expert Review of Neurotherapeutics. 2009;**9**(5):617-630

[75] Luchsinger JA, Tang MX, Stern Y, Shea S, Mayeux R. Diabetes mellitus and risk of Alzheimer's disease and dementia with stroke in a multiethnic cohort. American Journal of Epidemiology. 2001;**154**(7):635-641

[76] Iadecola C. The overlap between neurodegenerative and vascular factors in the pathogenesis of dementia. Acta Neuropathologica. 2010;**120**(3):287-296

[77] Takeda S, Sato N, Rakugi H, Morishita R. Molecular mechanisms linking diabetes mellitus and Alzheimer disease: Beta-amyloid peptide, insulin signaling, and neuronal function. Molecular BioSystems. 2011;**7**:1822-1827

[78] Wijesekara N, Ahrens R, Sabale M, Wu L, Ha K, Verdile G, et al. Amyloid-β and islet amyloid pathologies link Alzheimer's disease and type 2 diabetes

in a transgenic model. The FASEB Journal. 2017;**31**(12):5409-5418

[79] Oskarsson ME, Paulsson JF, Schultz SW, Ingelsson M, Westermark P, Westermark GT. In vivo seeding and cross-seeding of localized amyloidosis: A molecular link between type 2 diabetes and Alzheimer disease. The American Journal of Pathology. 2015;**185**:834-846

[80] Jackson K, Barisone GA, Diaz E, Jin LW, DeCarli C, Despa F. Amylin deposition in the brain: A second amyloid in Alzheimer disease? Annals of Neurology. 2013;**74**:517-526

[81] Fawver JN, Ghiwot Y, Koola C, Carrera W, Rodriguez-Rivera J, Hernandez C, et al. Islet amyloid polypeptide (IAPP): A second amyloid in Alzheimer's disease. Current Alzheimer Research. 2014;**11**:928-940

[82] de la Monte SM, Wands JR. Alzheimer's disease is type 3 diabetes-evidence reviewed. Journal of Diabetes Science and Technology. 2008;**2**(6):1101-1113

[83] Butterfield DA, Drake J, Pocernich C, Castegna A. Evidence of oxidative damage in Alzheimer's disease brain: Central role for amyloid beta-peptide. Trends in Molecular Medicine. 2001;**7**:548-554

[84] Lustbader JW, Cirilli M, Lin C, Xu HW, Takuma K, Wang N, et al. ABAD directly links abeta to mitochondrial toxicity in Alzheimer's disease. Science. 2004;**304**:448-452

[85] Martins RN, Harper CG, Stokes GB, Masters CL. Increased cerebral glucose-6-phosphate dehydrogenase activity in Alzheimer's disease may reflect oxidative stress. Journal of Neurochemistry. 1986;**46**:1042-1045

[86] Bhaskar K, Miller M, Chludzinski A, Herrup K, Zagorski M, Lamb BT. The PI3K-Akt-mTOR pathway regulates abeta oligomer induced neuronal cell cycle events. Molecular Neurodegeneration. 2009;**4**:14

[87] Fuentealba RA, Farias G, Scheu J, Bronfman M, Mar-zolo MP, Inestrosa NC. Signal transduction during amyloid-beta-peptide neurotoxicity: Role in Alzheimer disease. Brain Research. Brain Research Reviews. 2004;**2000**(47):275-289

[88] Mattson MP, Tomaselli KJ, Rydel RE. Calcium-destablizing and neurodegenerative effect of aggregated beta-amyloid peptide are attenuated by basic FGF. Brain Research. 1993;**621**:35-49

[89] Müller WE, Kirsch C, Eckert GP. Membrane-disordering effects of beta-amyloid peptides. Biochemical Society Transactions. 2001;**29**:617-623

[90] Kimura R, MacTavish D, Yang J, Westaway D, Jhamandas JH. Beta amyloid-induced depression of hippocampal long-term potentiation is mediated through the amylin receptor. The Journal of Neuroscience. 2012;**32**:17401-17406

[91] Jackson K, Barisone GA, Diaz E, Jin LW, DeCarli C, Despa F. Amylin deposition in the brain: A secondamyloid in Alzheimer disease? Annals of Neurology. 2013;**74**:517-526

[92] Götz J, Lim YA, Eckert A. Lessons from two prevalent amyloidosis-what amylin and Aβ have in common. Frontiers in Aging Neuroscience. 2013;**5**:38

[93] Verdile G, Fuller SJ, Martins RN. The role of type 742 2 diabetes in neurodegeneration. Neurobiology of Disease. 2015;**84**:22-38

[94] Grunberger G. Novel therapies for the management of type 2 diabetes mellitus: Part 1. Pramlintide and

bromocriptine-QR. Journal of Diabetes. 2013;**5**:110-117

[95] Zhu H, Wang X, Wallack M, Li H, Carreras I, Dedeoglu A, et al. Intraperitoneal injection of the pancreatic peptide amylin potently reduces behavioral impairment and brain amyloid pathology in 1murine models of Alzheimer's disease. Molecular Psychiatry. 2015;**20**:252-262

[96] Adler BL, Yarchoan M, Hwang HM, Louneva N, Blair JA, Palm R, et al. Neuroprotective effects of the amylin analogue pramlintide on Alzheimer's disease pathogenesis and cognition. Neurobiology of Aging. 2014;**35**:793-801

[97] Zhang Y, Zhou B, Deng B, Zhang F, Wu J, Wang Y, et al. Amyloid-β induces hepatic insulin resistance in vivo via JAK2. Diabetes. 2013;**62**:1159-1166

[98] Meakin PJ, Harper AJ, Hamilton DL, Gallagher J, McNeilly AD, Burgess LA, et al. Reduction in BACE1 decreases body weight, protects against diet-induced obesity and enhances insulin sensitivity in mice. The Biochemical Journal. 2012;**441**:285-296